Gérard Emilien
Cécile Durlach
Ulla Lepola
Timothy Dinan

Anxiety Disorders

Pathophysiology and Pharmacological Treatment

Springer Basel AG

Authors

Dr. Gérard Emilien
127 rue Henri Prou
78340 Les Clayes Sous Bois
France

Prof. Timothy Dinan
Department of Pharmacology and Therapeutics
University College Cork
Ireland

Dr. Ulla Marjatta Lepola
Kuopion Psykiatripalvelu Oy
Psychiatric Research Clinic of Kuopio
Asemakatu 46
FIN-70110 Kuopio
Finland

Dr. Cécile Durlach
23 Rue Raynouard
75016 Paris
France

A CIP catalogue record for this book is available from the Library of Congress, Washington D.C., USA

Deutsche Bibliothek Cataloging-in-Publication Data
Anxiety disorders : pathophysiology and pharmacological treatment /
written by Gérard Emilien .... - Basel ; Boston ; Berlin : Birkhäuser, 2002
ISBN 978-3-0348-9460-9 ISBN 978-3-0348-8157-9 (eBook)
DOI 10.1007/978-3-0348-8157-9

ISBN 978-3-0348-9460-9

Originally published by Birkhäuser Verlag, Basel, Switzerland in 2002
Softcover reprint of the hardcover 1st edition 2002
Printed on acid-free paper produced from chlorine-free pulp. TCF ∞
Cover design: Micha Lotrovsky, Therwil, Switzerland

ISBN 978-3-0348-9460-9

9 8 7 6 5 4 3 2 1 www.birkhasuer-science.com

Contents

Glossary

ACTH	Adrenocorticotropic hormone
ANF	Atrial natriuretic factor
APA	American Psychiatric Association
APD	Avoidant personality disorder
AQ	Avoidance questionnaire
ASI	Anxiety sensitivity inventory
BDZ	Benzodiazepine
BIS	Behavioural inhibition system
BIU	Behavioural inhibition to the unfamiliar
BPRS	Brief psychiatric rating scale
BSPS	Brief social phobia scale
cAMP	Cyclic adenosine monophosphate
CAPS	Clinician administered PTSD scale
CBF	Cerebral blood flow
CCK	Cholecystokinin
CCK_4	Cholecystokinin tetrapeptide
CCSQ	Confidence in coping strategies questionnaire
CFS	Conditioned fear stress
CGI	Clinical global impressions
CHRNA4	Neuronal nicotinic acetylcholine receptor $\alpha4$ gene
CISD	Critical incident stress debriefing
CNS	Central nervous system
CNV	Contingent negative variation
CPP	Comprehensive panic profile
CRF	Corticotropin-releasing factor
CRH	Corticotropin-releasing hormone
CSF	Cerebrospinal fluid
CSQ	Coping strategies questionnaire
DA	Dopamine
DES	Dissociative experience scale

DGRP	Duke global rating of PTSD
DHEA	Dehydroepiandrosterone
DID	Dissociative identity disorder
DMI	Desipramine
dPAG	Dorsoloateral periaqueductal gray
DSM	Diagnostic and statistical manual (of mental disorders)
DST	Dexamethasone suppression test
ECA	Epidemiological catchment area
EEG	Electroencephalogram
EMD-R	Eye movement desensitisation-reprocessing procedure
EMDR	Eye movement desesitisation and reprocessing
EMG	Electromyogram
EPM	Elevated plus-maze
ERP	Event-related potentials
ESR	Oestrogen receptor
FBA	Frontal brain asymmetry
FHPA	Fear of having a panic attack
FNES	Fear of negative evaluation scale
FPA	Frequency of panic attacks
FPS	Fear potentiated startle
FSS	Fear survey schedule
GABA	Gamma-aminobutyric acid
GAD	Generalized anxiety disorder
GH	Growth hormone
GP	General practitioner
HAM	Hamilton rating scale for anxiety
5-HT	5-hydroxytryptamine, serotonin
5-HTT	5-hydroxytryptamine transporter
HPA	Hypothalamic pituitary adrenal
HPS	Hypothalamic-pituitary-somatotropin
HRT	Hormone replacement therapy
i.c.v.	Intracerebroventricular
i.v.	Intravenous
ICD	International classification diagnostic
IES	Impact of event scale
KSP	Karolinska scales of personality
LSAS	Liebowitz social anxiety scale
MAOI	Monoamine oxidase inhibitor
MASC	Multidimensional anxiety scale for children
m-CPP	*m*-chlorophenylpiperazine
MD	Major depressive
MDTB	Mouse defence test battery
MHPG	3-methoxy-4-hydroxyphenylglycol
MINI	MINI International Neuropsychiatric Interview
MISS	Mississippi scale for posttraumatic stress disorder

MMPI	Minnesota multiphasic personality inventory
MRI	Magnetic resonance imaging
MRS	Magnetic resonance spectroscopy
NCS	National Comorbidity Study
NE	Norepinephrine
NIMH-OC	National Institute of Mental Health global obsessive compulsive scale
NK	Neurokinin
NMDA	N-methyl-D-aspartate
NPY	Neuropeptide Y
NSS	Neurologic soft sign
OCD	Obsessive-compulsive disorder
8-OH-DPAT	8-hydroxy-2-(di-n-propylamino)-tetralin
PACQ	Panic attack cognitions questionnnaire
PAG	Periaqueductal gray
PASQ	Panic attack symptoms questionnaire
PASS	Panic-associated symptom scale
PBR	Peripheral benzodiazepine receptor
p-CPA	p-chlorophenylalanine
PD	Panic disorder
PDSS	Panic disorder severity scale
PET	Positron emission tomography
PI-R	Padua inventory-revised
p.o.	Orally (per os)
p.r.n.	As occasion requires (pro re nata)
PSWQ	Penn State worry questionnaire
PTSD	Posttraumatic stress disorder
PTZ	Pentylenetetrazol
qd	Once a day
QOLI	Quality of life inventory
rCBF	Regional cerebral blood flow
RIMA	Reversible monoamine oxidase inhibitor
s.c.	Subcutaneous
SADS	Social avoidance distress scale
SAP	Stretched attend posture
SAS-A	Social anxiety scale for adolescents
SCARED	Screen for child anxiety related emotional disorders
SCVT	Stroop colour word test
SET	Social effectiveness therapy
SFS	Suffocation fear scale
SIAS	Social interaction anxiety scale
SP	Social phobia
SPAI	Social phobia & anxiety inventory
SPECT	Single photon emission computerized tomography
SPS	Social phobia scale
SSRI	Selective serotonin reuptake inhibitor

STAI	State-trait anxiety inventory
TCA	Tricyclic antidepressant
TCI	Temperament and character inventory
TFPP	Trifluoromethylphenylpiperazine
tid	Three times a day
TK	Tachykinin
TKS	Taijin-kyofu-sho
WHO QOL	World Health Organization Quality of Life
Y-BOCS	Yale-Brown obsessive compulsive scale

Introduction

Anxiety is a normal part of life. Anxiety, like depression, is both a normal emotion and a psychiatric disorder. The best way of conceptualising this may be to consider a graded progression of anxiety from normal to pathological degrees or of functionally useful arousal to disruptive and pathological anxiety. A certain amount of anxiety will improve our level of functioning and thereby enhance performance. However, some individuals experience high levels of anxiety that go beyond normal limits, either because of an abnormal reaction to 'normal' circumstances, or through reaction to abnormal circumstances. These people can be said to have an anxiety disorder. Although controversy continues regarding an acceptable definition of anxiety, it has been suggested that anxiety is an emotional state which is typified by a sense of impending catastrophe and includes feelings of uneasiness, apprehension, and tension (Jeffries, 1978). Symptoms of anxiety lie on a continuum of severity ranging from a short-lived, appropriate response to a chronic pathologic state that causes great distress and interferes with social and professional functioning. The term anxiety disorder is used to describe conditions in which pathological anxiety is the predominant factor. These conditions include phobic disorders, panic disorder (PD), generalised anxiety disorder (GAD), posttraumatic stress disorder (PTSD) and obsessive-compulsive disorder (OCD). Anxiety disorders have a high prevalence and constitute some of the most frequent psychological problems seen in medical practice. Some studies have begun to describe how difficult it is to ascertain the impact of prior trauma and stress among patients presenting with predominant panic, OCD, or other primary anxiety profiles. It has been suggested that the age-of-onset data of childhood anxiety disorders point to a developmental progression (simple phobia followed by separation anxiety, overanxiousness or GAD, OCD, social phobia (SP), and panic, with or without agoraphobia) (Last et al., 1992; Carter et al., 1995; Craske, 1997). This age-of-onset is mapped against a normative progression in fears and anxieties; it peaks during the second and third decades, and the disorders affect women twice as often as men (Kessler et al., 1994).

Anxiety disorders are generally classified by the nature of the object of concern or the focus that is associated with the high anxiety levels. In general, diagnostic systems determine five main types which are phobias, PTSD, PD, GAD and OCD (American Psychiatric Association (APA), 1994). Cognitive factors are regarded as extremely important in anxiety disorders. Phobias are conditions in which intense anxiety is associated with well-defined items or situations such as animals, open spaces or social situations. PTSD are similar to phobias in that pathological anxiety relates to specific events, but these tend to be abnormal environmental experiences such as car crashes or wars, in which the patient cannot fully process the memories of the event in a normal way. The trauma is instead re-experienced in a variety of ways including distressing recollections, dreams, and flashbacks. PD is an anxiety disorder characterised by spontaneous paroxysms of severe fear. The panic attack is a particularly well defined anxiety disorder with typical respiratory, perceptive and cognitive disturbances. GAD involves persistent levels of abnormal anxiety and worry with no apparent associated focus. It is chronic and its symptoms occur on most days for 6 months or more (APA, 1994). Finally, OCD involves abnormal focus on specific thoughts or actions that result in excessive anxiety, often with themes of contamination or doubt.

Genetic, familial-environment and individual-specific environmental risk factors can cause anxiety disorders (Kendler et al., 1995). Some family studies have shown a strong tendency toward familial aggregation of anxiety disorders and data on twins also suggest the importance of genetic factors in anxiety disorders (Andrews et al., 1990; Kendler et al., 1997). The largest and very informative twin study of anxiety disorders has provided estimates of the heritability of PD (44%), agoraphobia (39%), GAD (32%), animal phobias (32%) and SP (30%). A recent study that investigated the familial predisposition to PD examined the heritability of anxiety sensitivity through use of a twin group (Stein et al., 1999). Scores on the anxiety sensitivity index were analysed in a group of 179 monozygotic and 158 dizygotic twin pairs. It was shown that the broad heritability estimate of anxiety sensitivity index as a unifactorial construct was 45%. Thus this study suggests that one psychological risk factor for the development of PD-anxiety sensitivity may have a heritable component. These studies point to a genetic influence on the expression of these phenotypes, although environmental factors play a role (Kendler et al., 1992; 1993; 1995a). Anticipation (an increase in severity or a decrease in the age of onset inherent in the transmission of a disease gene from an affected parent to a child) has been reported in families with anxiety disorders. It is confirmed by other studies, trinucleotide repeat sequence may be considered to account for the familial aggregation of anxiety disorders (Ohara et al., 1999).

Understanding the effects of anxiogenic agents may clarify the mechanisms of anxiety. Yohimbine is a drug whose central nervous system actions include inducing amygdalar stimulation and behavioural indicators of anxiety. Much of the anxiogenic effect of yohimbine is thought to be caused by its pre-synaptic α_2-adrenergic antagonist activity, which enhances noradrenergic neurotransmission from the locus ceruleus to efferent central nervous system targets, notably including the amygdala (Bremner et al., 1996). This leads to noradrenergic stimulation of excitatory amygdalar output by acting on stimulatory β-adrenergic receptors (Ferry et al., 1997).

In vivo neuroimaging allows the investigation of brain circuits involved in the experience of anxiety and of receptor changes associated with anxiety disorders. Activation studies have revealed the involvement of many brain areas depending on the condition and the paradigm. However, the orbitofrontal cortex/anterior insula and the anterior cingulate were found to be involved in all the studies and may represent the nodal point between somatic and cognitive symptoms of any form of anxiety (Malicia, 1999).

Animal models of anxiety are an absolute requirement for both the identification of underlying biological mechanisms and the development of novel anxiolytics. Laboratory-based experimental research has led to an important breakthrough in our understanding and treatment of anxiety disorders as well as other types of psychopathology. Despite the importance of this work, the relevance of laboratory-based research using clinical and nonclinical populations has been underestimated, particularly given its importance and impact in the discovery of new treatments. Some of the most prominent behaviour therapy techniques, such as systematic desensitisation, were derived from basic experimental research with both humans and animals (Wolpe, 1958).

Management for anxiety disorders may involve physical treatments such as drugs, psychological treatments such as dynamic psychotherapy or behavioural cognitive therapy or a combination of both. The two approaches have advantages as well as disadvantages. Biofeedback techniques such as alpha, theta and alpha-theta enhancements have also been suggested to be potential effective treatments in some anxiety disorders. Regarding pharmacological innovations for potential anxiolytics, recent preclinical data support the hypotheses that selective agonists or antagonists for serotonin (5-HT_{1A}, 5-HT_{2A}, 5-HT_{2c}, 5-HT_3), cholecystokinin (CCK_B) and N-methyl-D-aspartate (NMDA) receptors are of potential interest for the development of new medicine. The development of newer drugs with improved safety and tolerability, such as the selective serotonin reuptake inhibitors (SSRIs) and reversible inhibitors of monoamine oxidase may also be an important step in the treatment of anxiety. It has been difficult to understand why the SSRIs work in several of these anxiety syndromes (PD, SP, GAD, PTSD). It is also clear that the SSRIs are effective in PD, SP, and probably in GAD and in parts of the PTSD syndrome. Imipramine, and more recently venlafaxine, is effective in GAD, and both affect serotonin and norepinephrine.

Psychiatric rating methods are used in many areas of psychopathological research and they are particularly indispensable in the testing of psychoactive drugs. The fact that rating systems lack a methodological basis is particularly likely to create additional problems in the clinical testing of new anxiolytics.

In this book, the discussion of the normal and pathological aspects of anxiety is critically examined. A chapter on the molecular basis of anxiety is included, outlining the potential of such approach in the discovery of novel effective pharmacological interventions. The face validity, predictability and usefulness of animal models, whether mouse mutants or behavioural, in the design of valid new efficacious products are discussed. Separate chapters dedicated to each particular type of anxiety such as GAD, SP, PTSD, PD and OCD as described by the revised Diagnostic and Statistical Manual (DSM-IV) and the International Classification (ICD-10, The ICD-10 Classification of Mental and Behavioural Disorders, 1992) criteria are included with particular attention to aetiology, differential diagnosis, epidemiology and both cognitive and pharmacological treatments. This book should be of benefit to psychiatrists, clinical psychologists, general practitioners, nurses, students and all those engaged in neuropsychiatric research.

The authors thank Professor Jeffrey Gray, Oxford, UK and Dr Loren Aguiar for reading and providing valuable and encouraging comments on the manuscript.

References

American Psychiatric Association. Diagnostic and Statistical manual of mental disorders (4th ed.). Washington, DC, 1994

Andrews G, Stewart G, Allen R, Henderson AS. The genetics of six neurotic disorders: a twin study. J Affect Disord 19, 2396, 1990

Bremner JD, Krystal JH, Southwick SM, Charney DS. Noradrenergic mechanisms in stress and anxiety: I. Preclinical studies. Synapse 23, 28–38, 1996

Carter AS, Pauls DL, Leckman JF. The development of obsessionally: Continuities and discontinuities. In: Cichetti D, Cohen DJ (eds): Developmental Psychopathology: Theory and Models. New York: Wiley, 609–632, 1995

Craske MG. Fear and anxiety in children and adolescents. Bull Menninger Clin 61 (2), A4–A36, 1997

Ferry B, Magistretti PJ, Pralong E. Noradrenaline modulates glutamate-mediated neurotransmission in the rat basolateral amygdala *in vitro*. Eur J Neuroscie 9, 1356–1364, 1997

Jeffries JJ. Anxiety: an attempt at definition. Canadian Pharmaceutical Journal 41, 1978

Kendler KS, Martin NG, Heath AC, Eaves LJ. Self-report psychiatric symptoms in twins and their non-twin relatives: are twins different? Am J Med Gen 60, 588–591, 1995

Kendler KS, Davis CG, Kessler RC. The familial aggregation of common psychiatric and substance use disorders in the National Comorbidity Survey: a family history study. Br J Psychiatry 170, 541–548, 1997

Kendler KS, Neale M, Kessler R, Heath A, Eaves L. Major depression and phobias: the genetic and environmental sources of comorbidity. Psychol Med 23, 361–371, 1993

Kendler KS, Neale MC, Kessler RC, Heath A, Eaves LJ. The genetic epidemiology of phobias in women. Arch Gen Psychiatry, 49, 273–281, 1992

Kendler KS, Walter EE, Neale MC, Kessler RC, Heath AC, Eaves LJ. The structure of the genetic and environmental risk factors for six major psychiatric disorders in women. Arch Gen Psychiatry, 152, 374–383, 1995a

Kessler RC. McGonagle KA. Zhao S. Nelson CB. Hughes M. Eshleman S. Wittchen H-U. Kendler KS. Lifetime and 12-month prevalence of DSM-III-R psychiatric disorders in the United States: Results from the National Comorbidity Survey. Arch Gen Psychiatry, 51, 8–19, 1994

Last CG, Perrin S, Hersen M, Kazdin AE. DSM-III-R anxiety disorders in children: sociodemographic and clinical characteristics. J Am Acad Child Adolesc Psychiatry 31, 1070–1076, 1992

Malizia AL. What do brain imaging studies tell us about anxiety disorders? J Psychopharmacol 13 (4), 372–378, 1999

Ohara K, Suzuki Y, Ochiai M, Yoshida K, Ohara K. Age of onset anticipation in anxiety disorders. Psychiatry Research 89, 215–221, 1999

Stein MB, Jang KL & Livesley WJ. Heritability of anxiety sensitivity: A twin study. Am J Psychiatry 156 (2), 246–251, 1999

The ICD-10 Classification of Mental and Behavioural Disorders. World Health Organization, 1992

Wolpe J. Psychotherapy by reciprocal inhibition. Stanford, CA: Stanford University Press, 1958

Chapter 1
Normal and pathological anxiety

1 What is anxiety?

The symptoms of "anxiety" are listed under two headings. Subjective ones (i.e. those felt as "psychological" experiences) include fear, emotional worries, feelings of terror, depersonalisation etc., and occasionally mental acts such as obsession-like thoughts concerning the safety of others, fear of dying etc. On the other hand, the "objective" symptoms of anxiety (also called "somatic" and later on "anxiety-equivalents") include abdominal pain, nausea, vertigo, dizziness, palpitations, dry mouth, hot flushes, hyperventilation, breathlessness, headache, restless legs, and other bodily experiences sometimes indistinguishable from complaints caused by physical disease. At the beginning of the 19th century, Landré-Beauvais (1813) defined "*anxieté*" as "a certain malaise, restlessness, excessive agitation" suggesting that these states may accompany "acute" and "chronic" diseases. With this approach, anxiety becomes a syndrome with both subjective and somatic components, and which can accompany diverse diseases.

The term anxiety is a shorthand term with a wide variety of meanings and manifestations. Semantic difficulties extend to the various meanings attached to similar terms in different languages. Anxiety may be defined as a psychophysiological phenomenon experienced as a foreboding dread or threat to a human organism whether the threat is generated by internal, real or imagined dangers. Whether this threat is conscious or unconscious or whether it is secondary to actual environmental threats of a biosocial, biophysical, or biochemical nature should also be considered (Lesse, 1970). Clinically anxious people, then, are to a large extent self-defined as those for whom anxiety has become extreme and for whom coping responses have become ineffective, leading them to seeking professional help (Lader, 1983).

Faithfully adhering to Freud's description of anxiety disorders, the term "Anxiety neurosis" was used in both *Diagnostic and Statistical Manual* (DSM-I) (APA, 1952) and DSM-II (APA, 1968). In DSM-III, the term "neurosis" was dropped and replaced by specific categories (APA, 1980). Anxiety neurosis was subdivided into PD and GAD. In DSM-III-R, diagnostic criteria for GAD were strengthened to increase clinical validity (APA, 1987). Also, agoraphobia was primarily considered a complication of PD. In DSM-IV, the subdivision of anxiety disorders into phobias and anxiety states was retained, the latter category now includes PD, GAD, OCD and PTSD (APA, 1994). Diagnostic criteria for panic attacks have remained largely unchanged, but the presence of psychological symptoms such as chronic anxiety between successive attacks is now required to diagnose PD (McNally, 1994). It is now widely acknowledged that specificity is a key issue in psychopathology and that classification systems such as the APA's *Diagnostic and Statistical Manual* are based on the idea that emotional disorders represent distinct nosological categories (i.e. that every disorder has its own specific features). Anxiety becomes pathological when it is more severe or more frequent than the individual can tolerate or is accustomed to experience (Lader & Marks, 1971). Thus, the term "anxiety disorders" is usually used to describe a heterogeneous group of disorders in which pathological anxiety is an important feature. The DSM-IV (1994) and the ICD-10 criteria describe several forms of anxiety disorders. Some differences in the number and duration of symptoms by disorder may be noted (see Table 1). In fact, considering the description of various types of anxiety, the definition states of anxiety do not concur. In the definitions of the state of GAD the revised International Classification (ICD-10) emphasises the somatic features of anxiety, whereas the revised DSM-IV emphasises excessive worry as the cardinal feature of the disorder.

Pathological anxiety is described primarily by high negative affect associated with a sense of uncontrollability (Barlow, 1988). It is characterised by hypervigilance suggesting a readiness to respond to danger or negative events. Cognitively, it is chronic hypervigilance biased to threatening stimuli, along with an inability to concentrate on normal daily tasks, that defines much of pathological anxiety (Eysenck, 1992; McNally, 1996). Behaviourally, readiness to respond to danger is increased. Indeed, manifestations of fear-related behaviours, such as exaggerated startle responses, are some symptoms of the anxiety disorders. Pathological anxiety may also involve other emotions such as guilt, shame, or anger (Izard & Youngstrom, 1996). The pathological anxiety is typically chronic and so severe that it disrupts one's ability to function in the tasks of daily living for long periods of time. There is also considerable comorbidity of anxiety disorders with major depression (Rapee & Barlow, 1991).

Anxiety disorders are extremely common, but often go unrecognised and untreated. In their diagnosis, a full assessment, which includes a history, physical examination and mental state, is mandatory. This is particularly relevant in anxiety disorders, which can have a number of possible aetiologies, both physical and psychological (Gelder et al., 1996). In general, anxiety disorders present with a number of non-specific symptoms, such as excessive fearfulness, sweating, fatigability, muscle tension, impaired concentration, irritability, increased sensitivity to noise and sleep disturbances. The National Comorbidity Study (NCS), using DSM-III-R criteria, estimated the frequency of diagnosable anxiety disorders to be 24.9% of the general population within their lifetime and 17.2% within the previous 6 months (Kessler et al., 1994). Approximately 3% of the population suffers from anxiety so severe that it disrupts routine life functions, and anxiolytics continue to be prescribed extensively (Kessler et al., 1994; Lépine et al., 1988). Phobic anxiety disorders are probably the most common owing to a high frequency of specific phobias, which affect up to 11.3% of the population in their lifetime, but which may not always require treatment (Kessler et al., 1994). Anxiety disorders have a mean age of onset in the 20s (Antony & Swinson, 1996). Left untreated, they tend to be chronic, with symptoms that are either continuous or episodic. At any age, anxiety disorders are more common in women than men. Better recognition and treatment

Table 1: Number and duration of symptoms by disorder for DSM-IV and ICD-10

Disorder	Number of symptoms		Duration of symptoms	
	DSM-IV	**ICD-10**	**DSM-IV**	**ICD-10**
Agora-phobia	–	Fear or avoidance in two or more of four situations. Two or more of 14 symptoms (with at least one of autonomic arousal)	–	Consistently manifest fear or avoidance.
PD	Four or more of 13 panic symptoms. One or more panic attacks followed by one or more of three symptoms.	Four or more of 14 symptoms (with at least one of autonomic arousal).	Panic symptoms develop abruptly and reach peak within 10 min. followed by at least 1 month of symptoms.	Moderate – four or more panic attacks in a 4-week period. Severe – four or more panic attacks per week over a 4-week period.
GAD	Three or more of six symptoms (with at least some present for more days than not).	Four or more of 22 symptoms (with at least one of autonomic arousal)	More days than not for at least 6 months.	Worry for at least 6 months.
SP	–	Two or more of 14 symptoms and one or more of three symptoms.	For persons under the age of 18, duration is at least 6 months.	–
Specific phobia	–	Two or more of 14 symptoms	–	Symptoms manifest for some time since onset of disorder.
OCD	–	–	Obsessions or compulsions take more than 1 hour a day.	Either obsessions or compulsions present on most days for at least 2 weeks.
PTSD	Traumatic event where both of two characteristics present. Event is re-experienced in one or more of five ways. Three or more of seven symptoms of avoidance and numbing. Two or more of five symptoms of increased arousal.	One or more of two symptoms (one of which requires two or more arousal symptoms).	Duration of disturbance is more than 1 month. Acute – Symptoms for less than 3 months. Chronic – Symptoms for more than 3 months. With delayed onset – onset of symptoms is at least 6 months after the stressor.	Symptoms must occur within 6 months of stressful event.

of anxiety disorders is an important public health issue. In people with anxiety disorders, functioning may be disturbed by high levels of arousal in conditions easily tolerated by others.

Public speaking typically elicits some fear or normal anxious behaviour that subsides once the presentation is underway or completed. Some people may actively try to reduce their feelings of threat by spending time in the lecture room before they give their talk. This differs from the pathological anxiety disorders in which the emotional responses are chronically dysfunctional. Individuals with public-speaking phobias will have a severe and debilitating autonomic, cognitive and somatic reaction to even the suggestion of giving a public presentation. The fear is so great that they will avoid speaking although this is detrimental to their career or self-esteem. Fear is one of the major normal precursors for the development of pathological anxiety disorders.

SP (social anxiety disorder) has been slower than other anxiety disorders to capture the attention of psychopathology researchers. One possible reason may be that SP is sometimes difficult to conceptualise as a form of psychopathology, given that up to 40% of the general population describe themselves as "shy" (Zimbardo et al., 1974). This is also reflected in the fact that SP was not an officially defined nosological category until the publication of the DSM-III (APA, 1980) and only a decade ago, SP was described as the "neglected" anxiety disorder (Liebowitz et al., 1985). Nevertheless, over the past several years, research into the nature and treatment of SP has increased dramatically. Recently, there seems to be a preference for the use of the term social anxiety disorder rather than SP as this term connotes a more pervasive and impairing disorder than is implied by the label "social phobia" (Liebowitz et al., 2000). It is suggested that switching to the alternative name of social anxiety disorder may be a good step in educating health professionals in both mental and primary care about the significant nature of this serious disorder.

Anxiety disorder is characterised by profound changes in autonomic functions that are usually related to an increase in the activity of the sympathetic nervous system (Szabadi & Bradshaw, 1988). However, more recent evidence indicates that apart from the sympathetic overactivity an inhibition of parasympathetic activity can also be detected in anxious patients. Thus, it was reported that patients suffering from PD show an attenuation of physiological heart rate variability, which is likely to reflect a reduction in vagal activity (Ewing et al., 1980; Yeragani et al., 1990). Of all the anxiety symptoms, OCD stands out as separate from the group in terms of the symptoms profile, biological markers of pathogenesis and treatment response. Many may argue that OCD is wrongly categorised among the anxiety disorders (Montgomery et al., 1994). Hypochondriasis may represent a variant of OCD. PD, which plays a fundamental role in the development of some forms of agoraphobia, also shows certain distinctive biological features. However, there may be more overlap with the other anxiety disorders and with depression than with agoraphobia (Montgomery et al., 1991).

Evidence regarding the structure of the anxiety disorders also has implications for theories that hypothesise a temperament or trait vulnerability to the development of anxiety disorders. Perhaps the most widely known theories of this sort are those proposed by these models: harm avoidance (Cloninger, 1986), neuroticism (Eysenck, 1967), trait anxiety (Gray, 1982), behavioural inhibition (Kagan, 1995), and negative affectivity (Tellegen, 1985). It may be important to distinguish trait and state anxiety (Lister, 1990). State anxiety is the emotion an individual experiences when confronted with a stressful stimulus, whereas trait anxiety is an enduring feature of a subject, that is, a stable trait (Spielberger, 1975). Therefore, state anxiety is that seen at any given time and when elevated is usually associated with a transient stressor. It remits once the stimulus is removed. Trait anxiety is a persistent, enduring feature of an individual which is a facet of the personality and which may have an inheritable component.

It may be assumed that the nature of anxiety is identical in children and older individuals. Although the field has made significant advances in understanding anxiety disorders, this information is based more on data derived from young adults. Whether these findings can be generalised to children and older population is unknown, although more and more research has started to carefully examine this topic.

1.1 Anxiety in children

Psychiatric investigators had virtually ignored the topic of childhood anxiety through the 1980s, possibly due to the mistaken impression that childhood anxiety is predominantly transient or unimpairing (Benjamin et al., 1990). Anxiety disorders are the most common psychiatric illnesses in children but most of them do not receive treatment (Pine, 1997). SP, separation anxiety disorder and GAD in children cause substantial distress and interfere with academic as well as social functioning (Ialongo et al., 1995; Hansen et al., 1998).

Longitudinal studies on the course of SP suggest involvement of common biological factors in childhood and adult SP (Schneier et al., 1992). Retrospective studies in adults note a particularly early onset for SP, as compared with other phobias, GAD or PD (Schneier et al., 1992). Probing neural circuits implicated in developmental aspects of SP, it was suggested that behavioural inhibition is a reflection of intrinsic hypersensitivity in a neural circuit centering the amygdala (Kagan, 1995, 1997). Taken together, longitudinal studies, family studies and studies of behavioural inhibition outline observable childhood precursors for adult SP. Amygdala sensitivity as assessed by magnetic resonance imaging may identify individuals most at risk for phobia. The amygdala exhibits a selective response to facial displays of aversive emotions, particularly fearful faces, even when they are presented below the levels of conscious perception (Breiter et al., 1996; Whalen et al. 1998). Adults with SP may exhibit an abnormal sensitivity to such facial displays of threat or fear, potentially manifested in physiological, cognitive, as well as brain imaging measures (Öhman, 1986). Using facial stimuli in an imaging study, preliminary evidence of such hypersensitivity in the amygdala of adults with SP was shown (Birbaumer et al., 1998). Hence, using imaging technology, it may be possible to examine amygdala sensitivity to social threat or fear cues in children and adults with SP. Such measure of amygdala-based hypersensitivity might then be used to identify phobic children most at risk for SP as adults.

Considering the relationship between anxiety in parents and their children, perhaps the most frequently noted association is between parental PD and childhood separation disorder (Capps et al., 1996; Warner et al., 1995; Weissman et al., 1984). Two studies note that first-degree relatives of patients with PD exhibit hypersensitivity to carbon dioxide inhalation (Coryell, 1997; Perna et al., 1995). Two other studies find that family loading for PD is concentrated in the relatives of panic patients with respiratory abnormalities (Perna et al., 1996; Horwath et al., 1998). These findings are consistent with theories implicating components of a common neural circuit in separation distress among animals and panic attacks among humans (Klein, 1993; Panksepp, 1998; Panksepp et al., 1992). Both phenomena are thought to involve components of the brain stem and hypothalamus. Both phenomena also involve fine-grained regulation of the respiratory system. Consistent with hypotheses in this realm, children with separation anxiety disorder exhibit many of the same respiratory abnormalities characteristic of adult PD (Pine et al., 1998a, 1998b). In particular, children with separation anxiety disorder exhibit more respiratory symptoms when breathing CO_2 relative to both psychologically healthy children as well as children with mood or other anxiety disorders. Given relationships among PD, separation anxiety disorder and respiratory dysfunction, these data may suggest that parents with PD might transmit a diathesis for certain forms of anxiety that is observable in the respiratory system. In some individuals, this diathesis may remain dormant whereas in others it may exhibit variable expressions across development, manifested as extreme degrees of separation distress during childhood or as panic attacks after puberty (Klein, 1993, Panksepp, 1998, Pine at al. 1998a, 1998b).

Children with GAD show high reassurance-seeking and a high comorbidity with separation anxiety disorder in childhood and with depressive disorders in adolescence (Masi et al., 1999). These findings have led to the formulation of the hypothesis of a developmental continuum, i.e. that the same children who meet the criteria for separation anxiety disorder when they were young (and cope through reassurance-seeking behaviour directed at a parent) may meet the criteria for GAD later if their anxiety persists while their coping responses become less parent-focused. The occurrence of different anxiety disorders in the same child over time is supported by a 4-year longitudinal study showing that while remission of initial anxiety disorders was common, 30% of anxious children had developed new psychiatric disorders, primarily anxiety disorders during the follow-up (Last et al., 1996).

Both in community and clinically based studies, children with an anxiety disorder typically present with other anxiety disorders as well as with depressive disorders (Gurely et al., 1996). In the NCS, GAD was the only childhood disorder besides major depression that retrospectively predicted adult episodes of major depression (Kessler & Walters, 1998). A similar strong association between GAD and major depression was noted in a prospectively assessed epidemiological cohort (Pine et al.,1998a). Based on results linking GAD and major depression in longitudinal or family studies, adverse life events are hypothesised to play a particularly strong role in the pathophysiology of GAD and depression. Hence, neural circuits involved in aspects of anxiety as well as depression may both involve the hippocampal formation. In anxiety, such involvement may derive through interactions with fear-relevant systems in the amygdala, while in depression, such involvement may derive through interactions with affect-relevant systems in the prefrontal cortex and striatum. Based on cognitive studies in children with anxiety disorders and adults at high risk for anxiety, anxiety-related cognitive biases and their associated hippocampal-amygdala abnormalities are thought to develop early in the course of a disorder (Daledin & Vasey, 1997; Williams et al., 1996). Such abnormalities may be potentially detectable using functional magnetic resonance imaging (MRI). For example, children with GAD are hypothesised to exhibit enhanced activity in the hippocampus and amygdala during certain cognitive tasks. These include navigation tasks that involve perception of dangerous contexts or orienting tasks that tap attentional biases (Maguire et al., 1998; Daledin & Vasey, 1997).

Research interest in the nature and underlying pathology of OCD has increased dramatically, particularly with respect to childhood-onset cases of the disorder. Once perceived to be rare in childhood, OCD is now recognised to be fairly common among children and adolescents, with estimated prevalence rates in the range of 1–3.6% (Flament et al., 1988; Valleni-Basile et al., 1994; Zohar et al., 1992). Current estimates suggest that between one third and one half of all adult cases of OCD have their onset in childhood or adolescence (Kolada et al., 1994; Noshirvani et al., 1991; Ristvedt et al., 1993).

Childhood anxiety disorders predict an increase by a factor of two to five in the risk of later anxiety disorders, major depression, suicide attempts, and hospitalisation for psychiatric illness (Pine et al., 1998a; Costello et al., 1999). Recent studies documenting the high degree of stress and impairment engendered by childhood anxiety disorders have further stimulated interest in pathophysiology (Benjamin et al., 1990; Ialongo et al., 1995)

1.2 Anxiety in the elderly

Although anxiety disorders in general are less prevalent among the elderly than among younger adults, they remain relatively common in late life (Flint, 1994). The Epidemiological Catchment Area (ECA) survey documented a once-month prevalence rate of 5.5% for all of the anxiety disorders in individuals aged 65 and older, which is lower than noted in younger adults (7.3%) (Regier et al., 1988). Although one could conclude from these figures that anxiety disorders may not represent a significant mental health problem in the elderly, this would not be accurate. For example, a survey conducted in Australia indicated a prevalence rate for anxiety disorders of 11.7% among nursing home residents based on responses to a self-report (Cheok et al., 1996). In general, one should be cautious in making assumptions about the prevalence of anxiety disorders in older adults. It is possible that anxiety disorders are associated with greater mortality and morbidity, which could explain the lower prevalence rates. Such speculation clearly may have differing implications for etiological theories of anxiety in the elderly.

Examination of the prevalence rates of specific anxiety disorders indicates that phobias (agoraphobia, SP and simple phobia) represent the most common of these disorders among older adults, with a rate of 4.8% (Flint, 1994). Much lower prevalence rates have been reported for OCD (0.8%), and PD (0.1%), although GAD appears to occur more frequently with a prevalence rate of 4.6%. Although specific prevalence estimates vary across studies, there is consensus that phobias are the most common anxiety disorders in the elderly, followed by GAD (Flint, 1994). Older women stand a much greater risk of experiencing an anxiety disorder relative to older men, with a documented 2:1 ratio (Regier et al., 1988; Weissman et al. 1985). Few studies have focused on worries in the elderly (Beck et al. 1996; Borkovec et al., 1983). The results suggest that the content of worry reflects developmentally appropriate themes across lifespan. Thus, older adults (ages 65 and up) reported more frequent worries about health, whereas younger adults (ages 25-64) reported more about family and finances. Although limited by methodological constraints, these data provide some important insights into the nature of worry in the elderly. In a study designed to examine the psychopathological features of GAD in older adults as compared to a matched community sample that was free of psychiatric diagnoses, it was shown that the GAD sample reported greater levels of worry, anxiety, social fears and depression with scores comparable to younger samples of GAD patients (Beck et al., 1996). This report indicated considerable similarity in the clinical characteristics of these two groups. New-onset anxiety in elderly people is often associated with depressive illness or medical disorders (Flint, 1994).

There is considerable consensus that most anxiety disorders begin before young adulthood (Barlow, 1988). It has been suggested that the specific age of onset for the various disorders might reflect developmental processes (Beidel & Turner, 1991). Thus, one could assume that most cases of anxiety disorders among older adults involve individuals who have experienced problems with anxiety for many years. In fact, the data are somewhat mixed on this issue. In considering specific phobia for example, some reports note a recent onset in older adults reporting this diagnosis while others suggest that phobias among older adults typically have been present since childhood (Eaton et al., 1989; Lindesay, 1991). The data regarding PD and OCD are somewhat confusing as well. Although both of these disorders do not appear to be prevalent in older adults, the ECA data suggest that when these diagnoses are noted, they are associated with an onset in young adulthood (Eaton et al., 1989). However, one study that examined anxiety disorders in elderly patients (ages 60 and older) observed a prevalence rate of 9.4% for PD, with over half of the sample reporting the onset of panic attacks after age 60 (Raj et al., 1993). Thus, this study showed that PD can begin in later life. In contrast, GAD appears to have a bimodal distribution of onset age. In the ECA study, 51.6% of the older participants who were diagnosed with GAD reported that the duration of their symptoms was less than five years (Blazer et al., 1991). The remainder of the sample reported that GAD symptoms had lasted for 21 years or longer. For the first group of GAD patients, it is possible that stressful life events may have precipitated the onset of excessive worry (Blazer et al., 1987, Ganzini et al., 1990). In particular, it has been observed that an increased incidence of GAD was reported in the 20 months following a catastrophic financial loss (Ganzini et al., 1990).

Anxiety is a common complaint in the elderly, but important questions about its nature and clinical significance need to be better understood (Sadavoy & LeClair, 1997). The prevalence of anxiety disorders in the elderly is thus high and merits clinical attention.

1.3 Personality and anxiety

Particular attention has been paid to relations between personality and anxiety (Gershuny & Sher, 1998). Gaining a better comprehension of personality-anxiety relations may be useful to the study of anxiety for several reasons which include that the aetiology of anxiety may be further elucidated and assessment of anxiety may be more comprehensive and illustrative. Treatments of anxiety may be better administered based on individual differences. Several studies have examined general relations between broad-band personality traits and anxiety. A recent study designed to assess personality traits in patients with a DSM-IV diagnosis of SP using the Karolinska Scales of Personality (KSP) showed that in total 59% of the volunteers had at least one personality disorder and 47% were diagnosed with an avoidant personality disorder (APD) (Schalling et al., 1987; Marteinsdottir et al., 2001). The results support the view that SP and APD reflect different aspects of a social anxiety spectrum. The typical SP patient, according to the traits identified by the KSP, is a hypersensitive, unconfident worrier who perceives autonomic disturbances and is unable to relax. This individual is easily fatigued, seems to lack self-assertiveness and avoid involvement with others. Furthermore, the low scores in socialisation and social desirability indicate problems with social adjustment.

Cross-sectional studies have revealed a positive relation between neuroticism and anxiety, and/or a negative relation between extraversion and anxiety (Trull & Sher, 1994; Zinbarg & Revelle, 1989). A recent study that examined personality differences between compulsive checkers, nonchecking anxious individuals and normal controls on five basic personality dimensions (emotional stability, extraversion, agreeableness, conscientiousness and intellect) showed that the combined group of all anxious individuals was less extraverted and less emotionally stable than nonchecking/nonanxious controls (Gershuny et al., 2000). The compulsive checkers were less emotionally stable and more conscientious than nonchecking anxious controls. It is possible that compulsive checkers depleted their cognitive and emotional resources more quickly during testing than the anxious and nonanxious controls. However, this hypothesis needs to be tested and confirmed by subsequent clinical research.

Attempts to demonstrate significant and consistent psychophysiological differences between subjects high and low in trait anxiety have in general been unsuccessful (Eysenck & Eysenck, 1985). However, consistent cognitive differences have been identified which are probably reflected in some aspects of brain function

(Eysenck, 1987). Nevertheless, even the most detailed model of the brain substrates of anxiety cannot incorporate such findings (Gray, 1982).

Individual differences in state or trait anxiety are important endogenous variables. The predominance of female patients being treated for anxiety disorders may reflect diagnostic biases, for instance in self-report, but equally, may represent real biological variation. By contrast, in the rat, it is the male that shows the greatest sensitivity to experimental manipulations of fear and to early environmental stress (Gray, 1971).

Some researchers have suggested that it is rather the way we lead our life that may have a significant influence on the risk for anxiety disorders. For example, some investigators have demonstrated that cigarette smoking is associated with anxiety disorders (Kandel et al., 1997; Brook et al., 1998). This is mainly due to factors including respiration and the presumed anxiogenic effects of nicotine. In support of this hypothesis, clinical studies have indicated that cigarette smoking preceded the onset of panic attacks among patients with PD (Breslau et al., 1991; Pohl et al., 1992).

1.4 Cognitive aspects of anxiety

An important aspect of the cognitive basis of anxiety is that it involves the selective processing of information perceived as signifying a threat or danger to one's personal safety or security (Beck et al., 1985). Cognitive theories have been proposed for a number of specific anxiety disorders including PD, SP, OCD and GAD (Clark, 1986, Sopa & Clark, 1993, Salkovskis, 1989; Wells, 1995). Although these theories differ slightly depending on the specific anxiety disorder, all consider a selective bias for threat information in attention, interpretation and memory a central characteristic that distinguishes anxious and non-anxious states.

An impressive amount of evidence for specific cognitive process variables in many anxiety disorders has been produced during these last few years. For example, an exaggerated responsibility as a key cognitive process variable in OCD has been identified (Salkovskis, 1985). It has been shown that a cognitive treatment that exclusively targets excessive responsibility leads to clinically significant therapy gains for patients with OCD (Ladouceur et al., 1996). Other anxiety disorder process variables that have been identified include anxiety sensitivity. After reviewing the empirical data on anxiety sensitivity, it has also been concluded that this variable is a specific marker of fear of anxiety and panic-related sensations (Taylor, 1996). Obviously, exposure to interoceptive cues, a key treatment component for PD, targets anxiety sensitivity (Barlow, 1988).

The cognitive model of anxiety is a schema-based information processing perspective that considers the erroneous or biased interpretation of stimuli as dangerous or threatening to an individual's physical or psychological well-being, a core feature of anxiety disorders (Beck et al., 1985). Along with the selective processing of threat or danger stimuli, the anxious individual underestimates personal coping resources and the safety or rescue features in the environment. Furthermore the distinction between normal and pathological anxiety is one of degree rather than kind because of the vital role that fear plays in the survival of an individual. The difference is that in pathological anxiety there is a biased or overestimated perception of danger that does not correspond to the exigencies of the internal or external environment, whereas in nonclinical anxiety states the estimation of threat corresponds more closely to the objective dangers in the environment.

A modern approach to the theory of anxiety must recognise three interrelated mental operations which are estimation of the nature and magnitude of external and internal dangers, emotional and physiological reaction and their regulation and finally the estimation of the type, degree and efficacy of protective intervention. Therefore, the cognitive model recognises that anxiety consists of a complicated pattern of cognitive, affective, physiological and behavioural changes (Beck et al. 1985). At the physiological level, one notes autonomic hyperarousal in preparation for flight, fight, freezing or fainting. At the behavioural level, one notes mobilisation in order to escape or defend oneself against the perceived danger, inhibition of risk taking behaviour in an attempt to maximise safety and deactivation of motor responses resulting in avoidance and feelings of helplessness. At the subjective level, the individual feels frightened or apprehensive. At the cognitive level, anxiety involves certain sensory-perceptual symptoms such as feelings of unreality, hypervigilance and self-consciousness, thinking difficulties such as poor concentration, inability to control thinking, blocking, difficulty of reasoning and conceptual symptoms like cognitive distortions, fear-related beliefs, frightening images and frequent automatic thoughts (Beck et al. 1985). These operations are strongly rooted in neurobiological development and experiential history.

In experimental studies, it is now well established that anxiety states are associated with increased attention to threat cues, and a greater likelihood of perceiving the threatening meaning of ambiguous events (Mathews & MacLeod, 1994). Relative to normal controls, anxiety-disordered populations show, in the modified Stroop task, greater colour-naming interference from threatening words (e.g. collapse, death, failure, stupid) and slower search times for neutral targets in the presence of threat distracters (Mathews et al., 1990; Williams et al., 1996). In contrast, they show relatively faster detection of probe stimuli appearing in the same location as threatening words or of angry faces in a set of happy faces (Byrne & Eysenck, 1995; Mogg et al., 1992). In general, when a task involves ignoring threatening cues, it seems that anxiety leads to a slowing of performance, but when attention to threat helps to locate a target, then performance is relatively speeded. Such findings suggest that anxiety-disordered individuals have their attention captured automatically by threat-related cues and meanings. A recent study designed to further clarify the emotional Stroop effect in anxiety disorders tested two different groups of anxiety patients, namely patients with GAD and patients with SP, most of whom were afraid of giving speeches as compared to non-anxious controls (Becker et al., 2001). Stimuli were of four kinds: GAD-related words, SP-related words, words with a neutral valence and words with a positive valence. Results of the Stroop task showed that patients suffering from GAD displayed an attentional bias. They took longer to name the print colour of GAD-related words than SP patients and controls. However, GAD patients also took longer than controls to name the colour of positive words and speech-related words. Colour naming times of the SP patients followed a different pattern. They showed longer naming times than controls only for the colour of speech-related words. There was no difference between SP patients and controls for the colour-naming times of GAD-related, neutral or positive words. Thus, GAD patients were slowed by all types of emotional words, while SP patients were distracted specifically by speech-related words.

In the model of attentional bias, two distinct pre-attentive processing stages are postulated (Williams et al., 1988). At the first stage, the threat value or negativity of a stimulus event is computed by an effective decision mechanism, with high levels of current state-anxiety increasing the resulting threat value output. If threat value is determined to be high enough, a secondary resource allocation mechanism is triggered, that is influenced by trait anxiety differences. High levels of trait anxiety lead to the allocation of attentional resources towards the stimulus. In contrast, low trait levels are reported to lead to attention being directed away from the threatening event. However, recent studies showed that low as well as high trait-anxious individuals were attentionally vigilant for threatening pictures, contrary to the model of Williams et al (Mogg & Bradley, 1998; Lang et al., 1995). These new data suggest that anxiety-related differences become apparent only with mild or ambiguous threats, such as words, faces, or slightly aversive pictures. The assumption of the model of Williams et al. that low trait-anxious individuals have a universal tendency to avoid attending to stimuli with a high threat value therefore needs to be clarified. Avoidance in low trait-anxious individuals may occur under relatively mild threat conditions; given severe enough threats they switch over to a pattern of attentional vigilance. The difference between high and low trait-anxious individuals thus resides in the threshold at which this switch to a vigilant mode occurs or the responsiveness of this switching mechanism to some attributes of threatening stimuli.

Another influential model of attentional bias termed the self-regulatory executive function attributed attentional bias to top-down processes, related to the individual's plans and goals (Wells and Matthews, 1994). In this model, phenomena such as emotional Stroop interference are attributed to a voluntarily executed plan, which specifies the monitoring of negative stimuli that intrude into awareness (Wells & Matthews, 1994). This model argues that the evidence for nonconscious emotional processing bias is not convincing and that, even if it was, top-down control might still indirectly influence the reaction to stimuli that cannot be reported. That is, when anxious individuals voluntarily adopt a threat-monitoring plan, the consequence is that all threatening stimuli attract attention, including those that do not succeed in reaching full subjective awareness. However, although simulations showed that his arrangement satisfactorily mimics emotional interference effects, its plausibility must rest on the voluntarily strategy assumption.

Another model of anxiety and attention is that described by Öhman (1993). In this account, incoming information is first analysed by feature detectors, before being passed on to a nonconscious "significance evaluating system". Biologically prepared or high intensity stimuli may result in feature detectors activating autonomic arousal, without need of further processing. Öhman's position thus partly resembles that of Wells and Matthews in that conscious expectation of threat can set up the conditions for attentional bias, but differs from it in that the significance evaluator responds to stimuli automatically and pre-attentively, without awareness or direct strategic control. Despite this, the model specifies that autonomic activation to threats is not produced directly by the significance evaluator, but only indirectly *via* conscious perception. Such a conclusion seems at odds with findings that conditioned or unconditioned threat stimuli that cannot be reported, can still produce autonomic responses.

There are a number of issues that can be raised about the cognitive basis of anxiety which include questions of whether selective processing of threat is specific to anxiety vs. other emotional states, whether threat bias is confined to certain cognitive processes or is it apparent at all stages of information processing and whether threat bias in anxiety should be considered a state or trait phenomenon. It was concluded that the processing bias in anxiety is automatic in terms of being involuntary and possibly unconscious but is not resource or capacity-free (McNally, 1995).

In a recent study designed to test a new six-system model which includes physiological, behavioural, cognitive, affective, trait and state components of anxiety and also differentiates between direct and mediated responses, the results highlight the importance of considering not only behavioural, somatic and cognitive systems but also an affective component in the study of anxiety (Wilken et al., 1999). Consistent with other research work, stressful affective stimuli are more potent when the emotional stimulus directly produces anxiety than when an external stimulus elicits arousal mediated by affect (Hubert & Jong-Meyer, 1990). The results also showed that personality traits have an important influence on the effects of stressors on behavioural and physiological responses. High-anxiety subjects reported similar subjective feelings of stress regardless of their stress condition, but low anxious subjects reported greater anxiety in the high-stress condition. This may be a result of the fact that low anxious subjects normally experience less stress and are further below their stress limit which allows external stressors to induce larger increments in felt anxiety. Therefore, high anxious subjects reported feeling more negative, less calm, and less relaxed than low anxious subjects. This finding demonstrates that trait anxiety is an important determinant of reported stress on the sensory-affective task.

1.4.1 Gray neuropsychological model of anxiety

The most comprehensive neuropsychological account of anxiety argues that a septo-hippocampal "behavioural inhibition system" (BIS) monitors environmental events and feedback from the animal's own responses, and is particularly sensitive to signals associated with novelty, non-reward or punishment (Gray, 1982). When these are detected, ongoing behaviour is suppressed, while attention and arousal are increased. Thus anxiety is activity in the BIS. It is hypothesised that anxiolytics act indirectly to impair the BIS through gamma-aminobutyric acid (GABA)-ergic modulation of the ascending noradrenergic and serotonergic pathways to the hippocampus, which are responsible for the registration and assessment of aversive stimuli.

1.5 Comorbidity of anxiety disorders

The term comorbidity indicates the presence of more than one disorder in a person in a given period of time (Wittchen & Essau, 1989). Once an anxiety disorder is suspected, it is important to investigate the cause. Anxiety disorders may be associated with other diagnoses, such as depression or physical illness (Kessler et al., 1994). Up to a half of those meeting lifetime criteria for major depression also meet the criteria for an anxiety disorder (Regier et al., 1998).

Since epidemiological studies have shown that psychiatric disorders frequently co-occur, comorbidity is more often addressed explicitly in research (Volrath & Angst, 1989). A major component of these comorbidity diagnoses consists of anxiety disorders, mood disorders and substance use disorders (Regier et al., 1990). In the ECA survey, it was observed that those with any anxiety disorder as compared to the rest of the sample had a 50% increase in the odds of being diagnosed with an alcohol disorder (odds ratio = 1.52; Regier et al., 1990). Similarly, the subsample with anxiety disorder had about a 70% increase in the odds of being diagnosed with any substance use disorder (odds ratio = 1.7). Further, because both anxiety disorders and substance use disorders are among the most common psychiatric conditions, these odds ratios indicate that the real number of comorbid cases is relatively high. Notably, PD presented an even greater increase in the odds of being diagnosed with alcohol or drug dependence (odds ratio = 3.3 and 4.4, respectively) than was true for the broader diagnostic categories (Regier et al., 1990). The same pattern held for the ECA subsample with OCD in which the odds ratios associated with alcohol and drug dependence were 2.5 and 3.6, respectively (Regier et al., 1990). Interestingly, panic and OCD were not significantly related to alcohol or drug abuse in the absence of dependence. However, a separate analysis for phobic disorders did not confirm the findings by Regier et al. (Himle & Hill, 1991). This re-analysis showed an approximate 2- to 2.5-fold increase in the likelihood of being diagnosed with alcohol abuse or dependence among those with agoraphobia and SP, respectively. However, an increased risk for alcohol abuse or dependence among those with simple phobia was not found. A causal explanation for the aetiology of comorbidity is that anxiety disorder or anxiety symptoms *per se* may serve to promote directly the pathological use of alcohol or drugs. This primary hypothesis, sometimes called "self-medication hypothesis" suggests that the pharmacological or psychological effects of alcohol and some drugs serve to decrease aversive anxiety symptoms, thereby promoting persistent and escalating use of alcohol and drugs. Studies in young populations suggest that patients with an anxiety disorder and comorbidity diagnoses such as depression, alcohol dependence and chronic benzodiazepine (BDZ) use are more severely and chronically ill and more disabled (Pasnau & Bystritsky, 1994; Van Balkom et al., 1996; Mulsant et al., 1996). They also utilise services more frequently and are more difficult to treat.

Anxiety often coexists with depression (Blazer et al., 1991). Major depression is present in up to 70% of older people with GAD and in quite a few people with phobias or PTSD (Manela et al., 1996; Lindesay, 1991). A study reported that one-third of an elderly population with phobic disorders and GAD also suffered from major depression (Lindesay et al., 1989). A recent study which investigated patterns of comorbidity among the anxiety disorders in a community-based older population in the Netherlands reported that 10% of the elderly with an anxiety diagnosis suffered from two or more anxiety disorders (Van Balkom et al., 2000). Major depression (13% vs. 3%), BDZ use (24% vs. 11%) and chronic somatic diseases (12% vs. 7%) were significantly more prevalent in respondents with an anxiety disorder than in respondents without anxiety disorders. When anxiety disorders are diagnosed in older individuals, there is a relatively high probability of comorbid conditions being present.

1.6 Anxiety scales

When measuring anxiety by a scale, one must be aware of the particular emphasis of the scale that one selects. The results of an investigation using one scale may have been very different if another scale had been used. Instruments used in research must be reliable and what they measure must be absolutely clear. Progress in research is hindered both by the varied meanings of the term "anxiety" and by the rating scales used to assess it. There is often a general assumption that all the anxiety scales assess the same construct of anxiety and that selection of a scale is purely a matter of personal preference or convenience. However, this is wrong. Some anxiety scales attempt complete coverage of all aspects of anxiety but many put major emphasis on one or another aspect. A problem with the attempted coverage of all aspects in a single scale is that it is unusual for all aspects of the anxiety states to be present to an equal degree in any one individual.

There are difficulties in the process of validation of scales that purport to assess anxiety. *Face validity* refers to whether the scale appears, on inspection, to assess the aspect of anxiety in which the clinician is interested. *Content validity* refers to whether the scale covers all aspects of the theoretical anxiety state but this may be less important as few individuals will experience the full gamut of symptoms of anxiety at any one time. *Concurrent validity* is the measure of how well the scale performs against some other criterion of severity but there can be no gold standard for the evaluation of such a diffuse and variable state of anxiety. *Reliability* of a scale refers to whether it consistently provides the same reading when applied under the same conditions. This measure causes problems with regard to a state that may vary in severity from one moment to another or from day to day. Although most users of anxiety scales will show evidence as to whether two raters arrive at the same score when utilising a scale (inter-rater reliability), such a procedure cannot be employed in the presentation of a self-assessment scale.

Examination of the anxiety scales used in the literature suggests considerable variation in construction and composition. Today, the original version of the Hamilton Anxiety Scale (HAM-A) is mainly used as the indicator for anxiolytic efficacy in nearly all evaluation studies with potential anxiolytic drugs. No rival observer scale for the severity of anxiety has so far received comparable acceptance. The HAM-A was designed for patients with a diagnosis of anxiety neurosis and the validation was mainly performed for this group of patients. However, diagnostic habits have changed and the concept of anxiety neurosis has been substituted by a new concept of anxiety disorders comprising PD, phobic disorders and GAD. The degree of overlap between the old and new concepts is limited and therefore the HAM-A is often applied beyond its intended scope. While the HAM-A is suitable for rating and assessing patients who have already been diagnosed as suffering from neurotic anxiety states, it is unsuitable for differential diagnosis (Hamilton, 1959; Beneke, 1987). The HAM-A focuses to a large extent on somatic symptoms and only the anxiety subscale of the Brief Psychiatric Rating Scale (BPRS) places a significant emphasis on the cognitive aspect of anxiety disorders. The HAM-A is dominated by the somatic correlates of anxiety; only six items relate unequivocally to the assessment of psychic phenomena. Hamilton advised that his scale should be employed for assessment of patients who had already received a diagnosis of an anxiety disorder; however, such caution is often disregarded. The subscale of somatic anxiety is strongly related to somatic side effects. Therefore, the applicability of the HAM-A in anxiolytic treatment studies is limited and more specific anxiety scales are needed for each specific anxiety disorder such as PD, PTSD and GAD. In the assessment of severity of symptoms of anxiety, a preference for a visual analogue scale (100 mm) has been suggested (Lader & Marks, 1974).

The State-Trait Anxiety Inventory (STAI) is a 40-item questionnaire in which physiological and subjective symptoms of anxiety are rated on a 4-point Likert scale (Spielberger et al., 1970). The A-state scale is comprised of items 1 through 20 and is designed to measure relatively transient anxiety that varies over time and context. Each item is rated on a 0 to 4 scale with scores on the A-state scale ranging from 20 to 80. Higher scores are indicative of higher levels of state anxiety. Prior research demonstrates that the STAI has adequate psychometric properties (internal consistency estimates that range from 0.83–0.92 and a test-retest reliability coefficient of 0.40 for the state version of the STAI) (Spielberger et al., 1970).

The measurement of anxiety in children is complicated by poor correspondence between children's self-reported anxiety ratings and ratings of their anxiety provided by other informants (Klein, 1991). Outcome-evaluation studies typically address this dilemma by reporting treatment-related changes separately for child, parent and clinician report. However, in clinical practice, major report discrepancies can result in confusion. Reporting differences also highlight the limitations of relying exclusively on symptoms checklists for assessing anxiety. Clinical interviews of parents and child are essential to a complete diagnostic evaluation in children. Despite these difficulties, several psychometrically sound measures of anxiety in children have recently become available (Greenhill et al., 1998). The Screen for Child Anxiety Related Emotional Disorders (SCARED) and the Multidimensional Anxiety Scale for Children (MASC) have the best empirical validation to date (Birmaher et al., 1997; March, 1998). The SCARED uses a 38-item Likert-type scale to assess anxiety factors: physical symptoms, panic, general anxiety, SP, and separation anxiety. The MASC uses a 39-item Likert type scale to assess anxiety factors: physical symptoms, social anxiety, harm avoidance, and separation anxiety. Both show high internal consistency, test-retest reliability, and discriminant validity with fair parent-child agreement. Scores on these instruments were recently reported to be highly correlated in a clinical population (Muris et al., 1998).

Some preliminary data have begun to consider the utility of the HAM-A for assessing the severity of anxiety symptoms, irrespective of psychiatric diagnosis in older individuals (Sheikh, 1991). The availability of a clinician-rated tool that provides symptom severity ratings to complement categorical diagnoses is particularly important in light of concerns about the relevance of current psychiatric nomenclature for classifying anxiety problems in late life. Therefore, this type of measure could be of particular use in assessing treatment outcomes.

The BPRS has been in use since 1962 but was developed primarily for controlled psychoactive drug trials and similar research (Overall & Gorham, 1962; Overall, 1974). Further refinement during its first 18 years of use, including questions of reliability and validity, has been summarised (Hedlund & Vieweg, 1980). It is a useful outcome measure. Subscale scores may provide more specific prediction of change and may help clarify outcome in individual patients who show insignificant change by total score.

Clinical observations may capture dimensions of behaviour that are not readily reduced to specific symptoms. Global assessment scales quantify such observations. The most widely used is the clinical global impressions (CGI) scale (Guy, 1976). The CGI asks the clinician to refer to his total clinical experience to assess the severity of the patient's current mental illness (1 item) and to evaluate improvement from the patient's baseline condition as previously observed (1 item). The CGI therefore captures and quantifies global improvement by the clinician regarding both severity and improvement. It offers a crude, yet very useful measure of change in patients with anxiety disorders.

2 Relevance of laboratory research on anxiety disorders

Experimental research is both relevant and indispensable for the continued advancement of our understanding and treatment of anxiety disorders. The clinical relevance of laboratory-based experimental research for understanding and treating anxiety-related problems has been questioned. Critics questioned the external validity, practical utility and value of experimental research for understanding the psychological processes that contribute to clinical problems in the natural environment. The issue of how laboratory experimentation can contribute to our understanding of the dysfunctional processes involved with anxiety disorders remains somewhat unclear (Cahill et al., 1998). In particular, it has been argued that the high degree of experimental control characteristic of laboratory-based research often fails to yield a rich source of clinically relevant information that can be employed in naturalistic conditions (Chlorpita, 1997). Due to the high degree of experimental control, laboratory-based studies have been useful in isolating many basic psychological processes that underlie, in part, the aetiology and maintenance of anxiety disorders. By using this information, psychological principles can be isolated and then effective psychosocial interventions that use these principles to correct faulty learning principles can be developed (Eifert et al., 1997).

Although naturalistic studies are advantageous in providing a large degree of scope and a wealth of clinically relevant data, such advantages often come at the expense of precision and control. Experimental research, on the other hand, strives to clarify the nature and parameters of psychological processes, thereby providing comprehensive explanations at different levels of analysis. The high degree of internal validity of laboratory studies increases their explanatory power, permitting causally oriented hypothesis testing.

External validity (i.e. generalizability) and ecological validity (i.e. the extent to which laboratory preparations represent stimuli in the natural environment) are related but also distinct concepts. Although high ecological validity is frequently related to high generalizability, tasks or stimuli with low ecological validity may still have high generalizability to real-world phenomena. For example, cognitive tasks such as dot probe and Stroop colour-word tests may be useful in detecting sensitivity to particular types of threat cues, but are low in ecological validity. Low ecological validity, however, does not necessarily limit the utility of such cognitive methods, especially when considering their high degree of generalizability to cognitive processes that occur in naturalistic contexts (McNally et al., 1989).

An example of an advantage of using nonclinical participants is research on individuals who experience panic attacks but do not seek treatment, probably because panic does not interfere sufficiently with their life functioning (Norton et al., 1999). Studying such individuals allows to examine mechanisms of panic that are relatively uncontaminated by other psychopathology and before individuals develop the full-blown pathology. This may provide clarification about mechanisms that are related to potential causes of panic attacks and their prevention.

3 Genetic factors and brain imaging

Genetic factors most likely play a role in pathological anxiety. Twin studies on anxiety disorders suggest that genetic factors do play a role in the aetiology of pathological anxiety (Kendler et al., 1995; Torgersen, 1997). The specific anxiety disorders do not seem to be genetically homogenous, but at the same time there is no discrete set of genetic factors for each disorder (Kendler et al., 1995). A study reported that about 10-15% of children seem to be born excessively shy with heightened levels of arousal and a propensity for exaggerated social wariness and behaviourally inhibited responses that persist at least into later childhood (Kagan et al., 1988).

Frontal brain asymmetry (FBA) represents a trait marker related to psychopathology as well as a state marker associated with acute emotional reactions (Davidson et al., 1990; Davidson & Nathan, 1989; Tomarken et al., 1992). Recent studies revealed FBA with a right frontal hyperactivation during rest in anxious, depressed patients while an inverse FBA was found in anxious undergraduate students (Bruder et al., 1997; Heller et al., 1997). Both studies also found relatively greater right than left parietal activation in anxious, depressed patients and anxious undergraduates during phases of anxious arousal. These posterior asymmetries are in line with the proposal that anxious arousal including panic should be associated with a relatively increased right parietotemporal activation, while anxious apprehension should be associated with a relatively increased left parietal activation (Heller et al., 1995; 1997).

OCD, PD and PTSD share many other clinical features such as anticipatory anxiety and depression. All three groups had similar levels of anxiety, which tends to increase regional cerebral blood flow (rCBF) (Lucey et al., 1995). A study which compared rCBF in OCD, PD and PTSD patients using DSM-III-R criteria showed that caudate and superior frontal cortical perfusion were reduced in both OCD and PTSD compared with PD and healthy controls (Lucey et al., 1997). Although OCD, PD and PTSD all had high levels of anxiety, caudate hypoperfusion was not seen in PD. It is possible that OCD and PTSD but not PD share mental activity (possibly obsessive thinking, intrusive imagery or resistance) which is associated with reduction in caudate perfusion.

4 Management

Two forms of treatment are generally thought to be effective in the treatment of anxiety disorders: drug treatment and behavioural therapy. Whereas drug treatment may be prescribed by a general practitioner, behavioural cognitive psychotherapy has been developed by psychiatrists and psychologists and is usually delivered at specialist centres. For most people, acute situational anxiety improves with support, reassurance and the passage of time. Formal psychotherapy and pharmacological interventions are used for individuals with pathologic anxiety, defined as anxiety persisting for more than several weeks or when the anxiety, regardless of its duration, is causing important distress or deterioration in daily normal function.

The premise of the cognitive model of anxiety is that it is not events *per se* but peoples' expectations and interpretations of events that are responsible for the anxiety. According to this hypothesis, anxious people overestimate the danger inherent in a situation, thereby causing an activation of autonomic and behavioural manifestations of anxiety. They then misinterpret these sensations as a further source of threat, leading to a vicious circle that maintains or deteriorates their anxiety disorder (Clark, 1989). Cognitive therapy involves identifying, evaluating, controlling and modifying these negative thoughts and cognitive distortions and attributions.

Cognitive therapy is consistently more effective than no therapy or placebo for PD with or without agoraphobia, GAD, PTSD and SP (Antony & Swinson, 1996). Exposure therapy is particularly useful for treating phobic avoidance and compulsive rituals (Antony & Swinson, 1996). Exposure therapy encourages patients to face feared situations or objects. Exposure usually occurs in a graded fashion over several weeks. Best results are obtained when exposure is prolonged rather than brief, takes place in real life rather than in fantasy, and is regularly practised by patients through self-exposure homework.

Following the younger adult literature, some case studies have suggested the utility of cognitive behaviour therapy for the reduction of anxiety in older adults. In fact, case reports have described the potential efficacy of a wide range of treatment approaches including exposure and response prevention, relaxation training, and cognitive therapy for older adults with GAD, PD, specific phobia and OCD (King & Barrowclough, 1991; Swales et al., 1996; Thyer, 1981, Junginger & Ditto, 1984).

Controlled trials involving patients of various ages have shown that several anxiety disorders respond to pharmacological treatment such as antidepressant medications, BDZs and buspirone (Antony & Swinson, 1996; APA, 1998, Ravizza, 1997, Steinberg, 1994).

Among medications prescribed for anxiety in late life, the BDZs are probably more prevalent. In fact, anywhere from 17% of older outpatients to 50% of nursing home patients are prescribed these medications (Salzman, 1991). Lower doses than those prescribed for younger adults also are usually recommended, and there clearly is the need to consider the impact of associated medical illness and prescription use on the effects of these medications (Stoudemire & Moran, 1993). Despite the frequency with which these medications are used in the elderly, the majority of the studies performed to assess the efficacy and safety of BDZs in this population were not well controlled and numerous difficulties characterised the identification and selection of patients (Salzman, 1991). The field remains in desperate need of well-controlled studies addressing the efficacy of BDZ treatment for late-life anxiety, especially since the long-term efficacy of these medications remains controversial (Lader, 1999). Given these concerns, some authors have suggested that psychosocial interventions be used as alternatives whenever possible (Wengel et al., 1993).

In a recent study designed to assess the efficacy and safety of serotonin-reuptake inhibitors in children with anxiety disorders, it was shown that fluvoxamine induces a significant improvement in children and adolescents with SP, separation anxiety disorder or GAD (The Research Unit on Pediatric Psychopharmacology Anxiety Study Group, 2001).

5 Discussion

There are positive features of anxiety. It can be conceptualised as a biological warning system that prepares the body to react mentally and physically to potentially dangerous situations. Moderate anxiety can be useful by directing the individual's attention to the danger and motivating coping behaviour. However, when anxiety is severe, it becomes disorganising and therefore counterproductive (Hoehn-Saric & McLeod, 1990). Research on anxiety based on a diagnostic or categorical approach should take into account the full spectrum of the anxiety variable. It is also important to assess anxiety using more than one method. In addition to self-report measures, one can use behavioural assessment techniques, physiological measures and ratings by trained experienced clinicians. With their high prevalence, anxiety disorders, more than any other mental disorders, cause many economic burdens, loss of productivity and suffering for the patients, family and carers. It is worth noting that anxiety disorders cause almost one-third of the total of economic costs created by mental disorder (Rice & Miller, 1998).

Both the ECA survey and the NCS provide evidence of an approximate doubling to quadrupling of risk for alcohol or drug dependence given the presence of most anxiety disorders (Kessler et al., 1997; Regier et al., 1990). However, simple phobia was not associated with alcohol disorders in the ECA survey but it was in the NCS. These prevalence data suggest that all or most anxiety disorders have a significant relationship to alcohol disorder. However, they do not clarify the nature of these relationships.

Biological research on separation anxiety disorder holds the hope of clarifying factors that influence the transmission of panic-related disorders from parents to children. Children born to parents with PD are hypothesised to exhibit abnormalities in respiratory regulation, particularly when they also show signs of separation anxiety disorder. During childhood, this form of anxiety disorder is associated with separation anxiety, whereas during adolescence, this form of anxiety is associated with spontaneous panic attacks that may eventually develop into PD.

The field is just beginning to collect accurate epidemiological data concerning the anxiety disorders in the older adults. Unfortunately, there is no epidemiological information about the prevalence of anxiety disorders among special populations, such as elderly who reside in residential care facilities and individuals who present to medical personnel. Preliminary reports suggest that individuals living in residential care facilities may report greater difficulties with anxiety relative to community-dwelling elderly (Bland et al., 1988). Individuals with medical problems also stand a greater risk for anxiety disorders. Another special population that has received little attention are individuals at risk for PTSD. In particular, individuals exposed to extreme traumas (such as combat, Holocaust, or being taken as a prisoner of war) may function adequately until they begin to age, at which point PTSD symptomatology may begin (Averill & Beck, 2000). Such phenomenon may be explained by increased psychological and physical vulnerability associated with ageing, exposure to an event which resembles the initial trauma and the reflective nature of many older adults, a propensity which is developmentally typical (Aarts & Op den Velde, 1996; Robinson et al., 1992). Thus, further research needs to be focused on older adults who were exposed to trauma as they may represent a special population with higher risk of anxiety disorders.

The progress in developing effective treatments for the five principal anxiety disorders (PD, SP, OCD, GAD and PTSD) in adults has been rapid in the past 15 years. There are now some well-controlled clinical studies documenting effective pharmacological and psychological treatments for all of these disorders, although generally the evidence is better developed for some disorders than for others particularly in adults. In the treatment of anxiety disorders, the long-term effects of cognitive behaviour therapy on developmental outcomes in anxious children and elderly remain to be elucidated since most studies follow children and elderly for less than a year. Further, the treatment's high reliance on verbal ability limits its utility in less verbal children and the transposition of cognitive behaviour therapy from academic centres to the community has not yet been fully demonstrated in psychiatric patients of all ages.

References

Aarts P & Op den Velde W. Prior traumatization and the process of aging. In: B Van der Kolk, A McFarlane & L Weisaeth (eds): Traumatic stress: The effects of overwhelming experience on mind, body, and society. New York, Guildford Press, 359–377, 1996

American Psychiatric Association. Diagnostic and statistical manual of mental disorders. First Edition, Washington DC, American Psychiatric Association, 1952

American Psychiatric Association. Diagnostic and statistical manual of mental disorders. Second Edition, Washington DC, American Psychiatric Association, 1968

American Psychiatric Association. Diagnostic and statistical manual of mental disorder (3rd edition). Washington, DC, 1980

American Psychiatric Association. Diagnostic and statistical manual of mental disorders. Third Edition, Revised. Washington DC, American Psychiatric Association, 1987

American Psychiatric Association. Practice guidelines for the treatment of patients with panic disorder. Am J Psychiatry 155, 1–34, 1998

American Psychiatric Association. Diagnostic and statistical manual of mental disorder (4th edition). Washington, DC, 1994

Antony MM & Swinson RP. Anxiety disorders and their treatment: a critical review of the evidence-based literature. Ottawa, Ont: Health Canada, 1996

Averill PM & Beck JG. Posttraumatic stress disorder in older adults: A conceptual review. J Anxiety Disord 14, 133–156, 2000

Barlow DH. Anxiety and its disorders: The nature and treatment of anxiety and panic. New York: Guildford Press, 1988

Beck JG, Stanley MA & Zebb BJ. Characteristics of generalized anxiety disorder in older adults: A descriptive study. Behav Res Ther 34, 225–234, 1996

Beck AT. Theoretical perspectives on clinical anxiety. In: AH Tuma & J Maser (eds): Anxiety and the anxiety disorders. Hillsdale NJ: Lawrence Erlbaum Associates, 183–196, 1985

Becker ES, Rinck M, Margraf J & Roth WT. The emotional Stroop effect in anxiety disorders. General emotionality or disorder specificity? J Anxiety Disord 15, 147–159, 2001

Beidel DC & Turner SM. Anxiety disorders. In: M Hersen & SM Turner (eds): Adult psychopathology and diagnosis. New York, Wiley, 226–278, 1991

Beneke M. Methodological investigations of the Hamilton Anxiety Scale. Pharmacopsychiatry 249–255, 1987

Benjamin RS, Costello EJ, Warren M. Anxiety disorders in a pediatric sample. J Anxiety Disord 4, 293–316, 1990

Birbaumer N, Grodd W. Diedrich O. Klose U. Erb M. Lotze M. Schneider F. Weiss U. Flor H FMRI reveals amygdala activation to human faces in social phobics. Neuroreport 9, 1223–1226, 1998

Birmaher B, Khetarpal S, Brent D, Cully M, Balach L, Kaufman J. The screen for child anxiety related emotional disorders (SCARED): screen construction and psychometric characteristics. J Am Acad Child Adolesc Psychiatry 36, 545–553, 1997

Bland RC, Newman SC & Orn H. Prevalence of psychiatric disorders in the elderly in Edmonton. Acta Psychiatrica (Supp) 338, 57–63, 1988

Blazer D, Hughes D & George LK. Stressful life events and the onset of a generalized anxiety syndrome. Am J Psychiatry 144, 1178-1183, 1987

Blazer D, George LK, Hughes D. Generalized anxiety disorder. In: Robins LN, Regier DA (eds): Psychiatric disorders in America: the Epidemiological Catchment Area Study. New York, NY: The Free Press, 1991

Borkovec TD, Robinson E, Pruzinsky T & DePree JA. Preliminary exploration of worry: Some characteristics and processes. Behav Res Ther 21, 9–16, 1983

Breiter HC, Etcoff NL, Whalen PJ, Kennedy WA, Rauch SL, Buckner RL, Strauss MM, Hyman SE, Rosen BR. Response and habituation of the human amygdala during visual processing of facial expression. Neuron 17, 875–887, 1996

Breslau N, Kilbey MM, Andreski P. Nicotine dependence, major depression, and anxiety in young adults. Arch Gen Psychiatry 48, 1069–1074, 1991

Brook JS, Cohen P, Brook DW. Longitudinal study of co-occurring psychiatric disorders and substance use. J Am Acad Child Adolesc Psychiatry 37, 322–330, 1998

Bruder GE, Fong R, Tenke CE, Leite P, Towey JP, Stewart JE, McGrath PJ, Quitkin FM. Regional brain asymmetries in major depression with or without anxiety disorder: a quantitative electroencephalographic study. Biol Psychiatry 41, 939–948, 1997

Byrne A & Eysenck MW. Trait anxiety, anxious mood, and threat detection. Cognition and Emotion 9, 549–562, 1995

Cahill SP, Carrigan MH & Evans IM. The relation between behavior theory and behavior therapy: Challenges and promises. In: JJ Plaud & GH Eifert (eds): From behavior theory to behavior therapy. Boston: Allyn & Bacon, 294–319, 1998

Capps L, Sigman M, Sena R, Henker B, Whalen C. Fear, anxiety, and perceived control in children of agoraphobic parents. J Child Psychol Psychiatry Allied Disc 37, 445–452, 1996

Cheok A, Snowdon J, Miller R & Vaughan R. The prevalence of anxiety disorders in nursing homes. Int J Geriatr Psychiatry 11, 405–410, 1996

Chlorpita BF. Since the operant chamber: Are we still thinking in Skinner boxes? Behavior Therapy 28, 577–583, 1997

Clark DM. A cognitive approach to panic. Behav Res Ther 24, 461–470, 1986

Clark MD. Anxiety states: panic and generalized anxiety. In: K Hawton, PM Salkovskis, J Kirk, DM Clark (eds): Cognitive behaviour therapy for psychiatric problems. Oxford, Eng: Oxford Medical Publications, 52–96, 1989

Cloninger CR. A unified biosocial theory of personality and its role in the development of anxiety states. Psychiatric Development 3, 167–226, 1986

Coryell W. Hypersensitivity to carbon dioxide as a disease-specific trait marker. Biol Psychiatry 41, 259–263, 1997

Costello EJ, Angold A, Keeler GP. Adolescent outcomes of childhood disorders: the consequences of severity and impairment. J Am Acad Child Adolesc Psychiatry 38, 121–128, 1999

Daledin EL & Vasey MW. An information-processing perspective on childhood anxiety. Clin Psychol Rev 17, 407–429, 1997

Davidson RJ, Ekman P, Saron C, Senulis JA, Friesen WV. Approach-withdrawal and cerebral asymmetry: emotional expression and brain physiology. I. J Pers Soc Psychol 58, 330–341, 1990

Davidson RJ, Nathan AF. Frontal brain asymmetry predicts infants" response to maternal separation. J Abnorm Psychol 98, 127–131, 1989

Eaton WW, Kramer M, Anthony JC, Dryman A, Shapiro S & Locke BZ. The incidence of specific DIS/DSM-III mental disorders: Data from the NIMH Epidemiologic Catchment Area Program. Acta Psychiatr Scand 79, 163–178, 1989

Eifert GH, Schulte D, Zvolensky MJ, Lejuez CW, Lau AW, Iwamasa GY & Orsillo SM. Manualized behavior therapy. Merits and challenges. Behaviour Therapy 28, 499–515, 1997

Eysenck HJ & Eysenck MW. Personality and individual differences. London: Plenum, 1985

Eysenck M. Anxiety: The cognitive perspective. Hillsdale, NJ: Erlbaum, 1992

Eysenck MW. Trait theories of anxiety. In: J Strelau & HJ Eysenck (eds): Personality dimensions and arousal. New York: Plenum, 79–97, 1987

Eysenck HJ. Biological bases of personality. Springfield, IL: Charles C. Thomas, 1967

Ewing DJ, Hume L, Campbell IW, Murray A, Neilson JMM, Clarke BF. Autonomic mechanisms in the initial heart rate response to standing. J Appl Physiol 49, 809–814, 1980

Flament MF, Whitaker A, Rapoport JL, Davies M, Berg CZ, Kalikow K, Sceery W & Shaffer D. Obsessive compulsive disorder in adolescence: An epidemiological study. J Am Acad Child Adolesc Psychiatry 27, 764–771, 1988

Flint AJ. Epidemiology and comorbidity of anxiety disorders in the elderly. Am J Psychiatry 151, 640–649, 1994

Hedlund JL & Vieweg BW. The Brief Psychiatric Rating Scale (BPRS): a comprehensive review. J Oper Psychiatry 11, 48–65, 1980

Ganzini L, McFarland BH & Culter D. Prevalence of mental disorders after catastrophic financial loss. J Nerv Ment Dis 178, 680–685, 1990

Gershuny BS, Sher KJ, Rossy L & Bishop AK. Distinguishing manifestations of anxiety: how do personality traits of compulsive checkers differ from other anxious individuals? Behav Res Ther 38, 229–241, 2000

Gelder M, Gath D, Mayou R, Cowen P. Oxford textbook of psychiatry, 3rd ed. Oxford: Oxford University Press, 1996

Gershuny BS & Sher KJ. The relation between personality and anxiety: Findings from a 3-year prospective study. J Abnorm Psychol 107, 252–262, 1998

Gray JA. The psychology of fear and stress. London: Weidenfeld & Nicolson, 1971

Gray JA. The neuropsychology of anxiety. Oxford: Oxford University Press, 1982

Greenhill LL, Pine D, March J, Birmaher B, Riddle M. Assessment issues in treatment research of pediatric anxiety disorders: what is working, what is not working, what is missing and what needs improvement. Psychopharmacol Bull 34, 155–164, 1998

Gurely D, Cohen P, Pine DS, Brook J. Discriminating anxiety and depression in youth: a role for diagnostic diagnostic. J Affect Disord 39, 191–200, 1996

Guy W. ECDEU. Assessment manual for psychopharmacology. US Dept Health, Education and Welfare publication (ADM) 76-338. Rockville, Md: National Institute of Mental Health, 218–222, 1976

Hamilton M. The assessment of anxiety by rating. Brit J Psychiatry Spec 32, 50–55, 1959

Hansen C, Sanders SL, Massaro S, Last CG. Predictors of severity of absenteeism in children with anxiety-based school refusal. J Clin Child Psychol 27, 246–254, 1998

Heller W, Etienne MA, Miller GA. Pattern of perceptual asymmetry in depression and anxiety: implications for neuropsychological models of emotion and psychopathology. J Abnorm Psychol 104, 327–333, 1995

Heller W, Nitschke JB, Etienne MA, Miller GA. Patterns of regional brain activity differentiate types of anxiety. J Abnorm Psychol 106, 376–385, 1997

Himle JA & Hill EM. Alcohol abuse and the anxiety disorders: Evidence from the Epidemiologic Catchment Area Survey. J Anxiety Disord 5, 237–245, 1991

Hoehn-Saric R & McLeod DR. Generalized anxiety disorder in adulthood. In: M Hersen, CG Last (eds): Handbook of child and adult psychopathology. New York: Pergamon Press, 247–260, 1990

Horwath E, Adams P, Wickramaratne P, Pine D, Weissman M. Panic disorder with smothering symptoms: evidence for increased risk in first degree relatives. Depress Anxiety 6, 147–153, 1998

Hubert W & Jong-Meyer R. Psychophysiological response patterns to positive and negative film stimuli. Biol Psychol 31, 73–93, 1990

Ialongo N, Edelsohn G, Werthamer-Larsson L, Crockett L, Kellam S. The significance of self-reported anxious symptoms in first grade children: prediction to anxious symptoms and adaptive functioning in fifth grade. J Child Psychol Psychiatry 36, 427–437, 1995

Izard CE & Youngstrom EA. The activation and regulation of fear and anxiety. In: DA Hope (ed): Nebraska Symposium of Motivation, Vol. 43. Perspectives on anxiety, panic and fear. Lincoln: University of Nebraska Press, 1–59, 1996

Junginger J & Ditto B. Multitreatment of obsessive-compulsive checking in a geriatric patient. Behav Modif 8, 379–380, 1984

Kagan J, Reznick JS & Snidman N. Biological bases of childhood shyness. Science 240, 167–171, 1988

Kagan J. Galen's prophecy. New York: Basic Books, 1995

Kagan J. Temperament and the reactions to unfamiliarity. Child Dev 68, 139–143, 1997

Kandel DB, Johnson JG, Bird HR et al. Psychiatric disorders associated with substance use among children and adolescents findings from the Methods for the Epidemiology of Child and Adolescent Mental Disorders (MECA) study. J Abnorm Child Psychol 25, 121–132, 1997

Kendler KS, Walter EE, Neale MC, Kessler RC, Heath AC & Eaves LJ. The structure of the genetic and environmental risk factors for six major psychiatric disorders in women. Arch Gen Psychiatry 52, 374–383, 1995

Kessler RC, Crum RM, Warner LA, Nelson CB, Schulenberg J & Anthony JC. Lifetime co-occurrence of DSM-III-R alcohol abuse and dependence with other psychiatric disorders in the National Comorbidity Survey. Arch Gen Psychiatry 54, 313–321, 1997

Kessler RC, Walters E. Epidemiology of DSM-IIIR major depression and minor depression among adolescents and young adults in the National Comorbidity Survey. Depress Anxiety 7, 3–14, 1998

Kessler RC, McGonagle KA. Zhao S. Nelson CB. Hughes M. Eshleman S. Wittchen H-U. Kendler KS. Lifetime and 12-month prevalence of DSMIII-R psychiatric disorders in the United States. Arch Gen Psychiatry 51, 8–19, 1994

King P & Barrowclough C. A clinical pilot study of cognitive-behavioral therapy for anxiety disorders in the elderly. Behav Psychother 19, 337–345, 1991

Klein RG. Parent-child agreement in clinical assessment of anxiety and other psychopathology: a review. J Anxiety Disord 5, 187–198, 1991

Klein DF. False suffocation alarms, spontaneous panics, and related conditions: an integrative hypothesis. Arch Gen Psychiatry 50, 306–317, 1993

Kolada JL, Bland RC & Newman SC. Obsessive-compulsive disorder. Acta Psychiatr Scand Suppl 376, 24–35, 1994

Lader MH & Marks IM. The rating of clinical anxiety. Acta Psychiatr Scand 50, 112–137, 1974

Lader M. Anxiety and depression. In: A Gale & JA Edwards (eds): Physiological correlates of human behaviour. Vol. III: Individual differences and psychopathology. London: Academic Press, 155–167, 1983

Lader M. Limitations on the use of benzodiazepines in anxiety and insomnia: are they justified. Eur Neuropsychopharmacol 9 (Suppl 6), S399–S405, 1999

Lader MH, Marks IM. Clinical anxiety. London: Heinneman Medical, 1971

Ladouceur R, Léger E, Rhéaume J & Dubé D. Correction of inflated responsibility in the treatment of obsessive-compulsive disorder. Behav Res Ther 34, 767–774, 1996

Landré-Beauvais AJ. 2nd ed. Sémiologie ou traité des signes des maladies. Paris: Brosson, 1813

Lang P, J, Bradley M & Cuthbert BN. International Affective Picture System (IAPS). Gainesville: NIMH Center for the Study of emotion and Attention, University of Florida, 1995

Last CG, Perrin S, Hersen M, Kazdin AE. A prospective study of childhood anxiety disorders. J Am Acad Child Adoles Psychiatry 37, 167–179, 1996

Lépine JP, Boulanger JP, Pariente P. Enquête nationale sur l'anxiété: Méthodologie et résultats préliminaires. Actual Med Intern Psychiatr 79 (Suppl), 11–18, 1988

Lesse S. Anxiety: its components, development and treatment. New York: Grune & Stratton, 1970

Liebowitz MR, Gorman JM, Fyer AJ & Klein DF. Social phobia: Review of a neglected anxiety disorder. Arch Gen Psychiatry 42, 729–736, 1985

Liebowitz MR, Heimberg RG, Travers J & Stein MB. Social phobia or social anxiety disorder: What's in a name? Arch Gen Psychiatry 57, 191–192, 2000

Lindesay J. Phobic disorders in the elderly. Br J Psychiatry 159, 531–541, 1991

Lindesay J, Briggs K, Murphy E. The Guy's/Age Concern Survey: prevalence rates of cognitive impairment, depression and anxiety in an urban elderly community. Br J Psychiatry 150, 815–823, 1989

Lister RG. Ethologically based animal models of anxiety disorders. Pharmacol Ther 46, 321–340, 1990

Lucey JV, Costa DC, Adshead G, Deahl M, Busatto G, Gacinovic S, Travis M, Pilowsky L, Ell PJ, Marks IM and Kerwin RW. Brain blood flow in anxiety disorders. Br J Psychiatry 171, 346–350, 1997

Lucey JV, Costa DC, Blanes T, Busatto GF, Pilowsky LS, Marks IM, Ell PJ & Kerwin RW. Regional cerebral blood flow in obsessive-compulsive disorder patients at rest. Differential correlates with obsessive-compulsive and anxious-avoidant dimensions. Br J Psychiatry 167, 629–634, 1995

Maguire EA, Burgess N, Donnett JG, Frackowiak RS, Frith CD, O'Keefe J. Knowing where and getting there: a human navigation network. Science 280, 921–924, 1998

Manela M, Katona C, Livingston G. How common are the anxiety disorders in old age? Int J Geriatr Psychiatry 11, 65–70, 1996
March J. Multidimensional Anxiety Scale for Children (MASC). Toronto: Multi-Health Systems, Inc, 1998
Marteinsdottir I, Furmark T, Tillfors M, Fredrikson M, Ekselius L. Personality traits in social phobia. Eur Psychiatry 16, 143–150, 2001
Masi G, Mucci M, Favilla L, Romano R, Poli P. Symptomatology and comorbidity of generalized anxiety disorder in children and adolescents. Compr Psychiatry 40, 210–215, 1999
Mathews A & MacLeod C. Cognitive approaches to emotion and emotional disorders. Ann Rev Psychol 45, 25–50, 1994
Mathews A, May J, Mogg K & Eysenck M. Attentional bias in anxiety: Selective search or defective filtering? J Abnorm Psychol 99, 166–173, 1990
McNally RJ. Phenomenology. In RJ McNally (ed): Panic disorder. A critical analysis. New York, NY: Guildford Press, 1–26, 1994
McNally RJ. Cognitive bias in the anxiety disorders. In DA Hope (ed): Nebraska Symposium of Motivation, Vol. 43. Perspectives on anxiety, panic and fear. Lincoln: University of Nebraska Press, 211–250, 1996
McNally RJ. Automaticity and the anxiety disorders. Behav Res Ther 33, 747–754, 1995
McNally RJ, Foa EB & Donnell CD. Memory bias for anxiety information in patients with panic disorder. Cognition and Emotion 3, 27–44, 1989
Mogg K, Mathews A & Eysenck M. Attentional bias to threat in clinical anxiety states. Cognition and Emotion 6, 149–159, 1992
Mogg K & Bradley. A cognitive-motivational analysis of anxiety. Behav Res Ther 36, 809–848, 1998
Montgomery SA, Roberts AG, Montgomery DB et al. Is obsessive compulsive disorder misclassified as an anxiety disorder (abstract)? Neuropsychopharmacol 10 (Suppl 3) (Pt 1), 377, 1994
Montgomery SA, Bullock T, Fineberg N. Serotonin selectivity for obsessive compulsive and panic disorders. J Psychiatr Neurosci 16 (2), Suppl 1, 30–35, 1991
Mulsant BH, Reynolds CF, Shear K, Sweet R, Miller M. Comorbid anxiety disorders in late-life depression. Anxiety 2, 242–247, 1996
Muris P, Gadet B, Moulaert V, Merckelbach H. Correlations between two multidimensional anxiety scales for children. Percept Mot Skills 87, 269–270, 1998
Norton GR, Pidlubny SR & Norton PJ. The use of nonclinical panickers to test a prediction. Behav Ther 30, 321–332, 1999
Noshirvani HF, Kasvikis Y, Marks IM, Tsakiris F & Monteiro WO. Gender-divergent aetiological factors in obsessive-compulsive disorder. Br J Psychiatry 158, 260–263, 1991
Öhman A. Fear and anxiety as emotional phenomena. In: M Lewis & J Haviland (eds): Handbook of emotions. New York: Guildford Press, 511–536, 1994
Öhman A. Face the beast and fear the face: animal and social fears as prototypes for evolutionary analyses of emotion. Psychophysiology 23, 123–145, 1986
Overall JE, Gorham DR. The Brief Psychiatric Rating Scale. Psychol Rep 10, 799–812, 1962
Overall JE. The Brief Psychiatric Rating Scale in psychopharmacology research. In: P Pichot (ed): Psychological measurement in psychopharmacology. Modern problems in pharmacopsychiatry, Vol. 7. Basel, Switzerland: Karger, 67–78, 1974

Panksepp J. Affective neuroscience: The foundations of human and animal emotions. New York: Oxford Press, 1998

Panksepp J, Newman JD, Insel TR. Critical conceptual issues in the analysis of separation-distress systems of the brain. In: KT Strongman (ed): International review of studies on emotion, Vol. 2. New York: Wiley, 51–71, 1992

Pasnau RO & Bystritsky A. On the comorbidity of anxiety and depression. In: JA Den Boer, JMA Sitsen (eds): Handbook of depression and anxiety. A biological approach. New York: Dekker, 45–56, 1994

Perna G, Cocchi S, Bertani A, Arancio C, Bellodi L. Sensitivity to 35% CO_2 in healthy first-degree relatives of patients with panic disorder. Am J Psychiatry 152, 623–625, 1995

Perna G, Bertani A, Caldirola D, Bellodi L. Family history of panic disorder and hypersensitivity to CO_2 in patients with panic disorder. Am J Psychiatry 153, 1060–1064, 1996

Pine DS. Childhood anxiety disorders. Curr Opin Pediatr 9, 329–338, 1997

Pine DS, Cohen P, Gurley D, Brook JS, Ma Y. The risk for early-adulthood anxiety and depressive disorders in adolescents with anxiety and depressive disorders. Arch Gen Psychiatry 55, 56–64, 1998a

Pine DS, Coplan JD. Papp LA. Klein RG. Martinez JM. Kovalenko P. Tancer N. Moreau D. Dummit III ES. Shaffer D. Klein DF. Gorman JM. Ventilatory physiology of children and adolescents with anxiety disorders. Arch Gen Psychiatry 55(2), 123–129, 1998.

Pohl R, Yeragani VK, Balon R, Lycaki H, McBride R. Smoking in patients with panic disorder. Psychiatry Res 43, 253–262, 1992

Raj BA, Corvea MH & Dagon EM. The clinical characteristics of panic disorder in the elderly. A retrospective study. J Clin Psychiatry 54, 150–155, 1993

Rapee RM & Barlow DH. Chronic anxiety: Generalized anxiety disorder and mixed anxiety-depression. New York: Guildford Press, 1991

Ravizza L. Paroxetine efficacy in the treatment of generalized anxiety disorder. Acta Psychiatr Scand 95, 444–450, 1997

Regier DA, Boyd JH, Burke JD, Rae DS, Myers JK, Kramer M, Robins LN, George LK, Karno M & Locke BZ. One-month prevalence of mental disorders in the United States: Based on five epidemiologic catchment area sites. Arch Gen Psychiatry 45, 977–986, 1990

Regier DA. Rae DS. Narrow WE. Kaelber CT. Schatzberg AF. Prevalence of anxiety disorders and their comorbidity with mood and addictive disorders. Br J Psychiatry 173 (Suppl 34), 24–28, 1998

Rice DP & Miller LS. Health economics and cost implications of anxiety and other mental disorders in the United States. Br J Psychiatry 173 (Suppl), 4–9, 1998

Ristvedt SL, Mackenzie TB & Christenson GA. Cues to obsessive-compulsive symptoms: Relationships with other patient characteristics. Behav Res Ther 31, 721–729, 1993

Robinson S, Netanel R & Rapaport J. Reactions of Holocaust survivors to the Gulf War and Scud missile attacks on Israel. In: S Robinson (ed): Echoes of the Holocaust (Vol. 1). Jerusalem: Talbieh Mental Health Center, 1–12, 1992

Sadavoy J, LeClair JK. Treatment of anxiety disorders in late life. Can J Psychiatry 42 (Suppl 1), 28S–34S, 1997

Salkovskis PM. Obsessional-compulsive problems: A cognitive-behavioral analysis. Behav Res Ther 23, 571–583, 1985

Salkovskis PM. Cognitive-behavioural factors and the persistence of intrusive thoughts in obsessional patients. Behav Res Ther 27, 677–682, 1989

Salzman C. Pharmacologic treatment of the anxious elderly patient. In: C Salzman & BD Lebowitz (eds): Anxiety in the elderly: Treatment and research. New York: Springer, 149-173, 1991

Schalling D, Asberg M, Edman G, Oreland L. Markers for vulnerability to psychopathology: temperament traits associated with platelet MAO activity. Acta Psychiatr Scand 76, 172–182, 1987

Schneier FR, Johnson J, Hornig CD, Liebowitz MR, Weissman MM. Social phobia: comorbidity and morbidity in an epidemiologic sample. Arch Gen Psychiatry 49, 282–288, 1992

Sheikh JI. Anxiety rating scales for the elderly. In: C Salzman & BD Lebowitz (eds): Anxiety in the elderly: Treatment and research. New York: Springer, 251–265, 1991

Spielberger CD, Gorsuch RL & Lushese RE. STAI: Manual for the State-Trait Anxiety Inventory. Palo Alto, CA: Consulting Psychological Press, 1970

Spielberger CD. The measurement of state and trait anxiety: conceptual and methodological issues. In: L Levi (ed): Emotions: their parameters and measurements. New York: Raven Press, 713–725, 1975

Steinberg JR. Anxiety in elderly patients. A comparison of azapirones and benzodiazepines. Drugs Aging 5, 335–345, 1994

Stopa L & Clark DM. Cognitive processes in social phobia. Behav Res Ther 31, 255–267, 1993

Stoudemire A & Moran MG. Psychopharmacologic treatment of anxiety in the medically ill elderly patient. Special considerations. J Clin Psychiatry 54, 27–33, 1993

Swales PJ, Solfvin JF & Sheikh JI. Cognitive-behavioral therapy in older panic disorder patients. Am J Geriatr Psychiatry 4, 46–60, 1996

Szabadi E & Bradshaw CM. Biological markers for anxiety states. In: K Granville-Grossman (ed): Recent advances in clinical psychiatry, Vol. 6. Edinburgh: Churchill Livingstone, 69–99, 1988

Taylor S. Nature and measurement of anxiety sensitivity: Reply to Lilienfeld, Turner, and Jacob (1996). J Anxiety Disord 10, 425–451, 1996

Tellegen A. Structures of mood and personality and their relevance to assessing anxiety, with an emphasis on self-report. In: AH Tuma & JD Maser (eds): Anxiety and the anxiety disorders. Hillsdale, NJ: Erlbaum, 681–706, 1985

The Research Unit on Pediatric Psychopharmacology Anxiety Study Group. Fluvoxamine for the treatment of anxiety disorders in children and adolescents. N Engl J Med 344, 1279–1285, 2001

Thyer BA. Prolonged *in vivo* exposure therapy with a 70-year old woman. J Behav Ther Exp Psychiatry 12, 69–71, 1981

Tomarken AJ, Davidson RJ, Wheeler RE, Doss RC. Individual differences in anterior brain asymmetry: emotional expression and brain physiology. J Pers Soc Psychol 62, 676–687, 1992

Torgersen S. Genetic basis of psychopathology. In: SM Turner & M Hersen (eds): Adult psychopathology and diagnosis (3rd ed.). New York: Wiley, 58–88, 1997

Trull TJ & Sher KJ. Relationship between the five-factor model of personality and Axis I disorders in a nonclinical sample. J Abnorm Psychol 103, 350–360, 1994

Yeragani VK, Balon R, Pohl R, Ramesh C, Glitz D, Weinberg P, Merlos B. Decreased R-R variance in panic disorder patients. Acta Psychiatr Scand 81, 554–559, 1992

Valleni-Basile LA, Garrison CZ, Jackson KL, Waller JL, McKeown RE, Addy CL & Cuffe SP. Frequency of obsessive-compulsive disorder in a community sample of young adolescents. J Am Acad Child Adolesc Psychiatry 33, 782–791, 1994

Van Balkom AJ, De Beurs E, Lange A, Koele P, Van Dyck R. Long-term benzodiazepine use is associated with smaller treatment gain in panic disorder with agoraphobia. J Nerv Ment Dis 184, 133–135, 1996

Van Balkom AJ, Beekman AT, de Beurs E, Deeg DJ, van Dyck R, van Tilburg W. Comorbidity of the anxiety disorders in a community-based older population in the Netherlands. Acta Psychiatr Scand 101, 37–45, 2000

Volrath M, Angst J. Outcome of panic and depression in a seven-year follow-up: Results of the Zurich study. Acta Psychiatr Scand 80, 591–596, 1989

Warner V, Mufson L, Weissman MM. Offspring at low and high risk for depression and anxiety: mechanisms of psychiatric disorder. J Am Acad Child Adolesc Psychiatry 34, 786–797, 1995

Weissman MM, Leckman JF, Merikanga KR, Gammon GD, Prusoff BA. Depression and anxiety disorders in parents and children. Arch Gen Psychiatry 41, 845–852, 1984

Wells A & Matthews G. Attentions and emotion: A clinical perspective. Hove, UK: Erlbaum, 1994

Wells A. Meta-cognition and worry: A cognitive model of generalized anxiety disorder. Behav Cogn Psychother, 23, 301–320, 1995

Weissman MM, Myers JK, Tischler GL, Holzer CE, Leaf PJ, Orvaschel H & Brody JA. Psychiatric disorders (DSM-III) and cognitive impairment among the elderly in a US urban community. Acta Psychiatr Scand 71, 366–379, 1985

Wengel SP, Burke WJ, Ranno AE & Roccaforte WH. Use of benzodiazepines in the elderly. Psychiatric Annals 23, 325–331, 1993

Whalen PJ. Rauch SL. Etcoff NL. Mclnerney SC. Lee MB. Jenike MA. Masked presentations of emotional facial expressions modulate amygdala activity without explicit knowledge. J Neurosci 18(1), 411–418, 1998

Williams JM, Mathews A & MacLeod C. The emotional Stroop task and psychopathology. Psychological Bulletin 120, 3–24, 1996

Wilken J, Smith BD, Tola K and Mann M. Anxiety and arousal: tests of a new six-system model. Int J Psychophysiol 33, 197–207, 1999

Wittchen HU & Essau CA. Comorbidity of anxiety disorders and depression: Does it affect course and outcome? J Psychiatry Psychobiol 4, 315–323, 1989

Zimbardo PG, Pilkonis PA & Norwood RM. The silent prison of shyness (Office of Naval Research Technical Report No. 2–17). Stanford, California: Stanford University, 1974

Zinbarg R & Revelle W. Personality and conditioning: A test of four models. J Pers Soc Psychol 57, 301–314, 1989

Zohar AH, Ratzoni G, Pauls DL, Apter A, Bleich A, Kron S, Rappaport M, Weizman A & Cohen DJ. An epidemiological study of obsessive-compulsive disorder and related disorders in Israeli adolescents. J Am Acad Child Adolesc Psychiatry 31, 1057–1061, 1992

Chapter 2
Biological basis of anxiety and strategies for pharmacological innovation

1 Introduction

Very little is known about the biological basis of anxiety disorder. Variance in personality traits, including those related to anxiety, is thought to be generated by a complex interaction of environmental and experiential factors with a number of gene products involving distinct brain systems such as the midbrain raphe serotonin (5-hydroxytryptamine, 5-HT) system (Loehlin, 1989; Plomin et al., 1994). Although twin studies have indicated that individual variation in measures of anxiety-related personality traits is 40–60% heritable, none of the relevant genes has yet been identified (Loehlin, 1989).

The BDZs are still extensively used in the symptomatic treatment of anxiety disorder. Although short-term efficacy is established, the long-term efficacy remains controversial, as relevant data are scanty and relapse, rebound and dependence or withdrawal not clearly distinguished (Lader, 1999). The failure of the BDZs to ameliorate major categories of anxiety disorders suggests that the endogenous BDZ system does not mediate all aspects of anxiety, and that the fear it appears to mediate is not central to all aspects of anxiety. The risk of BDZs comprises psychological and physical effects. Among the former are subjective sedation, paradoxical release of anxiety and/or hostility, psychomotor impairment, memory disruption, and the risks of accident. Physical effects include vertigo, dysarthria, and ataxia with falls, especially in the elderly. A follow-up of a survey in 1997 to a study of the recommendations of an international expert panel on the use of BDZs and other psychotherapeutic medications in the treatment of anxiety disorders suggests that the BDZs remain a mainstay of pharmacotherapy for most of these conditions (Uhlenhuth et al., 1999). Better understanding of the mechanisms of actions of BDZs may further clarify the neurophysiology underlying the anxiety disorders (Argyropoulos & Nutt, 1999). This, in turn, may lead to the development of new effective anxiolytic treatments, with fewer side effects compared to traditional BDZ compounds. It was expected that the SSRIs would replace the BZDs but it was observed instead that they replaced the tricyclics as the experts' first choice for the initial treatment of anxiety disorders. At the same time, the number of experts recommending antidepressants as a group increased from 1992 to 1997 for some disorders. Clearly, new effective pharmacological compounds without the side effects of the BDZs would be an obvious therapeutic advantage in the treatment of anxiety disorders. Such new agents are already available or at the closing stages of clinical trials.

Until recently, anxiety and depression have generally been considered to be distinct clinical dimensions, the former responding to BDZs, the latter to antidepressants. However, evidence from epidemiological, phenomenological and genetic-familial studies indicate that the boundary between these two disorders is not as clear as once thought (Goldberg et al., 1987; Leckman et al., 1983). In addition to the coexistence of anxiety and depression within the same individual and high frequency of both disorders within the same families, there is now evidence that certain biochemical abnormalities may be common to both disorders. Some antidepressants have been shown to be also effective in the treatment of some anxiety disorders. However, the mechanisms underlying the therapeutic efficacy of antidepressants in anxiety states are unclear. One speculation is that the anxiolytic activity of antidepressants is mediated *via* similar mechanisms as has been shown for BDZs and other anxiolytic compounds. Evidence supporting this hypothesis is provided by a number of neurochemical, behavioural and clinical findings, which indicate an involvement of the BDZ-GABA receptor complex in the action of antidepressants.

There is considerable interest in the development of new potential anxiolytics that have the efficacy of the BDZs but without their adverse effects. At present, buspirone, a 5-HT_{1A} agonist, is a non-BDZ marketed and approved treatment for some anxiety disorders (e.g. GAD); it causes limited discontinuation symptoms (Rickels et al., 1988). However, buspirone has a slow onset of anxiolytic action, and therefore does not lend itself well to short-term (1–2 weeks) treatment of acute anxiety symptoms. Imipramine, an antidepressant, is another drug with anxiolytic properties, but it also has a slow onset of action and many rather disturbing side effects (Kahn et al., 1986; Rickels et al., 1993).

In this chapter, we critically examine the status of the current knowledge on the biological basis of anxiety disorders and how far this contributes to the development of effective and safe medications in the treatment of anxiety. The preclinical and preliminary clinical data of various new pharmacological approaches including the cholecystokinins, opioids and neurosteroids in the treatment of anxiety are discussed.

2 Neurobiology of anxiety disorders

Anxiety disorders are hypothesised to be mediated by persistent alterations in neurotransmitter systems and in hypothalamic pituitary adrenal (HPA) axis systems implicated in the regulation of stress responses (Nemeroff, 1999). Patients with anxiety disorders show strong physiological reactions to stimuli that have been associated with pathological fear such as phobic stimuli. Psychophysiological examinations in the laboratory showed that GAD and PD patients have substantial and OCD patients borderline significant increases in muscle tension at rest, particularly in the forehead muscles (Hoehn-Saric & McLeod, 2000). Elevated muscle tension has been the most consistent finding in psychophysiological studies of patients with anxiety disorder. It probably represents a peripheral manifestation of central hyperarousal.

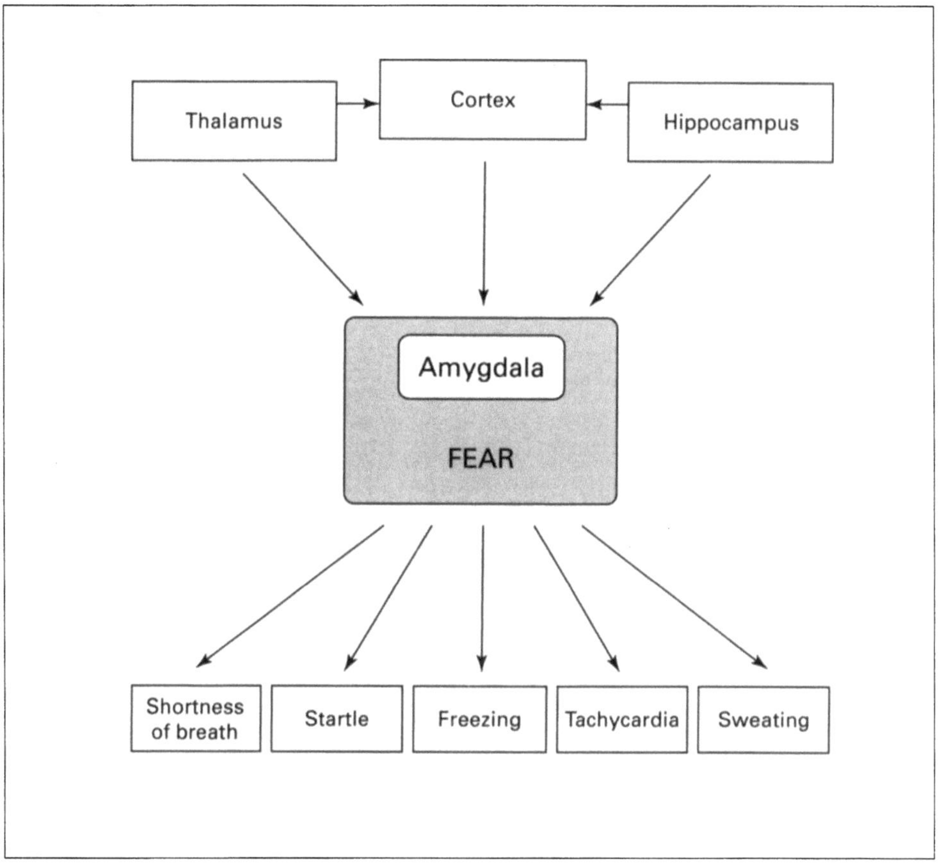

Figure 2.1
Simplified neural circuit mediating fear. The amygdala receives multiple inputs from various brain regions and organizes a coherent defensive strategy to threat. Examples of some somatic symptoms may include shortness of breath, startle, freezing, tachycardia and sweating.

The functional neuroanatomy of anxiety involves amygdala-based neurocircuits with critical reciprocal connections to the medial prefrontal cortex (Ninan, 1999; Hashimoto et al., 1999) (see Fig. 2.1). The amygdala is thus the brain organ that serves as the major interface between the sensory experiences, such as seeing a dangerous situation, and the biochemical and behavioural systems that ultimately respond to this information (Le Doux, 1990). Projections from the central amygdala to the nucleus of the stria terminalis initiate the HPA axis response (Roozendaal et al., 1992). Other brain systems postulated as central to the generation of fear and anxiety include the locus ceruleus and ascending noradrenergic system and the septohippocampal BIS. Conditioned fear stress-induced freezing behaviour in rats was attenuated by SSRIs and 5-HT_{1A} receptor agonists (Hashimoto et al., 1999). Furthermore, it has been shown that conditioned fear stress selectively increased 5-HT metabolism in the medial prefrontal cortex. These findings suggest that the brain, especially the medial prefrontal cortex serotonergic system, is deeply involved in the psychopathology of anxiety.

Basic and clinical investigations of the biochemistry of anxiety have generated hypotheses regarding the role of norepinephrine (NE), 5-HT, BDZs, endogenous opioids, purines and GABA in the aetiology and treatment of anxiety disorders.

5-HT and in particular 5-HT_{1A} receptors are thought to play an important role in the control of neuroendocrinological, emotional and behavioural functions, as well as in the adaptational responses to stress (Chaouloff, 1995; De Vry, 1995). Experimental research suggests that dysregulated 5-HT_{1A} receptors may contribute to the pathogenesis of psychiatric disorders (De Vry, 1995; 1996). This central role of 5-HT_{1A} receptors may be related to the particular distribution of these receptors in the brain. In the brain, 5-HT_{1A} receptors are located presynaptically as somatodendritic receptors on 5-HT neurons and postsynaptically in particular limbic and cortical regions. Although it is generally accepted that presynaptic 5-HT_{1A} receptors control 5-HT neuronal activity, recent evidence shows an additional role of postsynaptic 5-HT_{1A} receptors in the cortex as part of a negative feedback. Thus, 5-HT_{1A} receptors are localised both presynaptically on the soma and dendrites of the 5-HT neurons projecting to the forebrain, and postsynaptically, in particular in the limbic structures, such as the hippocampus, the hypothalamus and particular frontal cortical areas. Somatodendritic 5-HT_{1A} receptors in the raphe nuclei of the brain stem function as autoreceptors and regulate the activity of the 5-HT neurons, thereby allowing a general control of serotonergic tonus.

Considerable evidence indicates that increased serotonergic neurotransmission, which would be an evident consequence of the reduced 5-HT uptake capacity found in individuals with the short allele of the 5-HT transporter (5-HTT) polymorphism, is anxiogenic in animal models as well as in humans (Cloninger, 1987; 1988; Griebel, 1995; Handley, 1995). At the clinical level, reduced 5-HT uptake or reduced inhibitor binding to 5-HTT has been one of the most consistent biological findings in individuals with depression and several anxiety disorders (Owens & Nemeroff, 1994; Faludi et al., 1994). A study that investigated the association of anxiety-related traits with polymorphism in the 5-HTT gene regulatory region reported that the 5-HTT polymorphism accounts for 3–4% of total variation and 7–9% of inherited variance in anxiety-related personality traits in individuals as well as sibships (Lesch et al., 1996).

The heritability of interindividual variation in anxiety and other aspects of personality argues for variants of genes influencing these traits. In the tridimensional theory of personality, each of three personality dimensions is postulated to be related to the primary action of one neurotransmitter system: novelty seeking to dopamine activity, harm avoidance to serotonin activity, and reward dependence to NE activity (Cloninger, 1986; 1987; Joffe et al., 1993). Among the three dimensions, harm avoidance is most closely akin to anxiety, being influenced by anxiety state, anxiety trait, and sex. Individuals scoring higher than average in harm avoidance are characterised by anxiousness and shyness, and high harm avoidance scores are found in patients with GAD (Brown et al., 1992; Starcevic et al., 1996; Svrakic et al., 1992). Recently, a functional polymorphism in the promoter of the human serotonin transporter gene (SLC6A4*C) was identified and found to be linked to an anxiety-related personality trait, neuroticism (Lesch et al., 1996; Collier et al., 1996). The polymorphism affects gene transcription and ultimately, gene function. A study using sibpair linkage and association analysis in 655 Finns confirmed the relationship of SLC6A4*C to anxiety by sibpair but found no evidence of association, raising the question whether SLC6A4*C locus is itself affecting anxiety or is linked to a yet unidentified variant (Mazzanti et al., 1998). Further studies of the molecular of the role of serotonin polymorphism in anxiety-related traits are needed for clarification.

Anticipation, an increase in severity or a decrease in the age of onset inherent in the transmission of a disease gene from an affected parent to a child (a phenomenon related to trinucleotide repeat expansion diseases), is being increasingly described in human studies (Harper et al., 1996; Paulson & Fischbeck, 1996). Several family studies have shown a strong tendency toward familial aggregation of anxiety disorders and data on twins also suggest the importance of genetic factors in anxiety disorders (Andrews et al., 1990; Kendler et al., 1997). A recent clinical trial, which investigated a group of 350 patients with anxiety disorders, reported a significant age of onset anticipation in anxiety disorders (Ohara et al., 1999). The mean/median age of onset in the offspring generation was significantly lower than that in the parental generation. If this is confirmed by other studies, trinucleotide repeat sequences may be considered to account for the familial aggregation of anxiety disorders.

Abnormal response of the HPA axis has emerged as a pathologic marker in anxiety disorders due to the important and replicable findings of a blunted growth hormone (GH) response to infusion of the α_2-adrenergic antagonist clonidine in PD patients (Coplan et al., 1995; Nutt, 1989). Blunted GH secretion in response to clonidine has also been observed in GAD, SP, depression but not in OCD and schizophrenia (Abelson et al., 1991; Hollander et al., 1991; Matussek et al., 1980; Tancer et al., 1993). It has been postulated that a blunted GH response reflects a subsensitivity of postsynaptic α_2-adrenoceptor receptors (Siever et al., 1982). GH response to apomorphine, a dopaminergic agonist, is intact in PD patients and not significantly different from healthy controls, which is in contrast to the blunted response to apomorphine in major depressives (Pichot et al., 1995). These studies indicate a complex, and as yet unclear, interplay of factors modulating GH release in mood and anxiety disorders. The interaction between the hypothalamic-pituitary-somatotropin (HPS) and HPA axes is of particular interest as corticotropin-releasing factor (CRF) is known to be dysregulated in mood and anxiety disorders. CRF challenge and dexamethasone suppression studies have revealed HPA axis abnormalities similar, though less robust, to those observed in depression (Coryell et al., 1989).

Until recently, atrial natriuretic factor (ANF) has appeared to be a hormone involved in psychiatric illness (MacMillan & Steiner, 1994). It was recently demonstrated that PD patients who had panic attacks in response to lactate infusion had more pronounced surges in ANF than nonpanicking controls (Kellner et al., 1995). A possible role of ANF in the termination of panic attacks by a hypothetical antagonism of extrahypothalamic CRF, as ANF has been found to be present in the locus ceruleus, may be envisaged. Thus ANF might attenuate overactivation of the locus ceruleus by CRF while simultaneously suppressing the pituitary-adrenal system (Sullivan et al., 1998).

To test for the potential contribution of genetic variations in hormone receptors, the association between the alleles of the dinucleotide repeat of the oestrogen receptor 1 gene (ESR1) and the nine subscores and total score of the SCL-90 was recently examined (Comings et al., 1999). This study showed that the ESR1 gene accounted for 7% of variance of the anxiety score, 5.4% of the total symptom score and 3.9% of the phobic anxiety score. The anxiety and total symptoms score were significant. Since oestrogen levels are much higher in women than in men, these results might explain the higher frequency of anxiety disorders in women. Replication studies using both the SCL-90 and cases of primary GAD, PD or agoraphobia based on DSM-IV criteria would be desirable.

2.1 Generalised anxiety disorder (GAD)

Excessive anxiety and worry occurring frequently for at least 6 months characterise GAD (APA, 1994). The anxiety, worry, or physical symptoms cause clinically significant distress and impairment in social and occupational functioning. Kinetic binding properties of peripheral benzodiazepine receptor (PBR) density and PBR mRNA were significantly decreased in untreated GAD patients as compared to controls by 45 and 70%, respectively, using binding of [^{3}H]Pk 11195, a ligand for receptor assay (Rocca et al., 1998).

2.2 Panic disorder (PD)

PD is an anxiety disorder characterised by spontaneous paroxysms of severe fear (APA, 1994). It has a prevalence of 1–2% and results in considerable morbidity and increased mortality (Weissman et al., 1997; Katerndahl & Realini, 1993; Katon, 1996). Pharmacologic and metabolic probes have revealed that alterations of serotonergic, noradrenergic, GABA-ergic, and brain CCK function characterise this disorder. Corticosteroid dysregulation as well as increased sensitivity to the anxiety provoking effects of carbon dioxide and lactate have been noted (Lesch et al., 1992; George et al., 1995; Nutt, 1989; Bradwejn et al., 1992; Abelson & Curtis, 1996; Gorman et al., 1991; Reschke et al., 1995). Platelet PBR density was found to be significantly reduced in PD patients compared with normal controls (Marazziti et al., 1994).

PD as well as other anxiety disorders have recently been found to be significantly associated with low voltage electroencephalogram (EEG) characteristics (Enoch et al., 1995). A gene responsible for about one third of the cases of low voltage EEG was genetically mapped to 30q13.2–q13.3 (Steinlein et al., 1992). In the same chromosomal region, the gene for neuronal nicotinic acetylcholine receptor α4 subunit (CHRNA4) has been located. However, such findings need to be confirmed by other investigators.

Yohimbine (an α_2-adrenergic antagonist), which stimulates firing of the locus ceruleus, has been observed to induce more frequent panic attacks in PD patients than normal controls, though this has not been a consistent finding (Albus et al., 1992; Gurguis & Uhde, 1990). Panic responses to yohimbine appear specific to PD and PTSD, and there is an absence of yohimbine-induced panic response in patients with depression, schizophrenia, GAD and OCD (Heninger et al., 1988). Yohimbine can also induce an anxiety reaction in normal controls (Charney et al, 1983).

A positron emission tomography (PET) study shows that there is a global reduction in BDZ site binding throughout the brain in patients with PD compared with controls (Malizia et al., 1998). In addition, the loci with the largest regional decrease in binding (right orbitofrontal cortex and right insula) were areas thought to be essential in the central mediation of anxiety. This study highlights the case that abnormalities in basal or adaptive inhibitory neuro-modulation are of pathologic significance in this condition.

2.3 Social phobia (SP)

Patients with generalised SP have a persistent and excessive fear of one or more social or performance situations in which the person is exposed to unfamiliar people or to possible scrutiny by others (APA, 1994). Exposure to the feared social situation provokes anxiety, which may be similar to situationally predisposed panic attack. An abnormally low number of platelet PBRs (36%) have been demonstrated in generalised SP patients (Johnson et al., 1998).

A study designed to examine patterns of regional brain function has been conducted with social phobics (Birbaumer et al., 1998). Increased activation of the amygdala with functional MRI in response to neutral faces in social phobics compared to controls was reported. Both groups showed comparable activation of the amygdala in response to aversive odours. A recent study designed to assess regional brain and autonomic function in social phobics performed measurements of EEG, heart rate and blood pressure from SP patients and controls who anticipated making a public speech, as well as immediately after the speech was made (Davidson et al., 2000). Social phobics showed a marked increase in right-sided activation in the anterior temporal and lateral prefrontal scalp regions. Heart rate was also elevated in the phobics relative to controls in most conditions. These heart rate and EEG changes together accounted for >48% of the variance in negative affect during the anticipation phase. These findings support the hypothesis of right-sided anterior cortical activation during anxiety in SP.

2.4 Post-traumatic stress disorder (PTSD)

PTSD is a severe anxiety disorder that may occur after the exposure to a traumatic event (APA, 1994). The traumatic event is persistently re-experienced, and persistent avoidance of stimuli associated with the trauma, numbing of general responsiveness, and symptoms of increased arousal are present. Platelet PBRs were assessed in drug-free PTSD patients. Decreased platelet PBR density (62%) was observed in the PTSD patients compared with the control group. The reduction in PBR density in the PTSD patients was more prominent in men than in women (Gavish et al, 1996).

2.5 Obsessive-compulsive disorders (OCD)

The few studies that have been conducted, although far from conclusive, suggest that different neurotransmitters and brain regions may be implicated in child and adult onset OCD. One of the neurotransmitters implicated in the pathophysiology of OCD is serotonin. Specifically, it has been proposed that OCD may be the result of an oversensitivity or overactivity of specific central nervous system serotonergic pathways (Henin & Kendall, 1997). Both pre-and postsynaptic 5-$HT_{1B/D}$ receptors could be supersensitive in OCD. The therapeutic actions of SSRIs would be to down-regulate these presynaptic autoreceptors allowing increased synaptic levels of serotonin, possibly resulting in a subsequent down-regulation of postsynaptic 5-HT receptors. These postsynaptic receptors may be of the 5-$HT_{1B/D}$, 5-HT_{2c} or another subtype. Antagonists of the 5-$HT_{1B/D}$ receptor are thus likely to be potent and reliable anti-obsessive medications.

The available research suggests that patients with child-onset OCD are less responsive to treatment with SSRIs administered in isolation than individuals with adult-onset OCD, and may require the addition of neuroleptics to manage symptoms (Ackerman et al., 1994; McDougle et al., 1994). This difference in treatment response may be indicative of underlying differences in pathophysiology of child *versus* adult-onset OCD. These data suggest that dopaminergic as well as serotonergic functioning may be involved in OCD in child child-onset cases.

Clomipramine is superior to the SSRIs in the treatment of OCD (Trappler, 1999; Pigott & Seay, 1999). Although relatively pure noradrenergic re-uptake inhibitors such as desipramine are inactive in OCD, compounds inhibiting the re-uptake of both serotonin and noradrenaline, such as venlafaxine and milnacipran, may be superior to the SSRIs in OCD (Feighner, 1999; Westenberg, 1999). Clearly placebo-controlled studies are warranted to demonstrate the potential of SNRIs in OCD.

3 Recent development and future anxiolytics

3.1 5-HT receptors

At least ten subtypes of 5-HT receptors have been discovered to date, and it is not clear which of these subtypes is involved in, or is critical for the therapeutic efficacy of SSRIs (Hoyer et al., 1994). Among the newly cloned receptors, the 5-HT_7 subtype is characterised by a relatively high affinity for 8-hydroxy-2-(di-n-propylamino) tetralin (8-OH-DPAT), an aminotetralin derivative, leading to the proposal that the anxiolytic-like action of this drug might not depend solely on its known interaction with 5-HT_{1A} receptors (Ruat et al., 1993). In addition, the 5-HT_6 receptor is recognised by relatively low concentrations (10–100 nM) of various psychotropic drugs, such as the tricyclic antidepressants, with known efficacy in preventing anxiety-driven behaviour in animals and in reducing the frequency of panic attacks in humans (Monsma et al., 1993). Nevertheless, to date, the most convincing evidence of the potential interest of 5-HT receptor ligands in the treatment of anxiety disorders concerns 5-HT_{1A} receptor agonists and 5-HT_{2A} and 5-HT_{2c} receptor antagonists (Misane & Ogren, 2000).

Activation of the 5-HT_{1A} receptor by agonists results in an anxiolytic effect (Lucki et al., 1994; De Vry, 1995). Correlations were noted among the time and dose dependency of the anxiolytic effect, the inhibition of serotonergic firing in the dorsal raphe nuclei, and the inhibition of 5-HT release after systemic administration of agonists (Jolas et al., 1995; Sommermeyer et al., 1993). The 5-HT_{1A} receptor partial agonist buspirone and a series of congeners also produce this neurochemical effect and are used clinically for the treatment of anxiety. Based on these findings, it has been proposed that 5-HT_{1A} receptor agonists stimulate presynaptic receptors, which inhibit 5-HT release and consequently reduce 5-HT signalling at a multitude of diverse target receptors (De Vry, 1995). Because of the role of presynaptic 5-HT_{1A} receptors in regulating the 5-HT system, blockade of the receptor by antagonists is expected to increase central 5-HT function. However, microdialysis studies showed no detectable increase of 5-HT neurotransmission by 5-HT_{1A} receptor antagonists under normal condition (Kreiss & Lucki, 1994). At the behavioural level, the effect of 5-HT_{1A} receptor antagonists is controversial. Antagonists, such as pindolol, exhibit a biphasic dose-response curve with an initial anxiolytic effect that converts to an anxiogenic effect at high doses (Fletcher et al., 1996; Critchley & Handley, 1987). However, pindolol is also an adrenoceptor antagonist, and this activity may confound the drug's effect on the 5-HT_{1A} receptor. The more selective recently discovered phenylpiperazine silent antagonist 5-HT_{1A} receptor antagonist, WAY-100635, induced anxiolytic-like effects in the light/dark box anxiety model with no anxiogenic effect at high doses (Sanchez, 1995).

The development of highly selective and potent 5-HT_{1A} receptor ligands has helped to clarify the neurobiological function of these receptors (Glaser & De Vry, 1992). Among these are the full agonists 8-OH-DPAT and BAY r 1531 (a tetrahydropiperazine D_2 receptor), the pyrimidinylpiperazine partial agonists buspirone, ipsapirone and gepirone and the silent antagonist 5-HT_{1A} receptor antagonist WAY-100635 (Ennis, 1993; Forster et al., 1995). A preclinical study reported that pretreatment with WAY-100635 was able to potentiate the anxiolytic-like profile of SSRIs in the mouse marble-burying paradigm (McNicoll et al., 1995). This suggests the involvement of different 5-HT_{1A} receptor populations in the anxiolytic and antidepressant effects of SSRIs. The 5-HT_{1A} compounds buspirone, ipsapirone, indorenate, and 8-OH-DPAT share with BDZs the ability to reduce anxiety, but lack some of the adverse effects such as tolerance, dependence, and motor disruptions (Lopez-Rubalcava et al., 1992; Mattila et al., 1986).

Electrophysiological data show that chronic administration of azapirone drugs leads to desensitisation of 5-HT_{1A} autoreceptors in the dorsal raphe nucleus, with no change in 5-HT_{1A} receptor activity in the hippocampus (Schechter et al., 1990). A recent study designed to investigate the chronic buspirone treatment on 5-HT_{1A} receptor function demonstrated region-specific alterations in 5-HT_{1A} and $GABA_B$ receptor-activated G-proteins which may contribute to the clinical effects of this drug (Sim-Selley et al., 2000). Net 8-OH-DPAT-stimulated [^{35}S]GTPγS binding in the dorsal raphe nucleus and septum in brain sections from chronic buspirone-treated animals was noted. In contrast, the only significant difference in baclofen-stimulated [^{35}S]GTPγS binding between control and buspirone-treated animals was found in the hippocampus (26% increase in $GABA_B$ receptor-stimulated [^{35}S]GTPγS binding). The increase in $GABA_B$ receptor-mediated G-protein activation may result from chronic buspirone-induced alterations in 5-HT neurotransmission.

The development of high affinity and selective receptor agonists and antagonists for 5-HT_{2c} (previously called 5-HT_{1c}) receptors has generated great interest in the therapeutic potential of selective 5-HT_{2c} receptor ligands as anxiolytics (Martin et al., 1995). The presence of 5-HT_{2c} receptors in limbic and cortical regions is consistent with a possible important role in neuropsychiatric diseases such as anxiety and/or depression. In a study which investigated the effects of 5-HT_{2c} receptor agonists in a model of panic-like anxiety in rats (aversive stimulation of the dorsolateral periaqueductal gray), it was observed that the selective activation of 5-HT_{2c} receptors by Ro 60-0175, Org 12962 or Ro 60-0332 induced effects analogous to those observed following BDZ receptor activation by antipanic medications such as clonazepam, alprazolam and fluoxetine (Jenck et al., 1998). On the other hand, 5-HT_{2C} antagonists such as SB-2006646A have been reported to be anxiolytic in conflict models and the social interaction test in rodents whereas they are inactive in tests indicative of antipanic or anti-OCD activity. These results are consistent with the hypothesis that 5-HT has a dual action on the neural mechanism of anxiety by facilitating or inhibiting different kinds of anxiety in different brain regions (Graeff et al., 1996). These data also suggest that the 5-HT_{2c} receptor subtype plays a major role in the therapeutic properties of SSRIs. Clinical studies with selective 5-HT_{2c} agonists and antagonists will probably clarify their therapeutic potential. Deramciclane is a novel 5-HT_{2C} receptor antagonist with anxiolytic properties in phase II trials. Animal data suggest that it does not potentiate the effects of alcohol and improves sleep (Detari et al., 1999).

Compared to the established anxiolytics, 5-HT_3 receptor antagonists such as tropisetron, granisetron and ondansetron display a different profile (Lee et al., 1993; Yarker & McTavish, 1994; Wilde & Markham, 1996). They are anxiolytic in a limited number of animal anxiety models. If active, they are often very potent and display a bell-shaped dose-response curves, whereas the ratio between therapeutic activity and side effects appears remarkably large (Olivier et al., 2000). 5-HT_3 receptor antagonists remain active after chronic dosing and no indications for tolerance, dependence or rebound effects were reported which seems to suggest that these drugs may be an attractive alternative to the BDZs. However, human data are controversial and suggest that 5-HT_3 receptor antagonists may not represent a breakthrough in the treatment of various anxiety disorders as was initially thought (Olivier et al., 2000).

3.2 GABA receptors

GABA is the most widely distributed inhibitory neurotransmitter in mammalian brain (Sivilotti & Nistri, 1991). Initially, GABA was noted to activate bicuculline-sensitive Cl^- channels and subsequently, GABA-mediated activation of cation channels was discovered (Bormann, 1988; Bowery, 1989). GABA receptors in the brain have been classified as $GABA_A$, $GABA_B$ and $GABA_C$ (Bowery et al., 1980; 1981). The $GABA_A$ receptor directly gates a Cl^- ionophore and has modulatory bindings sites for BDZs, barbiturates, neurosteroids and ethanol (Borman, 1988; Macdonald & Olsen, 1994) (see Figs. 2.2a & 2.2b). It was recognised that additional isoforms of its subunits and subtypes of these isoforms exist. Six isoforms (α, β, γ, δ, ε, π) and 15 subtypes have been reported (Sieghart, 1995). It is not known which of these interact *in vivo* to form an ion channel, but it is assumed that $\alpha1\beta2\gamma2$ represents the major adult isoform (Schofield et al., 1987). By contrast, $GABA_B$ receptors couple to Ca^{2+} and K^+ channels *via* G-proteins and second messenger systems. They are activated by baclofen and are resistant to drugs that modulate $GABA_A$ receptors (Bormann, 1988; Bowery, 1989). A third type of GABA receptors designated as $GABA_C$ are Cl^- pores that are insensitive to both bicuculline and baclofen (Johnston, 1996). Several lines of evidence now indicates that $GABA_C$ receptors are composed of ρ-subunits (Feigenspan & Bormann, 1998; Enz & Cutting, 1998).

GABA-mediated neurotransmission in the CNS can be differentially modulated by diverse compounds that bind to allosteric modulatory sites named benzodiazepines/ϖ (BDZ/ϖ) sites associated with $GABA_A$ receptors (Barnard et al., 1998). BDZ and non-BDZ ligands that are currently in clinical use, such as diazepam, act as positive allosteric modulators of GABA-gated Cl^- channels, enhance GABA-ergic transmission and produce both anxiolytic and anticonvulsant effects on behaviour (Haefely, 1986). On the other hand, compounds acting as negative allosteric modulators, such as β-carboline FG 7142, which also bind to BDZ/ϖ sites but inhibit, rather than enhance $GABA_A$ receptor function, are referred to as inverse agonists and exhibit anxiogenic and proconvulsant activity (Corda et al., 1985; Dorow et al., 1983).

There is considerable evidence that specific, high-affinity BDZ receptors in brain mediate the pharmacological actions of BDZs, the most commonly used anxiolytic compounds. Central BDZ receptors have been shown to be linked to the $GABA_A$ receptor unit, a supramolecular structure comprising a chloride channel and GABA and barbiturate recognition sites (Haefely & Pole, 1983). The BDZs as well as the barbiturates have been found to increase the affinity of the GABA receptor for GABA, facilitating the action of this inhibitory neurotransmitter (Guidotti et al., 1978). Thus, the common action of the anxiolytics may lie in their facilitation of GABA-mediated inhibition. The $\alpha1$-subunit has been described as the main subunit that is photoaffinity labelled by BDZ [^{3}H]flunitrazepam (Duncalfe et al., 1996; DeLorey & Olsen, 1992; Gavish et al., 1992).

The use of mouse molecular genetics to study the target for BDZ action has been proposed (Rudolph et al., 1999). This work sets the example for developing BDZ-like drugs that ease anxiety, but without its deleterious side effects. Using the tech-

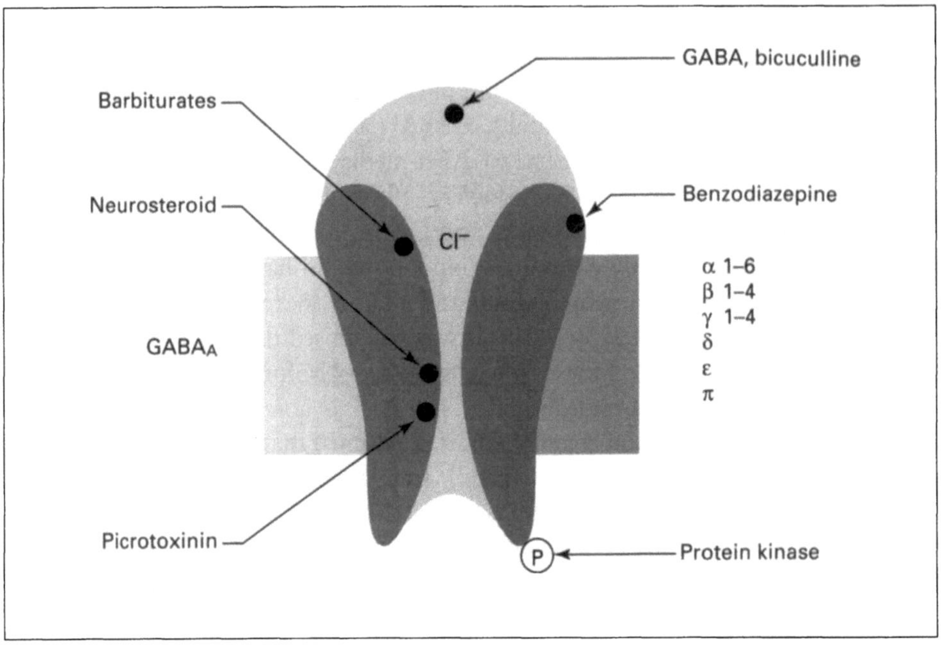

Figure 2.2a
Multiplicity of ionotropic GABA receptors. The $GABA_A$ receptor is a Cl^- pore with 5 Å diameter and modulatory binding sites for benzodiazepines, barbiturates and neurosteroids. The most abundant $GABA_A$ receptor in the brain is the $\alpha 1\beta 2\gamma 2$ isoform.

nique of homologous recombination, α1(H101R) mutant mice were engineered in which residue 101 in the α1 subunit is mutated from histidine to arginine. When the mutant mice received diazepam, they did not show sedation (measure of spontaneous locomotion in novel environment) or memory impairment (memory of discharge of electric shock in a dark chamber). However, the anxiolytic effects of diazepam were as strong in the α1(H101R) mutant mice as in controls. This study therefore highlights the importance of α1-containing $GABA_A$ receptors in the control of arousal and certain types of memory. It indicates novel opportunities of developing drugs that are specific for $GABA_A$-receptor subtypes and the discovery of novel anxiolytics without the adverse effects on sedation and memory.

A recent study suggests that the sedative, amnesic and possibly ataxic and, in part, anticonvulsive actions appear to be mediated by α1-subunit-containing receptors, whereas anxiolytic actions seem to be mediated by receptors that contain α2-, α3-, α5-subunits (McKerman et al. 2000). Another study demonstrated that the anxiolytic action of diazepam was absent in mice with the α2(H101R) point mutation but present in mice with the α3(H126R) point mutation (Löw et al., 2000). These results suggest that the anxiolytic effect of BDZ drugs is mediated by α2 $GABA_A$ receptors but not by α3 $GABA_A$. This conclusion was supported by studies using L838417, a novel BDZ-site ligand with a so far unique $GABA_A$ receptors sub-

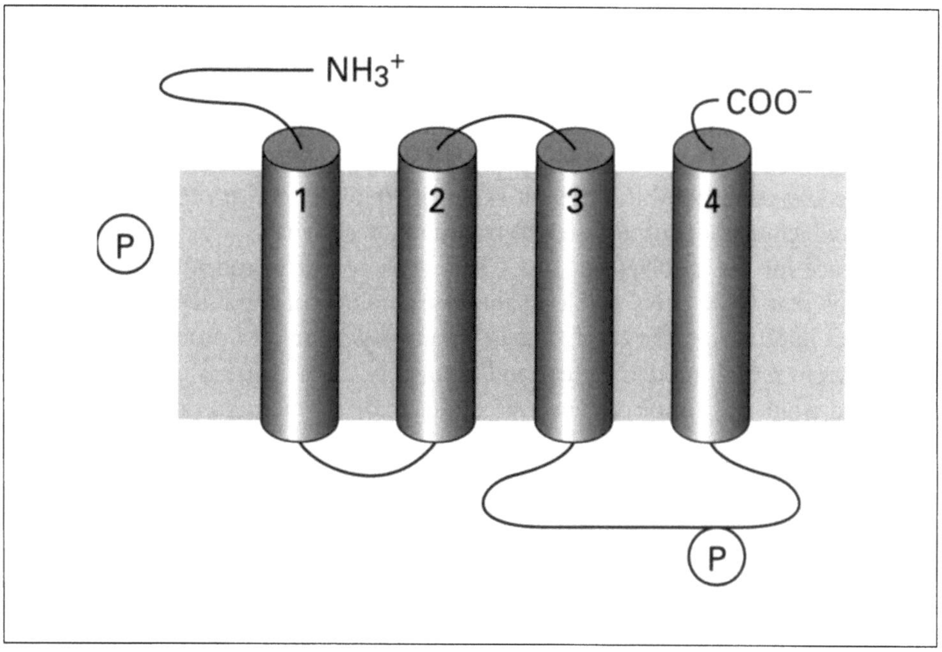

Figure 2.2b
Each subunit comprises four transmembrane domains (TM1–TM4). The large intracellular loop between TM3 and TM4 contains consensus sites for phosphorylation by protein kinases (P). The amphiphilic TM2 provides the lining of the Cl^- pore intrinsic to the pentameric structure.

type selectivity. Although this compound weakly enhances GABA-evoked currents at $GABA_A$ receptors that contain α2-, α3- or α5-subunits, it does not alter such currents in receptors that contain the α1-subunit. Indeed, L838417 in wild-type animals produced anxiolytic-like activity in the elevated plus maze and fear-potentiated startle test without causing sedation or ataxia. Much evidence seems to suggest that the α2 $GABA_A$ receptors are highly specific targets for the development of future selective anxiolytic drugs.

3.3 Neuropeptide (CCK, CRF, NPY and NK) receptors

Preclinical research with neuropeptides in anxiety disorders has involved the study of the effects of CCK, CRF, neuropeptide Y (NPY), tachykinins (TKs, substance P) and neurokinin (NK) A and B.

CCK is recognised as the most widely distributed neuropeptide in the brain and the most promiscuous of the co-existing peptides, living with dopamine, vasoactive intestinal peptide, NPY, GABA, Substance P and 5-HT (Hokfelt et al., 1985; Fuxe et al., 1980; Van Megen et al., 1996). CCK receptors, as agonists acting at CCK_B receptors have anxiogenic-like effects in various animal tests. These effects might involve the excitation of neurons in the nucleus tractus solitarius, therefore leading to neurovegetative disturbances, such as those occurring during a panic attack. Until now, only two types of CCK receptors have been cloned, CCK_A and CCK_B (the gastrin receptor seems to be identical to the brain CCK_B receptor) (Lee et al., 1993; Wank et al., 1994). The two binding sites for CCK_B receptor, designated CCK_{B1} and CCK_{B2}, could correspond to different states of coupling to G-proteins of the same receptor which might lead to different transduction systems.

Evidence for the involvement of CCK in anxiety/fear in rodents reinforces the hypothesis that CCK plays a role in the neurobiology of these disorders. Indeed, peripheral injection of various CCK_B antagonists was able to produce anxiolytic-like effects in several models of fear and/or anxiety. These various models were the black and white box in mice, the elevated plus maze in mice and rats, fear-potentiated startle paradigm, social interactions in rats, in a marmoset "human threat" model, in conflict tests and after stimulation in the dorsal periaqueductal gray matter in rats (Chopin & Briley, 1993; Costal et al., 1991; Dooley & Klamt, 1993; Daugé et al., 1993; Fink et al., 1994). Moreover, the involvement of CCK-B receptors was emphasised by the anxiogenic-like effects produced by peripheral or intracerebral injection of CCK_B agonists (Boc-CCk4, BC197 and pentagastrin, respectively) (Fink et al., 1994; Rex et al., 1994; Singh et al., 1991; 1991a). However, the effects of CCK_B antagonists are less potent compared to those of BDZs, especially in models such as conflict tests.

CCK_4 is known to elicit in normal subjects panic attacks that are both subjectively and quantitatively comparable to those naturally experienced by PD patients (de Montigny, 1989; Bradwejn et al., 1991; Jerabek et al., 1996). The anxiolytic-like action of recently developed CCK_B receptor antagonists, such as RB211, CI988 and L365260, probably involves the dorsal vagal complex at the bulbar level rather than the limbic structures (Harro et al., 1993). However, results obtained from preclinical studies with CCK receptor antagonists have been highly variable and clinical studies have also been unsuccessful. The reasons for this variability in drug effect in preclinical studies remain largely unknown but certainly include various factors such as experimental procedures, species and strain used. It is also likely that the classical animal models of anxiety are less sensitive to the action of CCK compounds and may be involved in a type of anxiety that is not assessed in these tests. Clinical trials with CCK_B antagonists in panic or GAD studies indicate that although the drugs are well tolerated, significant differences between placebo and drug could not be established (Kramer et al., 1995; Pande, 1997). It is possible that poor pharmacokinetic properties and inadequate dosage could account for these disappointing clinical results. Therefore, other clinical studies with novel CCK_B antagonists with better pharmacokinetic profile are necessary to demonstrate effective anxiolytic profile in patients suffering from anxiety.

CRF is a 41-amino acid peptide that plays a prominent role in endocrine, autonomic, behavioural and immune responses to stress (De Souza, 1995; Owens & Nemeroff, 1991). Evidence suggests that the actions of CRF are mediated through two G-protein-coupled seven-transmembrane domain receptor subtypes designated CRF_1 and CRF_2 (Chang et al., 1993; Chen et al., 1993; Perrin et al., 1995). These receptors exhibit distinct pharmacological profiles and unique distribution patterns in brain and peripheral tissues (Chalmers et al., 1995). A role for CRF in anxiety disorders has accumulated in recent years. Several lines of evidence suggest that the anxiety provoking behavioural effects of CRF involve CRF_1 receptors. CRF_1 knock-out mice show increased anxiolytic-like activity in the elevated plus maze and a tendency to enter the illuminated region of a light-dark box (Smith et al., 1998; Timpl et al., 1998). In addition, treatment with antagonists that selectively block CRF_1 receptor action was shown to promote anxiolytic responses in the elevated plus maze, the light-dark box, the mouse defence battery and the fear potentiated startle test (Griebel et al., 1998; Lundkvist et al., 1996; Okuyama et al., 1999; Schulz et al., 1996). Oral administration of the CRF_1 receptor antagonist antalarmin significantly decreased cerebrospinal fluid (CSF) CRF, pituitary-adrenal and autonomic responses to stress and inhibited behaviours indicative of fear and anxiety in adult primates (Habib et al., 2000). Interestingly, treatment of rats exposed to prenatal stress with CRF antagonists reverses the characteristic increases of fearful behaviour observed in these animals (Ward et al., 2000). In 9- to 11-day-old rat pups, the CRF_1 receptor antagonist CP 154,526 diminishes vocalisations indicative of anxiety in response to separation from their litters (Kehne et al. 2000). Concerning the role of CRF_2 receptors in anxiety behaviour, recent evidence seems to suggest that these receptors may also play an important role in the mediation of anxiety behaviour (Takahasti et al., 2001). Results obtained with CRF receptor antagonists in animal models of anxiety convincingly demonstrated that the blockade of central CRF receptors might yield anxiolytic-like activity. Clinical data also support the hypothesis of a role of CRF receptors in anxiety. Thus, CSF levels of CRF have been shown to be elevated in patients suffering from OCD and PTSD (Altemus et al., 1994; Stout et al., 1995). Given the integral role of CRF and its receptors in the mediation of stress and emotion, the CRF_1 receptor antagonists are being considered as novel anxiolytics as well as potentially preventive treatments for PTSD (Martin et al., 2000). The antidepressant and anxiolytic properties of the selective CRF_1 receptor antagonist R121919 was recently demonstrated in a clinical trial of depressed patients (Zobel et al., 2000). Given the fact that early life stress is related to substantial alterations in central CRF systems, it is plausible that CRF_1 receptor antagonists, once they are available, will represent the most direct treatment of symptoms related to early life stress in children and adults. NPY, a 36-amino acid peptide, has anxiolytic effects when administered centrally (Griebel, 1999). It has been proposed that endogenous NPY counteracts stress and anxiety (Heilig et al., 1994). The presence of NPY receptors in brain regions known to be activated in stress (e.g. amygdala, hypothalamus) has provided the rationale for studying NPY and related peptides in animal models of anxiety. Whereas a clinical study reported the lowest CSF NPY concentrations among depressed patients in those individuals with the most severe anxiety symptoms, another study observed higher plasma NPY-like immunoreactivity in patients with PD as compared with healthy volunteers (Widerlöv et al., 1988; Boulenger et al., 1996). There seems to be clear preclinical evidence that the central infusion of NPY and NPY fragments selective for the NPY-Y_1 receptor display anxiolytic-like effects in a variety of tests (Britton et al., 1997; Broqua et al., 1995). The data also suggest that the anxiolytic effect of NPY is mediated by the activation of NPY-Y_1 receptors in the central nucleus of the amygdala (Heilig, 1995). A recent preclinical study in rat showed that NPY in the lateral septum may act as an endogenous anxiolytic and antagonise corticotropin-releasing hormone (CRH) (stress)-induced anxiety (Kask et al., 2001). It was shown that bilateral microinjections of NPY into the dorsocaudal lateral septum but not into the intra-medial septum dose-dependently decreased anxiety in the social interaction test of rats, whereas the effects of CRH were opposite. Hence, this study demonstrated that NPY administered into the lateral septum has a potent and site-selective anxiolytic effect in the rat model of anxiety. The discovery of novel selective neuropeptide Y_1 receptor agonists/antagonists may hopefully provide new drugs for the treatment of anxiety disorders (Griebel, 1999).

Tachykinins refer to peptides sharing the common C-terminal amino acid sequence Phe-X-Gly-Leu-Met.NH_2. Substance P is the most potent TK for the TK NK_1 receptor, whereas neurokinin A exhibits the highest affinity for the TK NK_2 receptor and neurokinin B for the TK NK_3 receptor, respectively. All mammalian TKs have limited selectivity for a particular neurokinin receptor. The TK NK_1 receptor has been cloned from several species including man (Maggi et al., 1993; Regoli et al., 1994). The abundant distribution of TK NK_1 receptors in brain is reflected by a wide variety of behavioural changes after central administration of SP or selective TK NK_1 receptor agonists (Piot et al., 1995; Stoessl et al., 1995). A significant step forward concerning the involvement of TKs in anxiety and depression is a study which has provided evidence of a new specific, long-lasting and orally bioavailable TK NK_1 receptor antagonist, MK-869, in the reduction of vocalisation in guinea pig pups after maternal separation (Kramer et al., 1998). This behavioural response is sensitive to psychoactive drugs that alleviate not only symptoms of anxiety and depression in humans but also stress-induced vocalisations in mammals (Kramer et al., 1998). In a guinea pig model, a selective NK_1 receptor agonist induced vocalisations, which were inhibited by TK NK_1 receptor antagonists such as MK-869, as well as by antidepressants such as imipramine and fluoxetine. The mechanism of MK-869 is different from that of clinically used antidepressant and anxiolytic drugs. It may involve the integration of emotional responses to stress by the amygdala or related brain areas.

3.4 Glutamatergic pathways

Glutamate receptors have been subdivided into functional classes with increasing sophistication since the initial discovery of a general excitatory action of glutamate on nerve cells in the spinal cord of the cat in the late 1950s. NMDA receptors were named after the specific glutamate-like synthetic agonist NMDA which sets them apart from non-NMDA type glutamate receptors. All NMDA receptors appear to be highly permeable to Ca^{2+}, blocked in a voltage-dependent manner (at least to some degree) by Mg^{2+} binding in the channel, and appear to possess a binding site for the obligatory co-agonist glycine.

NMDA receptor antagonists have been shown to be anxiolytic in animal models of anxiety, although they have not been tested extensively (Wiley et al., 1990; 1995). Phencyclidine and other phencyclidine-like NMDA receptor antagonists have been shown to produce anxiolytic effects in a punishment procedure, although another study failed to find this effect (Porter et al., 1989; Sanger & Jackson, 1989). NMDA antagonists such as dizocilpine (MK-801, the only non-competitive phencyclidine-like), for example, have actions similar to clinically proven anxiolytics in the elevated plus maze, ultrasonic vocalisation and other models but not in a few others (Corbett & Dunn, 1991; Criswell et al., 1994; Dunn et al., 1989). In addition, compounds such as LY 354740 that inhibit the release of glutamate *via* presynaptic metabotropic glutamate receptors also exhibit a similar spectrum of anxiolytic activity. Overall, the effects of phencyclidine-like NMDA receptor antagonists do not appear to be as specific or as consistent as those of competitive NMDA receptor antagonists. Drugs that act at the phencyclidine site produce also phencyclidine-like discriminative stimulus effects (Balster & Willetts, 1988). Since substitution for phencyclidine in drug discrimination tasks is predictive of phencyclidine-like subjective effects in humans, it is unlikely that phencyclidine or dizocilpine would ever be used clinically as antianxiety drugs (Balster, 1990). Because of the risk of abuse, with phencyclidine-related drugs, antagonists such as HA966, that act at the glycine-modulatory site on the NMDA receptor seem promising in the development of future anxiolytics (Corbett & Dunn, 1991).

NMDA receptor antagonists may show promise as potential anxiolytic agents, but differences among antagonists acting at different cellular sites may be expected. Based on these data there are clearly several avenues for developing substances that limit glutamatergic transmission that may result in effective antianxiety medications.

3.5 Opioid receptors

Opioids exert their actions through three types of opioid receptor, μ, κ, and δ (Reisine & Pasternak, 1996). Thus, research into the mechanisms of opioid actions has focused on the function of each opioid receptor type and the functional interaction between the receptor types. It now seems clear that the μ-opioid receptor mediates most of the opioid actions, including analgesia, tolerance and reward (Reisine & Pasternak, 1996; Matthes et al., 1996; Zadina et al., 1997). Opiate agonists themselves do not reliably produce anxiolytic-like effects in animal models of anxiety although there is one report showing anxiolytic effect of the κ opioid agonist U50488H in the elevated plus-maze (Privette & Terrian, 1995; Pollard & Howard, 1990). However, another κ agonist, ethylketocyclazocine, has been reported to suppress punished responding in an operant model which suggests an anxiogenic effect (DeRossett & Holzman, 1985).

The opiate antagonist naloxone has been reported to block the anxiolytic effects of BDZs, barbiturates and meprobamate in several behavioural paradigms, one of which is the elevated plus-maze (Agmo et al., 1995; Belzung & Agmo, 1997; Duka et al., 1982). The antagonism is specific to anxiolytic-like actions, because motor incoordination, hypothermia or anticonvulsive effects of BDZs and pentobarbital are not blocked by the opiate antagonist (Agmo et al., 1995). In fact, the opiate antagonist does not bind to any significant degree to receptors that may be important for anxiolytic activity such as $GABA_A$, 5-HT_{1A} or dopamine receptors (Carlsson & Seeger, 1982; Martin et al., 1991). It is likely, then, that naloxone blocks anxiolytic activity through an action at opiate receptors. Hence, further research is required to establish the exact mechanism involved in the opioid receptors in anxiety.

3.6 Neurosteroids

Steroids that are formed within the brain from cholesterol are often defined as neurosteroids. The term neurosteroid was introduced by Baulieu in 1981 to designate a steroid hormone intermediate, dehydroepiandrosterone (DHEA) sulfate, that was found in brain at concentrations independent of its plasma levels (Beaulieu, 1981). DHEA sulfate is one of a variety of neurosteroids that includes pregnanolone sulphate, now thought to be formed *de novo* in mammalian brain *via* the classical mevalonate cholesterol pathway (Corpechot et al., 1983; Beaulieu & Robel, 1990).

There is now considerable evidence that these neuroactive steroids are potent positive allosteric modulators of $GABA_A$ receptors because they increase the frequency or duration of openings, or both, of the $GABA_A$-gated Cl^- channel (Paul & Purdy, 1992; Lambert et al., 1995). The neuroactive steroid allopregnanolone, like the BDZs, appears to bind with higher affinity to specific molecular forms of the $GABA_A$ receptor, possibly due to the presence of unique steroid recognition sites associated with one or more receptor subunits. In this way, it modulates GABA-ergic transmission. Thus, neurosteroids may be involved in a neuropsychiatric disorder such as anxiety. The stimulatory effects of 3α-reduced pregnane steroids or their precursor molecule, progesterone, at GABA receptors might exert anxiolytic effects in animals and humans (Patchev et al., 1997; Bitran et al., 1991). The administration of allopregnanolone (1.25, 5 and 10 mg, i.c.v) and pregnanolone (2.5, 5 and 10 mg, i.c.v.) elicited a significant anxiolytic effect in the plus-maze (Bitran et al., 1991). Whereas all doses of allopregnanolone increased the proportion of open arm entries, the proportion of time spent on the open arms was increased by 2.5 and 10 mg, but not 1.25 mg, of allopregnanolone. The anxiolytic potency of pregnanolone was lower, relative to allopregnanolone, as only higher doses of pregnanolone increased the proportion of entries into the open arms (2.5, 5 and 10 mg) and time spent on the open arms (5 and 10 mg). Neither allopregnanolone nor pregnanolone administration affected the total number of entries which suggests the anxiolytic specificity of the drug treatment. These results, therefore, demonstrate that intracerebroventricular (i.c.v.) injection of allopregnanolone resulted in anxiolytic activity in the rats. Preclinical work with DHEA also suggests that it may alter performance on cognitive tasks due to change in anxiety levels (Frye & Lacey, 1999).

Neuroactive steroids have shown efficacy in a number of preclinical models predictive of anxiolytic effects in patients (Beekman et al., 1998) (see Table 1). In general, the positive anxiolytic-like effects of neuroactive steroids are observed at doses below those that produce behavioural adverse effects such as sedation and response-rate decreases. The anxiolytic effects of BDZs can be increased by adjunctive treatment with neuroactive steroids (Vivian et al., 1997). Clinical evidence to date is supportive of these findings and indicates that neuroactive steroids are generally well tolerated. Further clinical studies are warranted to confirm their efficacy and safety.

3.7 Equilibrium between GABA-benzodiazepine and other receptors

Several results indicate a possible GABA-BDZ mediation of the anxiolytic action of various serotonergic drugs (Wright et al., 1992; Olsen & Venter, 1985). The BDZ receptor antagonist, flumazenil, and the $GABA_A$ receptor antagonist, bicuculline, counteracted the p-chlorophenylalanine (p-CPA)-induced anticonflict effect at doses not affecting the behaviour (Söderpalm & Engel, 1989). In a study designed to analyse the possible interaction between the serotonergic and GABA-ergic neurotransmitter systems in the anxiolytic action of 5-HT_{1A} agonists, the anxiolytic effect of buspirone (5 mg/kg), ipsapirone (5 mg/kg), indorenate (5 mg/kg) and 8-OH-DPAT (0.5 mg/kg) was established in the rat burying test (Fernandez-Guasti & Lopez Rubalcava, 1998). The data also showed that the GABA-BDZ antagonist flumazenil was able to prevent the anxiolytic action of ipsapirone, buspirone and 8-OH-DPAT, but not that of indorenate. These results confirm previous data that flumazenil effectively blocks the anxiolytic effects of serotonergic drugs in other anxiety paradigms such as the black and white transitions test and the modified Vogel conflict paradigm (Lopez-Rubalcava et al., 1992; Söderpalm & Engel, 1989). By contrast, the GABA antagonist bicuculline failed to block the anxiolytic effect of the serotonergic drugs. These data suggest that the BDZ rather than the GABA-ergic receptor is involved in the anxiolysis noted with the 5-HT_{1A} agonists. Since flumazenil blocked the antianxiety effects of the 5-HT_{1A} compounds, a possible interaction between the GABA-ergic and the serotonergic neurotransmitter systems can be proposed. However, there are also reports which indicate that flumazenil is unable to prevent the anxiolytic actions of the serotonergic compounds in other anxiety tests. Variations in the anxiolytic profile of these 5-HT_{1A} products among mice, rats, hamsters and pigeons have been demonstrated (Barret et al., 1986; Fernandez-Guasi & Hong, 1989; Fernandez-Guasi & Lopez-Rubalcava, 1995).

Preclinical work also showed that the combined administration of subthreshold doses of diazepam and the 5-HT_{1A} anxiolytics induced a potentiating anxiolytic effect in the burying behaviour paradigm (Fernandez-Guasti & Lopez-Rubalcava, 1998). These data support clinical studies which showed that buspirone and diazepam potentiate in their anxiolytic action, and that small doses of buspirone do not cause any additional decrement in the psychomotor performance induced by diazepam (Mattila et al., 1986). Taken together, these data may suggest that both

Table 2.1: Anxiolytic effects of some neuroactive steroids in some models of anxiety.

Drugs	Tests – Animals	References
Allopregnanolone (+), preganolone (+), CCD3693 (+)	Vogel conflict – mouse	Wieland et al., 1991
5α-THDOC (+)	Vogel conflict – rat	Crawley et al., 1986
Allopregnanolone (+), pregnanolone (+), CCD3693 (+)	Geller conflict – rat	Wieland et al., 1995 Brot et al., 1997 Edgar et al., 1997
Allopregananolone (+), pregnanolone (+), 5α-THDOC (+), CCD3693 (+)	Elevated plus maze – mouse	Wieland et al., 1995 Edgar et al., 1997 Rodgers & Johnson, 1998
Allopregnanolone (+), pregnanolone (+)	Elevated plus maze – rat	Bitran et al., 1991
Allopregnanolone (+), pregnanolone (+), 5α-THDOC (+)	Light-dark transition – mouse	Wieland et al., 1991 Wieland et al., 1995

5α-THDOC = 5α-tetrahydrodeoxy-corticosterone

GABA and 5-HT systems interact in the mediation of the anxiolytic action of the 5-HT_{1A} products. The nature of such interaction is yet unknown although anatomical experiments have shown that these two neurotransmitter systems are associated in brain areas with the modulation of anxiety (Gallager, 1978; Harandi et al., 1987).

It has also been demonstrated that the BDZ anxiolytic diazepam counteracts the anxiogenic effect of the non-peptide Y_1 receptor antagonist BIBP3226, suggesting that the equilibrium between GABA-ergic and NPY-ergic neurotransmission may be important for the regulation of an animal's emotional state (Kask et al., 1996). A recent study which used a transgenic mouse model expressing a mouse Y_1 receptor-β-galactosidase fusion gene (*Y1R/lacZ*) to study the effect of positive or negative modulators of $GABA_A$ receptors on Y_1 receptor gene expression also suggest that modulation of $GABA_A$ receptor function may regulate Y_1 receptor gene expression in medial amygdala (Oberto et al., 2000). The result of this study is consistent with the hypothesis that NPY-ergic and GABA-ergic systems are functionally coupled in the amygdaloid complex.

Recent studies have demonstrated that antidepressant drugs are actually more effective than BDZs in the treatment of anxiety states. A wide range of antidepressants elicits a reduction in BDZ receptors and displays anxiolytic effects within a conflict paradigm. The anxiolytic activity of antidepressants, however, does not appear to be mediated *via* the BDZ receptor, but possibly *via* another component of the complex such as the chloride channel associated with the $GABA_A$ receptor. The roles of two major neurochemical substrates that may be implicated in the anxiolytic activity of antidepressant are the BDZ-GABA receptor chloride ionophore complex and central serotonergic pathways. One critical feature of this GABA-mediated inhibition appears to involve the regulation of central monoaminergic response to aversive stimulation. Thus, anxiolytic agents block stress-induced increases in central NE, 5-HT and dopamine (DA) (Reinhard et al., 1982). In the light of these findings, the role of the BDZ-GABA receptor complex in the action of antidepressants is not really surprising. Additionally, as possible candidates for the mechanism of anxiolytic activity of these compounds, results of pharmacological, behavioural and clinical studies point to the importance of serotonin 5-HT_{1A} receptors and 5-HTT sites as targets for the action of antidepressants, triazolobenzodiazepines and anxioselective piperazine derivatives. Drugs combining several actions at different receptors might, therefore, be worth considering for the development of novel anxiolytics.

3.8 Use of mutant mice

The creation of mice heterozygous for the $GABA_A$-receptor γ_2 subunit has been helpful for the comprehension of the molecular basis of anxiety disorders and is probably one of the first genetic models of an emotional disorder (Crestani et al., 1999). These $\gamma_2^{+/-}$ mutant mice have reduced BDZ binding, indicating a reduction in the number of γ_2 subunits, and behave like patients suffering from anxiety disorders. They had as much as a 35% reduction in γ_2 subunits in areas such as the hippocampus, cingulate cortex and prefrontal cortex, but only about 5–15% in other brain areas. This suggests that the hippocampus is likely to mediate the increased anxiety in these mice. The $\gamma_2^{+/-}$ mice showed enhanced behavioural inhibition toward natural aversive stimuli and heightened responsiveness in trace fear conditioning and ambiguous cue discrimination learning. Like highly anxious people, the γ_2 heterozygous mice are more sensitive to the anxiolytic effects of the BDZ. However, the hippocampus is implicated only in the cognitive aspects of anxiety (autonomic changes and phenomena such as fear-potentiated startle are controlled separately by the amygdala) (Davis, 1992; McNaughton, 1997). The mice may therefore model only the cognitive hippocampal aspects of anxiety disorder. Nevertheless, regardless of the circuitry involved, they may represent a good model of some forms of anxiety predisposition because they are likely to overact to many anxiety-provoking situations. Such genetic models are important in improving our understanding of the study of innate contributors to anxiety disorders (Crestani et al., 1999; Heisler et al., 1998).

Another genetic animal model is the serotonin receptor 1A knockout mice technology; this approach demonstrates that mice without $5HT_{1A}$ receptors display decreased exploratory activity and increased fear of aversive environments (open or elevated spaces) (Ramboz et al., 1998; Parks et al., 1998). The data indicated that 5-HT_{1A} receptors are involved in the modulation of exploratory and fear-related behaviours and suggest that reductions in 5-HT_{1A} receptor density due to genetic defects or environmental stressors might result in increased anxiety. The absence of the 5-HT_{1A} receptor also appears to have a more pronounced effect in males than in females, particularly on some measures of anxiety.

Recent clinical investigations have also provided clearer understanding of the neurobiological deficits involved in some of the anxiety disorders such as GAD, PD and PTSD.

4 Discussion

Transgenic mice prove to be useful models for exploration of the pathogenesis of anxiety. These mice offer easily testable predictions about mutations that may be found in anxiety patients. The importance and usefulness of the mouse for quantitative trait analysis make it a valuable tool to investigate mouse models of human normal and pathological behaviour (Flint & Corley, 1996). One of the best-characterised anxiety phenotype in mice is that of "emotionality" which appears to be analogous to anxious temperament in humans (Flint & Corley, 1996). Today, investigation of animal behaviour has come to prominence in this area because of the ease with which specific genes can be inactivated. The promise of the mouse model is the relative ease with which sequences can be manipulated in the germ line. However, although the identification of genetic predisposing factors would certainly be a major advance, genes alone will not explain human anxiety. These mutant mice would only be a valuable model for testing hypotheses about how genes and environment interact to produce this anxiety condition.

5-HT_{1A} agonists are generally anxiolytics, whereas antagonists can have anxiogenic effects. However, there are exceptions, and not all antagonists induce anxiety. Potent SSRIs appear to have superior efficacy in many of the anxiety disorders, with indications that NE reuptake inhibitors have an advantage in severe types of anxiety. Medications with dual effects of blocking reuptake of both serotonin and NE, such as venlafaxine XR, have superior benefits in achieving remission in anxiety such as GAD. These pharmacological interventions may also provide a faster onset of action and be highly beneficial in comorbid anxiety with depression.

Unfortunately, relatively few studies have been devoted to the possible memory effects of non-BDZ anxiolytics. Nevertheless, animal data suggest that the 5-HT_{1A} receptor partial agonist buspirone also disrupts acquisition avoidance learning and retention, leading to the question of an unavoidable link between anxiety, memory and learning (Venault et al., 1986). Indeed, in contrast to anxiolytics, anxiogenic drugs, notably β-carbolines, promote learning capacity in rats (Bass et al., 1992).

The pharmacological, behavioural and molecular investigations of the peptide receptors (e.g. NPY-Y_1 and NK_1) have advanced remarkably the knowledge of neuropeptide receptors and function in general. This has led to the emergence of new compounds with potential clinical interest. Development has reached phase II clinical trials in the treatment of anxiety and depression for some of these compounds.

The novel manner in which neuroactive steroids are thought to transduce their effects in conjunction with their predicted efficacy and general lack of side-effects indicates these drugs as a novel class of $GABA_A$ receptor modulators and suggests additional clinical potential.

References

Abelson JL, Glitz D, Cameron OG, Lee MA, Bronzo M & Curtis GC. Blunted growth hormone response to clonidine in patients with generalized anxiety disorder. Arch Gen Psychiatry 48, 157–162, 1991

Ackerman DL, Greenland S, Bystritsky A, Morgenstern H & Katz RJ. Predictors of treatment response in obsessive-compulsive disorder: Multivariate analyses from a multicenter trial of clomipramine. J Clin Psychopharmacol 14, 247–254, 1994

Agmo A, Galvan A, Heredia A & Morales M. Naloxone blocks the antianxiety but not the motor effects of benzodiazepines and pentobarbital: experimental studies and literature review. Psychopharmacology 120, 186–194, 1995

Albus M, Zahn TP & Breier A. Anxiogenic properties of yohimbine: I. Behavioral, physiological and biochemical measures. Eur Arch Psychiatry and Clin Neurosci 241, 337–344, 1992

Altemus M, Swedo SE, Leonard HL, Richter D, Rubinow DR, Potter WZ & Papoport JL. Changes in cerebrospinal fluid neurochemistry during treatment of obsessive-compulsive disorder with clomipramine. Arch Gen Psychiatry 51, 794–803, 1994

American Psychiatric Association. Diagnostic and statistical manual of mental disorders, 4th ed. American Psychiatric Press, Washington, DC, 1994

Andrews G, Stewart G, Allen R & Henderson AS. The genetics of six neurotic disorders: a twin study. J Affect Disord 19, 2396, 1990

Balster RL. Perception of drug effects. In: MA Berkley & WC Stebbins (eds): Comparative perception, Vol. 1. New York: John Wiley and Sons, 127, 1990

Balster RL & Willetts. Receptor mediation of the discriminative stimulus properties of phencyclidine and sigma opioid agonists. In: FC Coplaert & RL Balster (eds): Transduction mechanisms of drug stimuli. Berlin: Springer-Verlag, 122, 1988

Barrett JE, Witkin JM, Mansbach RS, Skolnick P & Weissman BA. Behavioral studies with anxiolytic drugs. III. Antipunishment actions of buspirone in the pigeon do not involve benzodiazepine receptor mechanisms. J Pharmacol Exp Ther 238, 1009–1013, 1986

Barnard EA, Skolnick P, Olsen RW, Mohler H, Sieghart W, Biggio G, Braestrup C, Bateson AN & Langer SZ. International Union of Pharmacology XV, subtypes of γ-aminobutyric acidA receptors: Classification on the basis of subunit structure and receptor function. Pharmacol Rev 50 (2), 291–313, 1998

Bass EW Jr, Means LW & McMillen BA. Buspirone impairs performance of a three-choice working memory water escape task in rats. Brain Res Bull 28(3): 455–461, 1992

Baulieu EE. Steroid hormones in the brain: several mechanisms? In: K Fuxe, JA Gustafsson & L Wetterberg (eds): Steroid hormone regulation of the brain. Wenner-Gren Center International Symposium Series, Vol. 34. Oxford: Pergamon, 3–14, 1981

Baulieu EE & Robel P. Neurosteroids: a new brain function? J Steroid Biochem Mol Biol 37, 395–403, 1990

Beekman M, Ungard JT, Gasior M, Carter RB, Dijkstra D, Goldberg SR & Witkin JM. Reversal of behavioral effects of pentylenetetrazol by the neuroactive steroid ganaxolone. J Pharmacol Exp Ther 284(3): 868–877, 1998

Belzung C & Agmo A. Naloxone blocks anxiolytic-like effects of benzodiazepines in Swiss but not in BALB/c mice. Psychopharmacology 132, 195–201, 1997

Birbaumer N, Grodd W, Diedrich O, Klose U, Erb E, Lotze M et al. fMRI reveals amygdala activation to human faces in social phobics. Neuroreport 9, 1223–1226, 1998

Bitran D, Hilvers RJ & Kellogg CK. Anxiolytic effects of 3 alpha-hydroxy-5 alpha[beta]-pregnan-20-one: endogenous metabolites of progesterone that are active at the $GABA_A$ receptor. Brain Res 561(1): 157–161, 1991

Bormann J. Electrophysiology of $GABA_A$ and $GABA_B$ receptor subtypes. Trends Neurosci 11, 112–116, 1988

Boulenger JP, Jerabek I, Jolicoeur FB, Lavallee YJ, Leduc R & Cadieux A. Elevated plasma levels of neuropeptide Y in patients with panic disorder. Am J Psychiatry 153, 114–116, 1996

Bowery NG, Hill DR, Hudson AL, Doble A, Middlemiss DN, Shaw J & Turnbull MJ. (–)Baclofen decreases neurotransmitter release in the mammalian CNS by an action at a novel receptor. Nature 283, 92, 1980

Bowery NG, Doble A, Hill DR, Hudson AL, Shaw JS, Turnbull MJ & Warrington R. Bicuculline-insensitive GABA receptors on peripheral autonomic nerve terminals. Eur J Pharmacol 71, 53–70, 1981

Bowery NG. $GABA_B$ receptors and their significance in mammalian pharmacology. Trends Pharmacol Sci 10, 401–407, 1989

Bradwejn J, Koszycki D, Shriqui C. Enhanced sensitivity to cholecystokinin tetrapeptide in panic disorder: clinical and behavioral findings. Arch Gen Psychiatry 48, 603–610, 1991

Britton KT, Southerland S, VanUden E, Kirby D, Rivier J and Koob G. Anxiolytic activity of NPY receptor agonists in the conflict test. Psychopharmacology 132, 6–13, 1997

Broqua P, Wettstein JG, Rocher MN, Gauthiermartin B and Junien JL. Behavioral effects of neuropeptide Y receptor agonists in the elevated plus-maze and fear-potentiated startle procedures. Behav Pharmacol 6, 215–222, 1995

Brot MD, Akwa Y, Purdy RH, Koob GF & Britton KT. The anxiolytic-like effects of the neurosteroid allopregnanolone: interactions with GABA(A) receptors. Eur J Pharmacol 325 (1): 1–7, 1997

Brown SL, Svrakic MD, Przybeck TR & Cloninger CR. The relationship of personality to mood and anxiety states: a dimensional approach. J Psychiatry Res 26, 197–211, 1992

Carlsson KR & Seeger TF. Interaction of opiates with dopamine receptors: receptor binding and behavioral assays: Pharmacol Biochem Behav 16, 119–124, 1982

Chalmers DT, Lovenberg TW & De Souza EB. Localization of novel corticotropin-releasing factor (CRF2) mRNA expression to specific sub-cortical nuclei in rat brain: comparison with CRF1 receptor mRNA expression. J Neurosci 15, 6340–6350, 1995

Chang CP, Pearse II RV, O'Connell S & Rosenfeld MG. Identification of a seven transmembrane helix receptor for corticotropin-releasing factor and sauvagine in mammalian brain. Neuron 11, 1187–1195, 1993

Charney DS, Heninger GR & Redmond DE. Yohimbine induced anxiety and increased noradrenergic function in humans: Effects of diazepam and clonidine. Life Sci 33, 19–29, 1983

Chaouloff F. Regulation of 5-HT receptors by corticosteroids: Where do we stand? Fundam Clin Pharmacol 9, 219–233, 1995

Chen R, Lewis KA, Perrin MH & Vale WW. Expression cloning of a human corticotropin-releasing-factor. Proc Natl Acad Sci USA 8967–8971, 1993

Chopin P & Briley M. The benzodiazepine antagonist flumazenil blocks the effects of CCK receptor agonists and antagonists in the elevated plus-maze. Psychopharmacology 110, 409–414, 1993

Cloninger CR. A systematic method for clinical description and classification of personality variants. A proposal. Arch Gen Psychiatry 44 (6): 573–588, 1987

Cloninger CR. A unified biosocial theory of personality and its role in the development of anxiety states: a reply to commentaries. Psychiatric Developments 6 (2): 83–120, 1988

Collier DA, Stöber G, Li T, Heils A, Catalano M, Di Bella D, Arranz MJ, Murray RM, Vallada HP, Bengel D et al. A novel functional polymorphism within the promoter of the serotonin transporter gene: possible role in susceptibility to affective disorders. Mol Psychiatry 1, 453–460, 1996

Comings DE, Muhleman D, Johnson P & MacMurray JP. Potential role of the estrogen receptor gene (ESR1) in anxiety. Mol Psychiatry 4, 374–377, 1999

Coplan JD, Papp LA, Martinez J, Pine D, Rosenblum LA, Cooper T, Liebowitz MR & Gorman JM. Persistence of blunted human growth hormone response to clonidine in fluoxetine-treated patients with panic disorder. Am J Psychiatry Vol 152(4), 619–622, 1995.

Corbett R & Dunn RW. Effects of HA-966 on conflict, social interaction, and plus maze behaviors. Drug Development Research 24 (3), 201–205, 1991

Corda MG, Giorgio O, Gatta F & Biggio G. Long-lasting proconflict effect induced by chronic administration of the beta-carboline derivation FG 7142. Neurosci Lett 62, 237–240, 1985

Corpechot C, Synguelakis M, Talha S, Axelson M, Sjovall J, Vihko R, Baulieu EE & Robel P. Pregnenolone and its sulfate ester in the rat brain. Brain Res 270, 119–125, 1983

Coryell W, Noyes R Jr & Schlechte J. The significance of HPA axis disturbance in panic disorder. Biol Psychiatry 25, 989–1002, 1989

Costal B, Domemey AM, Hughes J, Kelly ME, Naylor RJ & Woodruff GN. Anxiolytic effects of CCK-B antagonists. Neuropeptides 19, 65–73, 1991

Crawley JN, Glowa JR, Majewska MD & Paul SM. Anxiolytic activity of an endogenous adrenal steroid. Brain Res 398 (2): 382–385, 1986

Crestani F, Loez M, Baer K, Essrich V, Benke D, Laurent JP, Belzung C, Fristchy J-M, Luscher B & Mohler H. Decreased GABAA-receptor clustering results in enhanced anxiety and a bias for threat cues. Nature Neurosci 2, 833–839, 1999

Criswell HE, DJ Knapp DH, Overstreet & GR Breese. Effects of ethanol, chlordiazepoxide and MK-801 on performance in the elevated-plus maze and on locomotor activity. Alcohol Clin Exp Res 18, 596, 1994

Critchley MA & Handley SL. Effects in the X-maze anxiety model of agents acting at 5-HT_1 and 5-HT_2 receptors. Psychopharmacology 93 (4): 502–506, 1987

Daugé V, Ladurelle N, Derrien M, Durieux C & Roques BP. Potential therapeutic application of CCK antagonists in anxiety and panic disorders. In: M Hamon, H Ollat, M-H Thiébot (eds): Anxiety: Neurobiology, clinic and therapeutic perspectives. Colloque INSERM, Vol. 232. John Libbey EuroText Ltd, 167–176, 1993

Davidson RJ, Marshall JR, Tomarken AJ & Henriques JB. While a phobic waits: Regional brain electrical and autonomic activity in social phobics during anticipation of public speaking. Biol Psychiatry 47, 85–95, 2000

Davis M. The role of the amygdala in fear-potentiated startle: implications for animal models of anxiety. Trends Pharmacol Sci 13, 35–41, 1992

DeLorey TM & Olsen RW. γ-Aminobutyric $acid_A$ receptor structure and function. J Biol Chem 267, 16747–16750, 1992

de Montigny C. Cholecystokinin tetrapeptide induces panic-like attacks in healthy volunteers: preliminary findings. Arch Gen Psychiatry 46, 511–517, 1989

DeRossett SE & Holzman SG. Effects of opiate antagonists and putative k agonists on unpunished and punished operant behavior in the rat. Psychopharmacology 86, 386–391, 1985

De Souza EB. Corticotropin-releasing factor receptors: physiology, pharmacology, biochemistry and role in central nervous system and immune disorders. Psychoneuroendocrinology 20, 789–819, 1995

Detari L, Szentgyorgyi V, Hajnik T, Szenasi G, Gacsalyi I & Kukorelli T. Differential EEG effects of the anxiolytic drugs, deramciclane (EGIS-3886), ritanserin and chlordiazepoxide in rats. Psychopharmacology 142 (3), 318–326, 1999

De Vry J. $5HT_{1A}$ receptor agonists: recent developments and controversial issues. Psychopharmacology 121, 1–26, 1995

De Vry J. $5HT_{1A}$ receptors in psychopathology and the mechanism of action of clinically effective therapeutic agents. Drug News Perspect 9, 270–280, 1996

Dorow R, Horowski R, Paschelke G, Amin M & Brarstrup C. Severe anxiety induced by FG 7142, a beta-carboline ligand for benzodiazepine receptor. Lancet 41, 98–99, 1983

Duncalfe LL, Carpenter MR, Smilie LB, Martin LL & Dunn MS. J Biol Chem 27, 9209–9214, 1996

Dunn RW, R Corbett & Fielding S. Effects of $5\text{-}HT_{1A}$ receptor agonists and NMDA receptor antagonists in the social interaction test and the elevated plus maze. Eur J Pharmacol 169, 1, 1989

Duka T, Millan MJ, Ulsamer B, Doenicke A. Naloxone attenuates the anxiolytic action of diazepam in man. Life Science, 31, 1833–1836, 1982

Dykstra LA, Preston KL & Bigelow GE. Discriminative stimulus and subjective effects of opioids with mu and kappa activity: data from laboratory animals and human subjects. Psychopharmacology 130 (1): 14–27, 1997

Edgar DM, Seidel WF, Gee KW, Lan NC, Field G, Xia H, Hawkinson JE, Wieland S, Carter RB & Wood PL. CCD-3693: an orally bioavailable analog of the endogenous neuroactive steroid, pregnanolone, demonstrates potent sedative hypnotic actions in the rat. J Pharmacol Exp Ther 282 (1): 420–429, 1997

Ennis MD. The therapeutic potential of $5\text{-}HT_{1A}$ agonists. Curr Opin Invest Drugs 4, 205–213, 1993

Davis EZ, Harris CR, Ellingson RJ, Andreason P, Moore V, Varner JL, Brown GL, Eckardt MJ & Goldman D. Relationship of genetically transmitted alpha EEG traits to anxiety disorders and alcoholism. Am J Med Genet Neuropsychiatric Genetics 60 (5), 400–408, 1995.

Enz R & Cutting GR. Molecular composition of GABAC receptors. Vis Res 38, 1431–1441, 1998

Faludi G, Tekes K & Tothfalusi L. Comparative study of platelet ^{3}H-paroxetine and ^{3}H-imipramine binding in panic disorder patients and healthy controls. J Psychiatry Neurosci 19 (2): 109–113, 1994

Feigenspan A & Bormann J. GABA-gated Cl^{-} channels in the rat retina. Prog Retinal Eye Res 17, 99–126, 1998

Feighner JP. Overview of antidepressants currently used to treat anxiety disorders. J Clin Psychiatry 60 (22):18–22, 1999

Fernandez-Guasti A & Hong E. Antianxiety effect of various putative S1 receptor agonists on the conditioned defensive-burying paradigm. In: P Evans, AR Archer, T Archer (eds): Behavioral pharmacology of 5-HT. Hillsdale, NJ: Lawrence Erlbaum, 377–382, 1989

Fernandez-Guasti A & Lopez-Rubalcava C. Modification of the anxiolytic action of 5-HT1A compounds by GABA-benzodiazepine agents in rats. Pharmacol Biochem Behav 60, 1, 27–32, 1998

Fernandez-Guasti A & Lopez-Rubalcava C. Action of ipsapirone and 8-OH-DPAT on exploratory behavior in hamsters (*Mesocricetus auratus*): Effects of antagonists and p-CPA. Pharmacol Biochem Behav 50, 375–382, 1995

Fink H, Rex A & Marsden CA. Behavioural and neurochemical effects of CCK-fragments in animal models of anxiety. Behav Pharmacol 5 (1), 30, 1994

Fletcher A, Forster EA, Bill DJ, Brown G, Cliffe IA, Hartley JE, Jones DE, McLenachan A, Stanhope KJ, Critchley DJ et al. Behav Brain Res 73, 337–353, 1996

Flint J & Corley R. Do animal models have a place in the genetic analysis of quantitative human behavioural traits. J Mol Med 74, 515–521, 1996

Forster EA, Cliffe IA, Bill DJ, Dover GM, Jones D, Reilly Y & Fletcher A. A pharmacological profile of the selective silent 5-HT_{1A} receptor antagonist WAY-100635. Eur J Pharmacol 281, 81–88, 1995

Frye CA & Lacey EH. The neurosteroids DHEA and DHEAS may influence cognitive performance by altering affective state. Physiol Behav 66 (1), 85–92, 1999

Fuxe K, Andersson K, Locatelli V, Agnati LF, Hokfelt T, Skirboll L & Mutt V. Cholecystokinin peptides produce marked reduction of dopamine turnover in discrete areas in the rat brain following intraventricular injection. Eur J Pharmacol 67, 329–331, 1980

Gallager DW. Benzodiazepines: Potentiation of a GABA inhibitory response in the dorsal raphe nucleus. Eur J Pharmacol 49, 133–143, 1978

Gavish M, Katz Y, Bar-Ami S & Weizman R. Biochemical, physiological, and pathological aspects of the peripheral aspects of the peripheral benzodiazepine receptor. J Neurochem 58, 1589–1601, 1992

Gavish M, Laor N, Bidder M, Fisher D, Fonia O, Muller U, Reiss A, Wolmer L, Karp L & Weizman R. Altered platelet peripheral-type benzodiazepine receptor in posttraumatic stress disorder. Neuropsychopharmacology 14, 181–186, 1996

George DT, Nutt DJ, Rawlings RR, Phillips MJ, Exkart MJ, Potter WZ & Linnoila M. Behavioral and endocrine responses to clomipramine in panic disorder patients with or without alcoholism. Biol Psychiatry 37, 112–119, 1995

Glaser T & De Vry J. Neurobiology of 5-HT_{1A} receptors. In: SM Stahl, M Gastpar, JM Keppel Hesselink & J Traber (eds): $Serotonin_{1A}$ receptors in depression and anxiety. New York: Raven Press, 35–53, 1992
Goldberg DP, Bridges P, Duncan-Jones P & Grayson D. Dimensions of neuroses seen in primary care settings. Psychol Med 17, 461–470, 1987
Graeff PG, Guimaraes FS, Andrade TC & Deaxin JF. The role of 5-HT in stress, anxiety and depression. Pharmacol Biochem Behav 54, 129–141, 1996
Griebel G. 5-Hydroxytryptamine-interacting drugs in animal models of anxiety disorders: more than 30 years of research. Pharmacol Ther 65 (3): 319–395, 1995
Griebel G, Perrault G & Sanger DJ. Characterization of the behavioral profile of the non-peptide CRF receptor antagonist CP-154, 526 in anxiety models in rodents. Psychopharmacology 138, 55–66, 1998
Griebel G. Is there a future for neuropeptide receptor ligands in the treatment of anxiety disorders? Pharmacol Ther 82, 1, 1–61, 1999
Guidotti A, Toffano G & Costa E. An endogenous protein modulates the affinity of GABA and benzodiazepine receptors in rat brain. Nature 275, 553–555, 1978
Habib KE, Weld KP, Rice KC, Pushkas J, Champoux M, Listwak S, Webster EL, Atkinson AJ, Schulkin J, Contoreggi C et al. Oral administration of a corticotropin-releasing hormone receptor antagonist significantly attenuates behavioral, neuroendocrine, and autonomic responses to stress in primates. Proc Natl Acad Sci USA 97 (11), 6079–6084, 2000
Haefely W & Pole C. Electrophysiological studies on the interaction of anxiolytic drugs with GABAergic mechanisms. In: JB Malick, SJ Enna & HI Yamamura (eds): Anxiolytics: Neurochemical, behavioural and clinical perspectives. New York: Raven Press, 113–115, 1983
Haefely W. biological basis of drug-induced tolerance, rebound and dependence. Contribution of recent research on benzodiazepines. Pharmacology 19, 353–361, 1986
Handley SL. 5-Hydroxytryptamine pathways in anxiety and its treatment. Pharmacol Ther 66 (1):103–48, 1995
Harandi M, Aguera M, Gamrani H, Didier M, Maitre M, Calas A & Belin MF. Gamma-aminobutyric acid and 5-hydroxytryptamine. Interrelationship in the rat nucleus dorsalis: Combination of radiographic and immunocytochemical technique at light and electron microscope levels. Neuroscience 21, 237–251, 1987
Harper PS, Harley HG, Reardon W & Shaw DJ. Anticipation in myotonic dystrophy: new light on an old problem. Am J Hum Genet 51, 10–16, 1992
Harro J, Vasar E & Bradwejn J. CCK in animal and human research on anxiety. Trends Pharmacol Sci 14 (6): 244–249, 1993
Hashimoto S, Inoue T & Koyama T. Effects of conditioned fear stress on serotonin neurotransmission and freezing behavior in rats. Eur J Pharmacol 378, 23–30, 1999
Heilig M, Koob GF, Ekman R & Britton KT. Corticotropin-releasing factor and neuropeptide Y: role in emotional integration. Trends Pharmacol Sci 17, 80–85, 1994
Heilig M. Antisense inhibition of neuropeptide Y (NPY)-Y_1 receptor expression blocks the anxiolytic-like action of NPY in amygdala and paradoxically increases feeding. Regul Pept 41, 61–69, 1995
Heisler LK, Chu HM, Brennan TJ, Danao JA, Bajwa P, Parsons LH & Tecott LH. Elevated

anxiety and antidepressant-like responses in serotonin 5-HT_{1A} receptor mutant mice. Proc Natl Acad Sci USA 95 (25):15049–15054, 1998

Henin A & Kendall PC. Obsessive-compulsive disorder in childhood and adolescence. In: TH Ollendick & RJ Prinz (eds): Advances in clinical child psychology, Vol. 19. New York: Plenum Press, 75–131, 1997

Heninger GR, Charney DS & Price LH. Alpha-2 adrenergic receptor sensitivity in depression. Arch Gen Psychiatry 45, 718–726, 1988

Hoehn-Saric R & McLeod DR. Anxiety and arousal: physiological changes and their perception. J Affect Disord 61, 217–224, 2000

Hokfelt T, Skirboll L, Everitt B, Meister B, Brownstein M, Jacobs T, Faden A, Kuga S, Goldstein M & Markstein R. Distribution of cholecystokinin-like immunoreactivity in the nervous system. Co-existence with classical neurotransmitters and other neuropeptides. Ann NY Acad Sci 448, 255–274, 1985

Hollander E, DeCaria C, Nitescu A, Cooper T, Stover B, Gully R, Klein DF & Liebowitz MR. Noradrenergic function in obsessive-compulsive disorder: Behavioral and neuroendocrine responses to clonidine and comparison to healthy controls. Psychiatry Res 37 (2), 161–177, 1991.

Hoyer D, Clarke DE, Fozard JR, Hartig PR, Martin GR, Mylecharane EJ, Saxena PR & Humphrey PPA. VII International Union of Pharmacology classification of receptors for 5-hydroxytryptamine (serotonin). Pharmacol Rev 46, 157–203, 1994

Jenck F, Moreau J-L, Berendsen HHG, Boes M, Broekkamp CLE, Martin JR, Wichmann J & Van Delft AML. Antiaversive effects of $5HT_{2c}$ receptor agonists and fluoxetine in a model of panic-like anxiety in rats. Eur Neuropsychopharmacol 8, 161–168, 1998

Jerabek I, Lavallée YJ, Jolicoeur FB & Boulenger J Ph. Cholécystokinine et anxiété. II. La CCK-4, modèle expérimental, des attaques de panique. Ann Psychiatr 11, 36–41, 1996

Johnson MR, Marazziti D, Brawman-Mintzer O, Emmanuel NP, Ware MR, Morton WA, Rossi A, Cassano GB & Lydiard RB. Abnormal peripheral benzodiazepine receptor density associated with generalized social phobia. Biol Psychiatry 43, 306–309, 1998

Jolas T, Schreiber R, Laporte AM, Chastanet M, De Vry J, Glaser J, Adrien J & Hamon M. Are postsynaptic 5-HT(1A) receptors involved in the anxiolytic effect of 5-HT(1A) receptor agonists and in their inhibitory effects on the firing of serotonergic neurons in the rat? J Pharmacol Exp Ther 272, 920–929, 1995

Johnston GAR. $GABA_C$ receptors: relatively simple transmitter-gated ion channels? Trends Pharmacol Sci 17, 319–323, 1996

Kahn RJ, McNair DM, Lipman RS, Covi L, Rickels K, Downing R, Fisher S & Frankenthaler LM. Imipramine and chlordiazepoxide in depressive and anxiety disorders. II. Efficacy in anxious outpatients. Arch Gen Psychiatry 43, 79–85, 1986

Kask A, Nguyen HP, Pabst R & Von Hörsten S. Neuropeptide Y Y_1 receptor-mediated anxiolysis in the dorsocaudal lateral septum: functional antagonism of corticotropin-releasing hormone-induced anxiety. Neuroscience 104, 799–806, 2001

Kask A, Rago L & Harro J. Anxiogenic-like effect of the neuropeptide Y Y1 receptor antagonist BIBP3226: antagonism with diazepam. Eur J Pharmacol 317, R3–R4, 1996

Katerndahl DA & Realini JP. Lifetime prevalence of panic states. Am J Psychiatry 150, 246–249, 1993

Katon W. Panic disorder: relationship to high medical utilization, unexplained physical symptoms, and medical costs. J Clin Psychiatry 57 (10), 11–18, 1996

Kehne JH, Coverdale S, McCloskey TC, Hoffman DC & Cassella JV. Effects of the CRF (1) receptor antagonist, CP 154,526 in the separation-induced vocalization anxiolytic test in rat pups. Neuropharmacology 39, 1357–1367, 2000

Kellner M, Herzog L, Yassouridis A, Holsboer F & Wiedemann K. Possible role of atrial natriuretic hormone in pituitary-adrenocortical unresponsiveness in lactate-induced panic. Am J Psychiatry 152, 1365–1367, 1995

Kendler KS, Davis CG & Kessler RC. The familial aggregation of common psychiatric and substance use disorders in the National Comorbidity Survey: a family history study. Br J Psychiatry 170, 541–548, 1997

Kramer MS, Cutler N, Feighner J, Shrivastava R, Carman J, Sramek JJ, Reines SA, Liu G, Snavely D, Wyatt KE et al. Distinct mechanism for antidepressant activity by blockade of central substance P receptors. Science 281, 1640–1645, 1998

Kramer MS, Cutler NR, Ballenger JC, Patterson WM, Mendels J, Chenault A, Shrivastava R, Matzurawolfe D, Lines C & Reines S. A placebo-controlled trial of L-365, 260, a CCKB antagonist, in panic disorder. Biol Psychiatry 37, 462–466, 1995

Kreiss DS & Lucki I. Differential regulation of serotonin (5-HT) release in the striatum and hippocampus by 5-HT_{1A} autoreceptors of the dorsal and median raphe nuclei. J Pharmacol Exp Ther 269 (3):1268–1279, 1994

Kumor KM, Haertzen CA, Johnson RE, Kocher T & Jasinski D. Human psychopharmacology of ketocyclazocine as compared with cyclazocine, morphine and placebo. J Pharmacol Exp Ther 238 (3): 960–968, 1986

Lader MH. Limitations on the use of benzodiazepines in anxiety and insomnia: are they justified? European Neuropsychopharmacology 9 (Suppl), S399–S405, 1999

Lambert JJ, Belelli D, Hill-Venning C & Peters JA. Neurosteroids and $GABA_A$ receptor function. Trends Pharmacol Sci 16 (9): 295–303, 1995

Leckman JF, Weissman M, Merikangask KR, Pauls DL & Prusoff BA. Panic disorder and major depression: Increased risk of depression, alcoholism, panic and phobic disorders in families of depressed probands with panic disorders. Arch Gen Psychiatry 40, 1055–1060, 1983

Le Doux JE. Information flow from sensation to emotion: plasticity in the neural computation of stimulus value. In: M Gabriel, J Moore (eds): Learning and computational neurosciences: Foundations of adaptive networks. Cambridge, Mass: MIT, 1990

Lee YM, Beinborn M, McBride EW, Lu M, Kolakowski LF Jr & Kopin AS. The human brain cholecystokinin-B/gastrin receptor. Cloning and characterization. J Biol Chem 268, 8164–8169, 1993

Lee CR, Plosker GL & McTavish D. Tropisetron. A review of its pharmacodynamic and pharmacokinetic properties and therapeutic potential as an antiemetic. Drugs 46, 925–943, 1993

Lesch KP, Wiesmann M, Hoh A, Muller T, Disselkamp Tietze J, Osterheider M & Schulte HM. $5HT_{1A}$ receptor effector system responsivity in panic disorder. Psychopharmacology (Berl), 106, 111–117, 1992

Lesch KP, Bengel D, Heils A, Sabol SZ, Greenberg BD, Petri S, Benjamin J, Müller CR, Hamer

DH & Murphy DL. Association of anxiety-related traits with a polymorphism in the serotonin transporter gene regulatory region. Science 274, 1527–1531, 1996

Loehlin JC. Partitioning environmental and genetic contributions to behavioral development. American Psychologist 44 (10):1285–1292, 1989

Lopez-Rubalcava C, Saldivar A, Fernandez-Guasti A. Interaction of GABA and serotonin in the anxiolytic action of diazepam ad serotonin in the anxiolytics. Pharmacol Biochem Behav 43, 433–440, 1992

Lucki I, Singh A & Kreiss DS. Antidepressant-like behavioral effects of serotonin receptor agonists. Neurosci Biobehav 18 (1): 85–95, 1994

Löw K, Crestani F, Keist R, Benke D, Brünig I, Benson JA, Fritschy J-M, Rülicke T, Bluethmann H, Möhler H & Rudolph U. Molecular and neuronal substrate for the selective attenuation of anxiety. Science 260, 131–134, 2000

Lundkvist J, Chai Z, Teheranian R, Hasanvan H, Bartfai T, Jenck F, Widner U & Moreau J-L. A non-peptidic corticotropin releasing factor receptor antagonist attenuates fever and exhibits anxiolytic-like activity. Eur J Pharmacol 309, 195–200, 1996

Macdonald RL & Olsen RW. $GABA_A$ receptor channels. Annu Rev Neurosci 17, 569–602, 1994

MacMillan H & Steiner M. A Atrial natriuretic factor. Does it have a role in psychiatry? Biol Psychiatry 35, 272–277, 1994

Maggi CA, Patacchini R, Rovero P & Giachetti A. Tachykinin receptors and tachykinin receptor antagonists. J Auton Pharmacol 13, 23–93, 1993

Malizia AL, Cunningham VJ, Bell CJ, Liddle PF, Jones T & Nutt DJ. Decreased brain $GABA_A$-benzodiazepine receptor binding in panic disorder. Arch Gen Psychiatry 55, 715–720, 1998

Martin A, Kaufman J & Charney D. Pharmacotherapy of early-onset depression. Update and new directions. Child Adolesc Psychiatr Clin N Am 9, 135–157, 2000

Mazzanti CM, Lappalainen J, Long JC, Bengel D, Naukkarinen H, Eggert M, Virkkunen M, Linnoila M & Goldman D. Role of the serotonin transporter promoter polymorphism in anxiety-related traits. Arch Gen Psychiatry 55, 936–940, 1998

Marazziti D, Rotondo A, Martini C, Giannaccini G, Lucacchini A, Panciolo-Guadagnucci ML, Diamond BI, Borison R & Cassano GB. Changes in peripheral benzodiazepine receptors in patients with panic disorder and obsessive-compulsive disorder. Neuropsychobiology 29, 8–11, 1994

Martin JR, Bös M, Jenck F, Köhler C, Moreau JL, Sleight A, Stadler H & Wichmann J. $5HT_{2c}$ receptor agonists and antagonists in animal models of anxiety. Eur Neuropsychopharmacol 5, 209, 1995

Martin DC, Introna RP & Aronstam RS. Fentanyl and sulfentanyl inhibit agonist binding to 5HT1A receptors in membranes from rat brain. Neuropharmacology 30, 323–327, 1993

Martin WR. Pharmacology of opioids. Pharmacol Rev 35 (4): 283–323, 1983

Matthes HW, Maldonado R, Simonin F, Valverde O, Slowe S, Kitchen I, Befort K, Dierich A, Le Meur M, Dolle P et al. Loss of morphine-induced analgesia, reward effect and withdrawal symptoms in mice lacking the mu-opioid-receptor gene. Nature 383 (6603): 819–823, 1996

Mattila M, Seppala T & Mattila MJ. Combined effects of buspirone and diazepam on objective and subjective tests of performance in healthy volunteers. Clin Pharmacol Ther 40, 620–626, 1986

Matussek N, Ackenheil M, Hippius H, Muller F, Schroder HT, Schultes H & Wasilewski B. Effect of clonidine on growth hormone release in psychiatric patients and controls. Psychiatry Res 2 (1): 25–36, 1980

McDougle CJ, Goodman WK, Leckman JF, Lee NC, Heninger GR & Price LH. Haloperidol addition in fluvoxamine-refractory obsessive-compulsive disorder: A double-blind, placebo-controlled study in patients with and without tics. Arch Gen Psychiatry 51, 302–308, 1994

McKerman RM et al. Sedative but not anxiolytic properties of benzodiazepines are mediated by the GABAA receptor $\alpha 1$ subtype. Nature Neurosci 3, 587–592, 2000

McNaughton N. Cognitive dysfunction resulting from hippocampal hyperactivity – a possible cause of anxiety disorder? Pharmacol Biochem Behav 56, 603–611, 1997

McNicoll C, Bill DJ & Fletcher A. Potentiation of SSRI-induced inhibition of mouse marble burying by a selective 5-HT_{1A} antagonist. J Psychopharmacol 9, A29, 1995

Misane I & Ogren SO. Multiple 5-HT receptors in passive avoidance: comparative studies of p-chloroamphetamine and 8-OH-DPAT. Neuropsychopharmacology 22 (2): 168–190, 2000

Monsma FJ Jr, Shen Y, Ward RP, Hamblin MW & Sibley DR. Cloning and expression of a novel serotonin receptor with high affinity for tricyclic psychotropic drugs. Mol Pharmacol 43 (3): 320–327, 1993

Nemeroff CB. The preeminent role of early untoward experience on vulnerability to major psychiatric disorders: The nature-nurture controversy revisited and soon to be resolved. Mol Psychiatry 4, 106–108, 1999

Ninan PT. The functional anatomy, neurochemistry, and pharmacology of anxiety. J Clin Psychiatry 60 (Suppl 22), 12–17, 1999

Nutt DJ. Altered central alpha-2 sensitivity in panic disorder. Arch Gen Psychiatry 46, 165–169, 1989

Oberto A, Panzica G, Altruda F & Eva C. Chronic modulation of the GABAA receptor complex regulates Y1 receptor gene expression in the medial amygdala of transgenic mice. Neuropharmacology 39, 227–234, 2000

Ohara K, Suzuki Y, Ochiai M, Yoshida K, Ohara K. Age of onset anticipation in anxiety disorders. Psychiatry Res 89, 215–221, 1999

Okuyama S, Chaki S, Kawashima N, Yoshiko S, Ogawa S-I, Nakazato A, Kumagai T, Ojubo T & Tomisawa K. Receptor binding, behavioral, and electrophysiological profiles of non-peptide corticotropin-releasing factor subtype 1 receptor antagonist CRA 1000 and CRF1001. J Pharmacol Exp Ther 289, 926–935, 1999

Olivier B, van Wijngaarden I & Soudijn W. 5-HT_3 receptor antagonists and anxiety: a preclinical and clinical review. Eur Neuropsychopharmacol 10, 77–95, 2000

Olsen RW & Venter JC. Benzodiazepine-GABA receptors and chloride channels: Structural and functional properties. New York: Alan R. Liss, 1985

Owens MJ & Nemeroff CB. Role of serotonin in the pathophysiology of depression: focus on the serotonin transporter. Clin Chem 40 (2): 288–295, 1994

Owens MJ & Nemeroff CB. Physiology and pharmacology of corticotropin-releasing factor. Pharmacol Rev 31, 425–473, 1991

Pande AC. Lack of efficacy of a cholecystokinin-B antagonist in anxiety disorders. Biol Psychiatry 42, 11–19, 1997

Parks CL, Robinson PS, Sibille E, Shenk T & Toth M. Increased anxiety of mice lacking the serotonin1A receptor. Proc Natl Acad Sci USA 95, 10734–10739, 1998

Patchev VK, Montkowski A, Rouskova D, Koranyi L, Holsboer F & Almeida OF. Neonatal treatment of rats with the neuroactive steroid tetrahydrodeoxycorticosterone (THDOC) abolishes the behavioral and neuroendocrine consequences of adverse early life events. J Clin Invest 99 (5): 962–966, 1997

Paul SM & Purdy RH. Neuroactive steroids. FASEB J 6 (6): 2311–2322, 1992

Paulson HL & Fischbeck KH. Trinucleotide repeats in neurogenetic disorders. Annu Rev Neurosci 19, 79–107, 1996

Perrin M, Donaldson C, Chen R, Blount A, Berggren T, Bilezikjian L, Sawchenko P & Vale W. Identification of a second corticotropin-releasing factor receptor gene and characterization of a cDNA expressed in heart. Proc Natl Acad Sci USA 92, 2969–2973, 1995

Pfeiffer A, Brantl V, Herz A & Emrich HM. Psychotomimesis mediated by kappa opiate receptors. Science 233 (4765): 774–776, 1986

Pichot W, Hansenne M, Gonzalez Moreno A & Ansseau M. Growth hormone response to apomorphine in panic disorder: comparison with major depression and normal controls. Eur Arch Psychiatry Clin Neuroscience 245 (6): 306–308, 1995

Pigott TA & Seay SM. A review of the efficacy of selective serotonin reuptake inhibitors in obsessive-compulsive disorder. J Clin Psychiatry 60 (2): 101–106, 1999

Piot O, Betschart J, Grall I, Ravard S, Garret C & Blanchard JC. Comparative behavioural profile of centrally administered tachykinin NK_1, NK_2 and NK_3 receptor agonists in the guinea-pig. Br J Pharmacol 116, 2496–2502, 1995

Pollard GT & Howard JL. Effects of drugs on punished behavior: pre-clinical tests for anxiolytics. Pharmacol Ther 45, 104–424, 1990

Porter JH, Wiley JL &d Balster RL. Effects of phencyclidine-like drugs on punished behavior in rats. J Pharmacol Exp Ther 248, 991, 1989

Plomin R, Owen MJ & McGuffin P. The genetic basis of complex human behaviors. Science 264 (5166): 1733–1739, 1994

Privette TH & Terrian DM. Kappa opioid agonists produce anxiolytic-like behaviors on the elevated plus-maze. Psychopharmacology 118, 444–450, 1995

Ramboz S, Oosting R, Amara DA, Kung HF, Blier P, Mendelsohn M, Mann JI, Brunner D & Hen R. Serotonin receptor 1_A knockout: An animal model of anxiety-related disorder. Proc Natl Acad Sci USA 95, 14476–14481, 1998

Regoli D, Boudon A & Fauchere JL. Receptors and antagonists for substance P and related peptides. Pharmacol Rev 46, 551–599, 1994

Reinhard JJ, Bannon MJ and Roth RH. Acceleration by stress of dopamine synthesis and metabolism in prefrontal cortex: antagonism by diazepam. Naunyn-Schmiedebergs Arch Pharmacol 318, 374–377, 1982

Reisine T & Pasternak G. In: JG Harman & LE Limbird (eds): Goodman and Gilman's The pharmacological basis of therapeutics. McGraw-Hill, 521–555, 1996

Rex A, Barth T, Voigt J-P, Domeney AM & Fink H. Effects of cholecystokinin tetrapeptide and sulfated cholecystokinin octapeptide in rat models of anxiety. Neurosci Lett 172, 139–142, 1994

Rickels K, Schweizer E, Csanalosi I, Case WG & Chung H. Long-term treatment of anxiety and risk of withdrawal: prospective comparison of clorazepate and buspirone. Arch Gen Psychiatry 45, 444–450, 1988

Rickels K, Downing R, Schweizer E & Hassman H. Antidepressants for the treatment of generalized anxiety disorder: a placebo-controlled comparison of imipramine, trazodone and diazepam. Arch Gen Psychiatry 50, 884–895, 1993

Rocca P, Beoni AM, Eva C, Ferrero P, Zanalda E & Ravizza L. Peripheral benzodiazepine receptor messenger RNA is decreased in lymphocytes of generalized anxiety disorder patients. Biol Psychiatry 43 (10), 767–773, 1998.

Rodgers RJ & Johnson NJ. Behaviorally selective effects of neuroactive steroids on plus-maze anxiety in mice. Pharmacol Biochem Behav 59 (1): 221–232, 1998

Roozendaal B, Koolhaas JM & Bohus B. Central amygdaloid involvement in neuroendocrine correlates of conditioned stress responses. J Neuroendocrinol 4, 46–52, 1992

Ruat M, Traiffort E, Leurs R, Tardivel-Lacombe J, Diaz J, Arrang JM & Schwartz JC. Molecular cloning, characterization, and localization of a high-affinity serotonin receptor (5-HT_7) activating cAMP formation. Proc Natl Acad Sci USA 90 (18): 8547–8551, 1993

Rudolph U, Crestani F, Benke D, Brunig I, Benson JA, Fritschy JM, Martin JR, Bluethmann H & Mohler H. Benzodiazepine actions mediated by specific gamma-aminobutyric acid(A) receptor subtypes. Nature 401 (6755): 796–800, 1999

Sanchez C. Serotonergic mechanisms involved in the exploratory behaviour of mice in a fully automated two-compartment black and white text box. Pharmacol Toxicol 77 (1): 71–78, 1995

Sanger DJ & Jackson A. Effects of phencyclidine and other N-methyl-D-aspartate antagonists on the schedule-controlled behavior of rats. J Pharmacol Exp Ther 248, 1215, 1989

Schechter LE, Bolanos FJ, Gozlan H, Lanfumey L, Haj-Dahmane S, Laporte AM, Fattaccini CM & Hamon M. Alterations of central serotonergic and dopaminergic neurotransmission in rats chronically treated with ipsapirone: biochemical and electrophysiological studies. J Pharmacol Exp Ther 255, 1335–1347, 1900

Schofield PR, Darlison MG, Fujita N, Burt DR, Stephenson FA, Rodriguez H, Rhee LM, Ramachandran J, Reale V & Glencorse TA. Sequence and functional expression of the GABA A receptor shows a ligand-gated receptor super-family. Nature. 328 (6127): 221–227, 1987

Schulz DW, Mansbach RS, Sprouse J, Braselton JP, Collins J, Corman M, Dunaiskis A, Farach S, Schmidt AW, Seeger T et al. CP-154,526: a potent and selective n on-peptide antagonist of corticotropin-releasing factor receptors. Proc Natl Acad Sci USA 93, 10477–10482, 1996

Siever LJ, Uhde TW, Silberman EK et al. Growth hormone response to clonidine as a probe of noradrenergic receptor responsiveness in affective disorder patients and controls. Psychiatry Res 6, 171–183, 1982

Sieghart W. Structure and pharmacology of g-aminobutyric $acid_A$ receptor subtypes. Pharmacol Rev 47, 181–233, 1995

Sim-Selley LJ, Vogt LJ, Xiao R, Childres SR & Selley DE. Region-specific changes in 5-HT1A receptor-activated G-proteins in rat brain following chronic buspirone. Eur J Pharmacol 389, 147–153, 2000

Singh L, Lewis AS, Field MJ, Hughes J & Woodruff GN. Evidence for an involvement of the brain cholecystokinin B receptor in anxiety. Proc Natl Acad Sci USA 88, 1130–1133, 1991

Singh L, Field MJ, Hughes J, Menzies R, Oles RJ, Vass CA & Woodruff GN. The behavioural properties of C1988, a selective cholecystokinin B receptor antagonist. Br J Pharmacol 104, 239–245, 1991a

Sivilotti L & Nistri A. GABA receptor mechanisms in the central nervous system. Prog Neurol 36, 35–92, 1991

Smith GW, Aubry J-M, Dellu F, Contrarino A, Bilezikjian LM, Gold LH, Chen R, Marchuk Y, Hauser C, Bentley CA et al. Corticotropin releasing factor receptor 1-deficient mice display decreased anxiety, impaired stress response, and aberrant neuroendocrine development. Neuron 20, 1093–1102, 1998

Söderpalm B & Engel JA. Does the p-CPA induced anticonflict effect involve activation of the $GABA_A$/benzodiazepine chloride ionophore receptor complex? J Neural Transm 76, 145–153, 1989

Sommermeyer H, Schreiber R, Greuel JM, De Vry J & Glaser T. Anxiolytic effects of the 5-HT_{1A} receptor agonist ipsapirone in the rat: neurobiological correlates. Eur J Pharmacol 240 (1): 29–37, 1993

Starcevic V, Uhlenhuth EH, Fallon S & Pathak D. Personality dimensions in panic disorder and generalized anxiety disorder. J Affect Disord 37, 75–79, 1996

Anokhin A, Yping M, Schalt E & Vogel F. Localization of a gene for the human low-voltage EEG on 20q and genetic heterogeneity. Genomics 12(1), 69–73, 1992

Stoessl AJ, Brackstone M, Rajakumar N & Gibson CJ. Pharmacological characterization of grooming induced by a selective NK1 tachykinin receptor agonist. Brain Res 700, 115–120, 1995

Stout SC, Kilts CD & Nemeroff CB. Neuropetides and stress: preclinical findings and implications for pathophysiology. In: MJ Friedman, S Charney, AY Deutsch (eds): Neurobiological and clinical consequences of stress: From normal adaptation to post-traumatic stress disorder. Philadelphia: Lippincott Raven, 1995

Sullivan GM, Copland JD & Gorman JM. Psychoneuroendocrinology of anxiety disorders. Psychoneuroendocrinology 21, 2, 397–412, 1998

Svrakic MD, Przybeck TR & Cloninger CR. Mood states and personality traits. J Affect Disord 24, 217–226, 1992

Tancer ME, Stein MB & Uhde TW. Growth hormone response to intravenous clonidine in social phobia: Comparison to patients with panic disorder and healthy volunteers. Biol Psychiatry 34, 591–595, 1993

Takahashi LK, Ho SP, Livanov V, Graciani N & Arneric SP. Antagonism of CRF2 receptors produces anxiolytic behavior in animal models of anxiety. Brain Res 902, 135–142, 2001

Timpl P, Spanagel R, Sillaber I, Kresse A, Reul JM, Reul HM, Stalla GK, Blanquet V, Stecker T, Holsboer F & Wurst W. Impaired stress response and reduced anxiety in mice lacking a functional corticotropin-releasing hormone receptor 1. Nat Genet 19, 162–166, 1998

Trappler B. Treatment of obsessive-compulsive disorder using clomipramine in a very old patient. Ann Pharmacotherapy 33 (6): 686–690, 1999

Uhlenhuth EH, Balter MB, Ban TA & Yang K. Trends in recommendations for the pharmacotherapy of anxiety disorders by an international expert panel, 1992–1997. Eur Neuropsychopharmacol 9 (6), S393–S398, 1999

Van Megen HJ, Westenberg HG, den Boer JA & Kahn RS. Cholecystokinin in anxiety. Eur Neuropsychopharmacology 6, 263–280, 1996

Venault P, Chapouthier G, de Carvalho LP, Simiand J, Morre M, Dodd RH & Rossier J. Benzodiazepine impairs and beta-carboline enhances performance in learning and memory tasks. Nature 321 (6073): 864–866, 1986

Vivian JA, Barros HM, Manitiu A & Miczek KA. Ultrasonic vocalizations in rat pups: modulation at the gamma-aminobutyric $acid_A$ receptor complex and the neurosteroid recognition site. J Pharmacol Exp Ther 282 (1): 318–325, 1997

Wank SA, Pisegna JR & de Weerth A. Cholecystokinin receptor family. Molecular cloning, structure and functional expression in rat, guinea pig and human. Ann NY Acad Sci 713, 49–66, 1994

Ward HE, Johnson EA, Salm AK & Birkle DL. Effects of prenatal stress on defensive withdrawal behavior and corticotropin releasing factor systems in rat brain. Physiol Behav 70, 359–366, 2000

Weissman MM, Bland RC, Canino GJ, Faravelli C, Greenwald S, Hwu H-G, Joyce PR, Karam EG, Lee C-K, Lellouch J et al. The cross-national epidemiology of panic disorder. Arch Gen Psychiatry 54, 305–309, 1997

Westenberg HG. Pharmacology of antidepressants: selectivity or multiplicity? J Clin Psychiatry 60 (17), 4–8; discussion 46–8, 1999

Widerlöv E, Lindstrom LH, Wahlestedt C & Ekman R. Neuropeptide Y and peptide YY as possible cerebrospinal fluid markers for major depression and schizophrenia, respectively. J Psychiatr Res 22, 69–79, 1988

Wieland S, Lan NC, Mirasedeghi S & Gee KW. Anxiolytic activity of the progesterone metabolite 5 alpha-pregnan-3-alpha-ol-20-one. Brain Res 565, 263–268, 1991

Wieland S, Beluzzi JD, Stein L & Lan NC. Comparative behavioral characterization of the neuroactive steroids 3 alpha-OH, 5 alpha-pregnan-20-one and 3 alpha-OH, 5 beta-pregnan-20-one in rodents. Psychopharmacology 118, 65–71, 1995

Wilde MI & Markham A. Ondansetron. A review of its pharmacology and preliminary clinical findings in novel applications. Drugs 52, 773–794, 1996

Willetts J, Balster RL & Leander JD. The behavioral pharmacology of NMDA receptor antagonists. Trends Pharmacol Sci 11, 423, 1990

Wiley JL, Cristello AF & Balster RL. Effects of site-selective receptor antagonists in an elevated plus-maze model of anxiety in mice. Eur J Pharmacol 294, 101–107, 1995

Wright IK, Upton N & Marsden CA. Effect of established and putative anxiolytics on extracellular 5-HT and 5-HIAA in the ventral hippocampus of rats during behavior on the elevated X-maze. Psychopharmacol (Berl) 109, 338–346, 1992

Yarker YE & McTavish D. Granisetron. An update of its therapeutic use in nausea and vomiting induced by antineoplastic therapy. Drugs 48, 761–793, 1994

Zadina JE, Hackler L, Ge L-J & Kastin AJ. A potent and selective endogenous agonist for the mu-opiate receptor. Nature 386 (6624), 499–502, 1997

Zobel AW, Nickel T, Kunzel HE, Ackl N, Sonntag A, Ising M & Holsboer F. Effects of the high-affinity corticotropin-releasing hormone receptor 1 antagonist R121919 in major depression: the first 20 patients treated. J Psychiatric Res 34 (3): 171–181, 2000

Chapter 3
Generalised anxiety disorder

1 Introduction

GAD is defined as anxiety, tension or worry associated with a considerable number of patients displaying a mix of somatic and psychological symptoms. The diagnostic definitions of GAD in various manuals, including ICD-10 and DSM-III/IV, differ in quality, number of symptoms, time frames and exclusion criteria. Consequently, lifetime prevalence rates vary between 1.2 and 6.4% in epidemiological surveys (Wittchen et al., 1994). Although the diagnostic reliability of GAD is comparatively low, the features constituting the diagnostic criteria have been noted to be reliable (Di Nardo et al., 1993). A study that compared the distribution of somatic symptoms associated with GAD in patients with "pure" GAD and patients with GAD plus comorbid current or lifetime psychiatric diagnoses showed that GAD is a distinct disorder that is relatively consistent in presentation in patients with or without other psychiatric disorders (Brawman-Mintzer et al., 1994). The hypothesis of the existence of distinct subtypes of GAD, i.e. a "pure" GAD and a "secondary" type with comorbid disorder, representing possibly a prodromal/residual state or an epiphenomenon associated with another disorder, was therefore not confirmed.

GAD is a chronic disorder that appears to have a bimodal distribution of onset age (Blazer et al., 1991). Age of onset varies between 2 and 61 years with a mean of 21 years (Yonkers et al., 1996). It typically occurs before 40 years of age, runs a chronic, fluctuating course and affects women twice as often as men (Walley et al., 1994; APA, 1994). The degree of comorbidity between GAD and other psychiatric disorders is high. Under DSM-IIIR and DSM-IV, however, it is accepted that GAD can exist independently of the anxiety that is related to the anticipation of panic or exposure to phobic or obsessional concerns (Barlow et al., 1986). Of particular interest has been the designation of worry or apprehensive expectation as the definitive feature of GAD. Sanderson and Barlow (1990) reported the comorbid characteristics of a sample of 22 patients meeting DSM-III-R criteria for GAD. About 59% met criteria for SP, and 27% met criteria for PD. Dysthymia was reported by 27% and depression by 14% of patients. This disorder occurs in all age cohorts with substantial prevalence, with at least a twofold higher prevalence in women compared to men (Beck et al., 1996; Brawman-Mintzer & Lydiard, 1996). In particular, GAD represents the least common anxiety disorder in mental health care settings, whereas it is the most common anxiety disorder in primary health care settings (Barlow, 1988). A recent study which explored the frequency and associated social disability of GAD and examined whether the ICD-10 definition of this disorder is appropriate reported that GAD is common in primary health care in nearly all countries (mean 1 month, prevalence rate 7.9%) with about 25% of these cases presenting with GAD in the absence of any comorbid psychiatric disorder (Maier et al., 2000). This study questions the clinical utility of the current ICD-10 diagnosis of GAD defining 6 months as a minimum duration and requiring at least 4 associated symptoms for diagnosis. With such definition, a substantial proportion of patients characterised by anxiety, tension and worrying remain undetected, and possibly not treated. The definition of GAD by ICD-10 was not found to be completely appropriate in this treatment setting, as the diagnostic threshold defined by ICD-10 was too restrictive. As the DSM-IV definition of GAD is even more restrictive, this conclusion may extend to the DSM-IV definition (Wacker et al., 1992).

2 Diagnostic

Diagnosis of this disorder has been difficult for several reasons. Considering that the diagnostic criteria for GAD have undergone significant change over the past 10 years (i.e. excessive worry was first identified as the key feature in GAD in DSM-III-R, unrealistic worry was replaced by uncontrollable worry in DSM-IV), it is not surprising that cognitive process variables for GAD have only recently begun to be identified.

A diagnosis of GAD refers to the presentation of a patient with an unexplained generalised increase in anxiety. There may be predominantly physical or emotional symptoms, which may persist or occur episodically. Any particular object, situation or thought not precipitated by any obvious life event should not provoke the anxiety. It differs from PD in that the symptoms are pervasive and do not occur as discrete episodes. Since the publication of DSM-IV, other changes have been suggested in order to increase the specificity of GAD diagnostic criteria without decreasing their sensitivity (Brown et al., 1995). In DSM-III-R, the diagnostic criteria for GAD included a list of 18 physical symptoms. In DSM-IV, the GAD physical symptom list was reduced to 6 in order to eliminate symptoms such as shortness of breath and tachycardia, which are more characteristic of PD and thus provide greater specificity to the definition of GAD (APA, 1994; Starcevic et al., 1994). The nosological status of GAD diagnostic entity is often critically discussed because of the very high rate of comorbidity with other psychiatric disorders, the assumed low degree of social disability in the absence of other disorders, and an ambiguous definition. The most frequent comorbid disorders were major depression, PD and agoraphobia.

A study which examined the numbers and types of symptoms in a sample of 90 patients with GAD and 77 patients with PD indicated that GAD and PD patients reported remarkably similar numbers of explained and unexplained medical symptoms (Barbee et al., 1997). PD patients reported higher numbers of cardiopulmonary and conversion complaints (p = 0.0276 and 0.0091) than GAD patients, and women reported higher numbers of sexual and generic complaints than men. The number of reported pain symptoms increased with age (p = 0.0001). However, none of the patients qualified for a diagnosis of somatization disorder based upon the application of all of these criteria to each symptom. Research with both DSM-III-R and DSM-IV has shown the diagnosis of GAD is reliable, although lower than other anxiety disorders (Di Nardo et al., 1993; Brown et al., 1994). It is important to consider that full-blown DSM-III-R GAD is rare in the young, with an estimated rate around 2% between 15 and 24 years of age (Wittchen et al., 1994).

3 The phenomenon of worry

Although worry can be found across the range of anxiety and depressive disorders in the general population, it represents the definitive feature of GAD under DSM-IV. What makes the worry pathological in GAD is not its content or the degree to which the worry is recognised as unreasonable, but is rather the perception that the worry is excessive and uncontrollable (Barlow & Wincze, 1998).

A model of GAD that includes four cognitive process variables, namely poor problem orientation, intolerance of uncertainty, cognitive avoidance and faulty beliefs about worry has been presented (Dugas et al., 1998). The first feature of the model is the central role given to intolerance of uncertainty, defined as the way an individual perceives information in uncertain or ambiguous situations and responds to this information with a set of cognitive, emotional and behavioural reactions. It has been suggested that intolerance of uncertainty is a key process variable in GAD that can exacerbate initial "what if...?" questions and even generates these questions in the absence of an immediate stimulus. The model also underscores the contribution of beliefs about worry to GAD. Another feature of the model is poor problem solving. Problem solving may be defined as a set of metacognitive processes that reflect awareness and appraisal of everyday problems and one's own problem-solving ability (Maydeu-Olivares & D'Zurilla, 1996). An effective cognitive-behavioral treatment package, based on the model, has been tested in single-case and randomised controlled trials (Ladouceur et al., 1997). Intolerance of uncertainty, cognitive avoidance, and faulty beliefs about worry also distinguish GAD patients from nonclinical moderate worriers and significantly contribute to identifying GAD patients and nonclinical control subjects (Ladouceur et al., 1998; Dugas et al., 1998). Intolerance of certainty may be defined as the way an individual perceives information in uncertain or ambiguous situations and responds to this information with a set of cognitive, emotional, and behavioural reactions (Ladouceur et al., 1997). In a study which aimed to test the broad specificity of GAD symptom and process variables, four groups of participants (patients with primary GAD, patients with secondary GAD, other anxiety disorders and nonclinical control volunteers) were examined from a structured interview and a series of standardised questionnaires (Ladouceur et al., 1999). The results indicate that DSM-IV GAD symptoms such as worry, physical symptoms and interference due to worry and anxiety distinguish GAD patients from those with other anxiety disorders. The two other variables of problem orientation and intolerance of uncertainty also differentiated GAD patients from other anxiety disorder patients. Overall this study supports the DSM-IV definition of GAD and indicates that problem orientation and intolerance of uncertainty are not only sensitive but specific GAD process variables.

The role of belief about worry is central to the cognitive model of GAD developed by Wells (Wells & Carter, 1999). This study shows that the results of a series of regression analyses support the hypothesis that pathological worry is directly associated with type 2 (meta-worry) rather than type 1 worry.

4 Neurobiology

Physiological studies suggest there is a diminished range of autonomic reactivity in response to psychological stress in GAD, although this pattern is not specific to GAD (Connor & Davidson, 1998; Hoehn-Saric, 1998).

Studies utilising various challenge paradigms, which examine the functional or dynamic aspects of the adrenergic system, found several differences between GAD patients and controls. A blunted GH response to clonidine (α_2-partial agonist) stimulation in GAD patients (also found in PD and major depression), suggesting a possible decrease in the sensitivity of α_2-adrenergic receptors in these patients, was reported (Abelson et al., 1991). However, no differences in blood pressure, heart rate, or 3-methoxy-4-hydroxyphenylglycol (MHPG) levels between GAD patients and controls after clonidine challenge were found. These results are further supported by studies that found a decrease in platelet α_2-adrenoreceptor binding site (B_{max}) in GAD patients compared with normal subjects (using the α_2 antagonist yohimbine or clonidine as a ligand), suggesting a possible decrease in the number of catecholamine receptors in GAD patients (Sevy et al., 1989; Cameron et al., 1990). In contrast, another study failed to find differences between GAD patients and controls in cardiovascular responses such as blood pressure and heart rate, self-rated anxiety, changes in plasma MHPG and cortisol after yohimbine challenge (Charney et al., 1989). However, an attenuated increase in MHPG in patients with GAD *versus* normal controls, which is consistent with the possibility that GAD patients may have presynaptic α_2-receptor hyposensitivity, was observed. In summary, baseline resting levels of catecholamine in patients with GAD appear to be normal, but the available data suggest that GAD patients may have subtle abnormalities such as reduced receptor sensitivity in the adrenergic system.

Challenge paradigms used to examine HPA axis reactivity in GAD patients (such as the Dexamethasone Suppression Test (DST)) suggested evidence of potential abnormalities. Indeed, a more abnormal escape from dexamethasone, which was not attributable to the presence of depression in DSM-III, diagnosed GAD patients *versus* normal controls was reported. A study found a nonsuppression rate of 38% in GAD patients (by using a cutoff of $\geq$0.4 ng/dL as nonsuppression), which was significantly higher than that for patients with depression (13%) (Avery et al., 1985). Another study reported a nonsuppression rate (by using a cutoff of $\geq$5 ng/dL) of 27% in GAD patients (Tiller et al., 1988). These data suggest possible abnormalities in the regulatory mechanisms of the HPA axis in GAD patients, possibly associated with abnormal stress response in these individuals.

A study evaluated the response of patients with GAD to the administration of sodium lactate (Cowley et al., 1988). It was found that patients with GAD (who

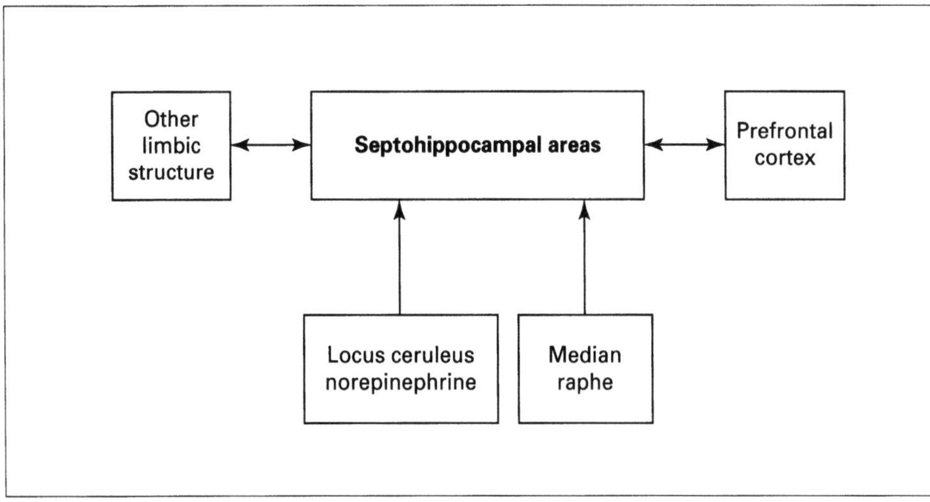

Figure 3.1
Neuroanatomical model of generalised anxiety disorder: behavioural inhibition system

never had panic attacks) panicked at a lower rate (11 vs. 41%) after lactate infusion than patients with PD. However, GAD patients were significantly more likely to report increased anxiety symptoms than nonpsychiatric controls. Unlike PD patients, patients with GAD also have very low rates of panic attacks in response to CO_2 inhalation (Gorman et al., 1988). GAD patients appear to resemble normal controls with respect to a panic challenge paradigm (e.g., fewer or no panic attacks) but appear more sensitive than normal controls in terms of number of symptoms and symptom intensity. This body of evidence further supports GAD as a biologically distinct disorder at least with respect to PD.

Several unifying neuroanatomic models of persistent anxiety states such as GAD have been proposed. Gray developed an elegant model (the BIS) for the neuroanatomic circuit that modulates responses to threat in animal models and potentially persistent anxiety states in humans (see Fig. 3.1) (Gray 1988). The BIS includes the septohippocampal areas and its connected structures including the noradrenergic and the 5-HT afferents. Gray hypothesised that in animals the septohippocampal areas are responsible for the processing of threat-relevant stimuli, such as signals of punishment, nonreward, or novel stimuli. The assessment of the presence of danger activates the BIS, which results in increased arousal and the inhibition of the entire regular, ongoing behaviours. Noradrenergic and serotonergic stimulation of the septohippocampal area further activates this system. This state of increased vigilance/scanning and hyperarousal mimics persistent anxiety states, such as GAD. Thus, it is possible that certain anxiolytic drugs may exert their effects *via* reduction of the noradrenergic or the serotonergic inputs into the septohippocampal areas.

It may be argued that biological research on GAD holds the hope of clarifying factors that influence comorbidity in the anxiety disorders. Relationships between

GAD and major depression may be hypothesised to involve abnormalities in brain systems involved in stress mediation, most notably components of the limbic system, including systems based in the hippocampal formation. As such, underlying abnormalities in such stress-sensitive systems are hypothesised to identify children most at risk for developing GAD during adolescence and major depression during adulthood.

4.1 Imaging studies

Regional differences in brain activity were also noted in patients with GAD. A study evaluated 18 patients who met DSM-III criteria for GAD by using PET measurements of cerebral glucose metabolism at baseline (during a passive avoidance task), after a cognitive vigilance task designed to stimulate anxiety, and after 3 weeks of treatment with BDZs or placebo (Wu et al., 1991). Higher relative metabolic rates for GAD patients in parts of the occipital, temporal (right posterior temporal lobe), frontal lobes (left inferior frontal gyrus), and the cerebellum relative to normal control subjects during a passive viewing task were observed. A decrease in absolute metabolic activity in the basal ganglia, temporal lobes, and cingulate gyrus in GAD patients was also found. The available imaging studies in patients with GAD suggest potential changes in brain activity in this population. A recent clinical trial that studied 10 drug-naive women with GAD and 10 age- and gender-matched healthy volunteers with MRI and with single photon emission computerized tomography (SPECT) images showed that the BDZ receptor-binding radioligand, NNC 13-8241, was significantly higher in the left temporal pole among patients with GAD (Tiihonen et al., 1997).

4.2 Genetics

Genetic factors, rather than environmental factors, may be particularly important in determining liability for developing GAD in women. Similar genetic factors appear to enhance vulnerability for developing major depressive disorder and GAD. It is hypothesised that specific and distinct environmental risk factors mediate expression of the specific phenotype (GAD vs. major depressive disorder) if this phenotype is present (Kendler et al., 1992).

In a large twin study that included 1033 female twin pairs, it was found that genetic factors appear to play a significant, but not overwhelming role in the aetiology of GAD (Kendler et al., 1992b). The heritability of GAD is estimated at around 30% in comparison to 70% heritability in major depression. In addition, it is also pointed out that the vulnerability to GAD and major depression is influenced by the same genetic factors (Kendler et al., 1992a). The available data suggest at least a modest genetic contribution to the development of GAD. These results also suggest that women with GAD are more likely to develop comorbid conditions. The presence of such coexisting diagnoses may reduce the likelihood of remission.

Table 3.1: Symptoms of GAD

Somatic	
Musculoskeletal	Restlessness or inability to relax
	Muscle aching or tension
	Easy fatigability
Gastrointestinal	Constipation/diarrhoea
	Difficulty swallowing ("lump in throat")
Psychic	
Anxiety	Excessive worry and anxiety that patient finds difficult to control.
	Anticipation of the worst.
	Fearful anticipation.
	Irritability
Depressed	Sleep difficulties
Cognitive	Difficulty concentrating
Other	Feelings of restlessness or jumpiness

5 Physiopathology

The low rate of endorsement of autonomic symptoms by GAD patients, together with the finding that symptoms within the motor tension and scanning and vigilance clusters are more closely associated with independent measures of GAD than symptoms from the autonomic activity cluster, support the recent exclusion of autonomic symptoms from the DSM-IV (Brown et al., 1995; Marten et al., 1993) (see Tab. 3.1). There appears to be a diminished vagal (or parasympathetic) tone associated with worry, rather than the sympathetic activity (dry mouth, sweating, urination) that is usually classed under the construct of autonomic activity (Thayer et al., 1996). Analysing symptoms reported by anxiety patients, Hamilton (1959) found two factors that he called psychic and somatic anxieties. Not only do patients with GAD differ considerably in psychic and somatic factors, but also each factor may be affected differentially by psychological and pharmacological interventions. Anxious individuals engaged in physical exercise classes reported more cognitive than somatic anxiety but those who practised passive meditation rated themselves equal on both dimensions (Schwartz et al., 1978).

In a study that examined the relationship between self-reports and psychophysiological recordings in patients suffering from GAD, it was found that although no systematic correlations were noted between patient ratings and physiological measures of somatic symptomatology during periods of rest or psychological stress (Stroop Test), parallel directional changes in the two sets of measures were observed upon exposure to stress (McLeod et al., 1986). This may indicate that patients could accurately report the direction, but not the degree, of changes of physical symptoms of anxiety. Therefore, patient's report and assessment of physical symptoms such as sweating and rapid heart rate can be useful in clinical evaluation and guidance for pharmacological treatment administration. Another more recent study which assessed the specificity of somatic symptoms that are associated with GAD according to the DSM-IV indicate that only muscle tension showed a unique relation to pathological worry (Joormann & Stöber, 1999). In contrast, difficulty of concentrating was exclusively related to depression symptoms. These data suggest that elevated muscle tension is a specific characteristic of pathological worry and that attention to these somatic symptoms should clarify the boundary between the diagnosis of GAD and depression. Symptoms such as restlessness, tendency to be easily fatigued, irritability and sleep disturbance seemed to be common features of pathological worry and depressive symptomatology.

6 Epidemiology and natural course

GAD is the second most common anxiety disorder among the elderly. Period prevalence rates range from 0.7 to 7.1% with a median rate of 2.2% (Blazer et al., 1991; Lindesay et al., 1989). It predominantly affects women, and typically has a chronic course, with periodic exacerbation. Epidemiological survey of DSM-III-R psychiatric disorders in a representative national sample (n = 8098) found that the prevalence rates in the total sample were 1.6% for current GAD (present for past 6 months), 3.1% for 12-month GAD, and 5.1% for lifetime GAD (Kessler et al., 1994; Wittchen et al., 1994).

A 5-year follow-up study of patients with GAD and PD who had originally participated in drug trials reported that although the GAD sample had milder symptoms than the PD at intake, fewer patients with GAD were in remission from their disorder at follow up (18 vs. 45%) (Woodman et al., 1999). Half of the GAD sample remained moderately impaired at the follow up which suggests that GAD is a chronic and disabling disorder.

Several clinical features appear to distinguish women from men with GAD. Dysthymia may be more likely to develop in women with GAD (Robins et al., 1984). The presence of a comorbid diagnosis is associated with a worsened prognosis and reduced remission rates compared with those in patients with GAD alone (Yonkers et al, 1996).

7 Treatment

7.1 Psychological

There is some evidence for the effectiveness of supportive therapy and cognitive-behavioral approaches with older people. A randomised, clinical trial compared 14 sessions of group cognitive-behavioral therapy with breathing, relaxation, cognitive techniques, and imaginal and *in vivo* exposure components to a supportive therapy condition with 48 older adults (ages 55–81) (Stanley et al., 1996). Both conditions led to comparable improvements in worry, anxiety and depression. By the end of treatment, 28% of the cognitive-behavioral participants and 54% of the supportive therapy participants were classified as treatment responders; this difference was not statistically significant. Only a small number of participants in either condition achieved high end-state functioning, defined as anxiety and depression scores in the nonclinical range, but gains in both conditions were generally maintained or increased by the 6-month follow-up.

7.2 Biofeedback

In a biofeedback study which used alpha-enhancement and alpha-suppression procedure to decrease anxiety in volunteers, 89 subjects who scored highest on trait anxiety (mean score 27.4) were compared with 8 others which scored lowest (4.3) (Hardt & Kamiya, 1978). There were 7 eyes-closed training sessions in 7 days. As training progressed, alpha-enhancement and state anxiety reduction became more strongly associated. The two best alpha-enhancers reduced trait anxiety scores to below average. Anxiety increased with alpha-suppression at the occipital but not the central sites, suggesting that the location of the alpha-measurement is important. The benefits of alpha-enhancement were more apparent after 2 h of training which suggests that the duration of training is also important. It is suggested that at least 5 h are needed.

Another study was performed in 45 patients who suffered from GAD for an average of 3.8 years (Rice et al., 1993). The patients were randomly assigned to frontal electromyogram (EMG) feedback, EEG alpha-increase feedback, EEG alpha-decrease feedback, pseudo-medication or waiting list control. The results showed that only EMG and alpha-increase groups improved significantly on the Welsh Anxiety Scale. Only alpha-increase resulted in reductions of heart rate reactivity to stress. In contrast, alpha-suppression caused the heart rate to be more reactive. Improvements in anxiety were maintained 6 weeks after treatment.

7.3 Pharmacological

Higher levels of psychic anxiety might tend to predict a more favourable response to serotonergic drugs such as buspirone or antidepressants such as imipramine and venlafaxine (Rickels et al., 1982; 1993; Haskins et al., 1997). Prominent somatic anxiety, especially in the absence of any subsyndromic depressive symptoms, might tend to predict a more favourable response to a benzodiazepine.

Psychic and somatic anxieties may respond differently to pharmacological interventions. Psychic symptoms of patients with GAD respond better to imipramine and somatic symptoms of such patients respond better to alprazolam (Hoehn-Saric et al., 1988). However, patients taking imipramine had significantly more side effects than those taking alprazolam throughout the study. Because of imipramine's side effects, it is necessary to explore the anxiolytic potential of other anxiolytics that are better tolerated. In a clinical study which examined two groups of chronically anxious patients (one suffering mainly from somatic anxiety and one suffering mainly from psychic anxiety), it was found that diazepam was more effective than placebo in both groups but that propranolol was superior to placebo only in the group with somatic anxiety, not in the group with psychic anxiety (Tyrer & Lader, 1974).). In a study which compared patients with GAD who had high levels of cardiovascular complaints with those who had low levels of cardiovascular complaints on rating instruments, it was found that the two groups differed on somatic but not psychic symptoms (Hoehn-Saric et al., 1989). Patients with high levels of cardiovascular symptoms had higher levels of cardiac lability and required higher doses of alprazolam (2.8 ± 1.3 vs. 1.8 ± 0.9 mg/day). These findings suggest that GAD patients with comparable levels of psychic anxiety may differ in levels of physical symptoms and require different pharmacological treatment and dose levels.

7.3.1 *Benzodiazepines (BDZs)*

BDZs are effective in the acute treatment of GAD. They all seem to have about the same efficacy (Hollister et al., 1993). GAD tends to be chronic and thus BDZ treatment tends to be long term. Management of BDZ discontinuation in long-term BDZ users includes gradual rather than abrupt discontinuation, use of cognitive therapy and the concomitant prescribing of other pharmacological medications (Rickels et al., 1990; Schweizer et al., 1990; Hegel et al., 1994). The results of a study performed in patients with GAD who had been long-term BDZ users (average duration of use of 8.5 years) suggest that management of BDZ discontinuation can be facilitated significantly by co-prescribing imipramine before and during the BDZ taper (Rickels et al., 2000).

7.3.2 *Buspirone*

Buspirone has demonstrated efficacy for the treatment of GAD (Boehm et al., 1990; Enkelmann, 1991). Although efficacy comparable to the BDZs was initially demonstrated with relatively low doses of buspirone (5 mg three times a day (tid)), at least 30 to 60 mg/day is now considered a more standard therapeutic dose (Enkelman, 1991; Lydiard et al., 1996). In contrast to the almost immediate effects of the BDZs, the onset of action of buspirone generally does not occur for 2 weeks and in some patients only after 3–6 weeks (Sussman, 1987).

Prior treatment with a BDZ might predict a reduced response to buspirone. In a study which divided patients into three groups (no prior BDZ treatment, recent: < 1 month; remote: > 1 month), it was suggested that initiation of buspirone therapy in GAD patients who have only recently terminated BDZ treatment should be undertaken cautiously and combined with appropriate patient education (DeMartinis et al., 2000). Discontinuation rates, adverse events and efficacy ratings all support the fact that buspirone patients who only recently stopped BDZ therapy did less well on all three measures. As experience has accumulated, enthusiasm has waned somewhat, primarily because of the slow onset of action and concerns about its level of potency.

7.3.3 Venlafaxine

The antidepressant venlafaxine has been shown in placebo-controlled trials to be effective for the treatment of GAD, and has received approval from the US Food and Drug Administration for this indication (Davidson et al., 1999). Venlafaxine effects were observed after one week to be greater than placebo, and these improvements were maintained throughout the remainder of the trials (Haskins et al., 1999). It has also the advantage of having no significant impact on driving ability (O'Hanlon et al., 1998). Short-term randomised clinical trials in 782 patients and 6-month trials in 595 patients showed significant reductions in GAD with daily doses of venlafaxine ranging from 37.5 to 225 mg (Hackett et al., 1999). A dose-response relationship was apparent, the highest doses produced significantly improved self-ratings of social adjustment (Hackett et al., 1999). A recent randomised controlled trial designed to compare the 6-month efficacy and safety of a flexible dosage of venlafaxine extended-release capsules in non-depressed outpatients with GAD showed that venlafaxine extended release is an effective, rapidly acting, safe, once-daily medication for both the short- and long-term treatment of anxiety (Gelenberg et al., 2000). The main outcome measures were changes from baseline in the HAM-A total score, the HAM-A psychic anxiety factor score, and the CGI scale severity of illness and Global Improvement scores, compared by intervention group. The results showed that during weeks 6 through 28, response rates in the venlafaxine group were 69% or higher compared with rates of 42–46% in the placebo group. Venlafaxine extended release may provide an important alternative to currently available anxiolytics.

7.3.4 SSRIs

In a recent comparative study, paroxetine and imipramine were compared with the BDZ 2'-chlordesmethyl-diazepam, and all three treatments appeared to be effective (Rocca et al., 1997). In this study, the BDZ had an earlier onset of action, but by study end, all treatments were equally efficacious. A placebo-controlled 8-week, flexible-dosage trial of paroxetine in GAD showed paroxetine in doses of 20 to 50 mg once daily to be effective in the treatment of patients with GAD (Pollack et al., 2001).

7.3.5 Tricyclics

A study assessed the effects of the tricyclic antidepressant clomipramine (50– 250 mg/day) in 10 patients with GAD (Wingerson et al., 1992). Those who remained in treatment experienced significant improvement. Because of intolerable side effects, only 5 patients completed the study. This report demonstrates the tolerability limitations due to side effects of the tricyclics when taken over the long-term.

7.3.6 *Other drugs*

Some open-label data for other antidepressants such as nefazodone suggest that it may also be an effective treatment for GAD, but further study is warranted (Hedges et al., 1996).

Newer products that show promise for GAD treatment include tropisetron, a receptor 5-HT_3 antagonist, serazopine, a 5-HT_2 receptor antagonist, ipsapirone, a 5-HT_{1A} partial agonist, suriclone, a cyclopyrrolone non-benzodiazepine GABA agonist and abecarnil, a partial BDZ agonist (Lecrubier et al., 1993; Katz et al., 1993; Cutler et al., 1993; Ansseau et al., 1991; Ballenger et al., 1991).

7.3.7 *Algorithm for treatment*

One approach for the treatment strategies of GAD is to use treatment algorithms. In the case of GAD, where there is no generally accepted treatment plan, an algorithm can serve as a basis for additional research.

There is some evidence to suggest that milder forms of GAD may respond to psychotherapy (see Fig. 3.2). Mild to moderate anxiety (usually defined as a HAM-A score of less than 20) appears to respond to treatment with both cognitive and relaxation psychotherapy (Borkovec & Costello, 1993; Barlow et al., 1992; Durham & Allan, 1993). Psychoanalytic psychotherapy may perhaps be helpful (Luborsky, 1984). For patients who do not respond to psychotherapy or have a more severe illness, pharmacotherapy is the treatment of choice (see Fig. 3.3). The patients who have a comorbid personality disorder, such as dependent or borderline, would benefit from a more psychotherapeutic approach.

For patients who have been exposed to long-term BDZs, initial treatment again should be with BDZs. For uncomplicated GAD, one strategy is to start with 5 mg per day of diazepam and titrate up to 5 mg per day every 2 to 3 days until remission of the anxiety or maximum dose of 60 mg per day is reached. This maximum dose is rarely needed to treat GAD.

Anxious patients who had previous treatment with a BDZ were five times more likely not to respond to buspirone than patients who had never been treated with a BDZ (Schweizer et al., 1986). Because of this preliminary evidence that BDZ-treated patients may become more resistant to buspirone, this algorithm proposes initiating treatment of BDZ-naïve GAD patients with buspirone. Treatment begins with 5 mg tid titrated 5 mg per day every 2 to 3 days until treatment response or maximum dose of 60 mg per day (20 mg tid) is attained. It was recommended that after 4 months of treatment, the BDZ should be slowly tapered to evaluate their continued need (Shader & Greenblatt, 1993). Because of the tolerance developed, there can be withdrawal symptoms (Rickels et al., 1988). This algorithm suggests tapering every 4 to 6 months after full treatment response. The patients who have GAD re-emergence can be maintained on either buspirone or BDZ. There should also be a greater emphasis on medications with shorter half-lives.

Antidepressants have been shown to be equal in efficacy to BDZs but the therapeutic effect usually requires 3 to 4 weeks. Tricyclic antidepressants like imipramine or SSRIs like fluvoxamine have been shown to be effective in the anxiously

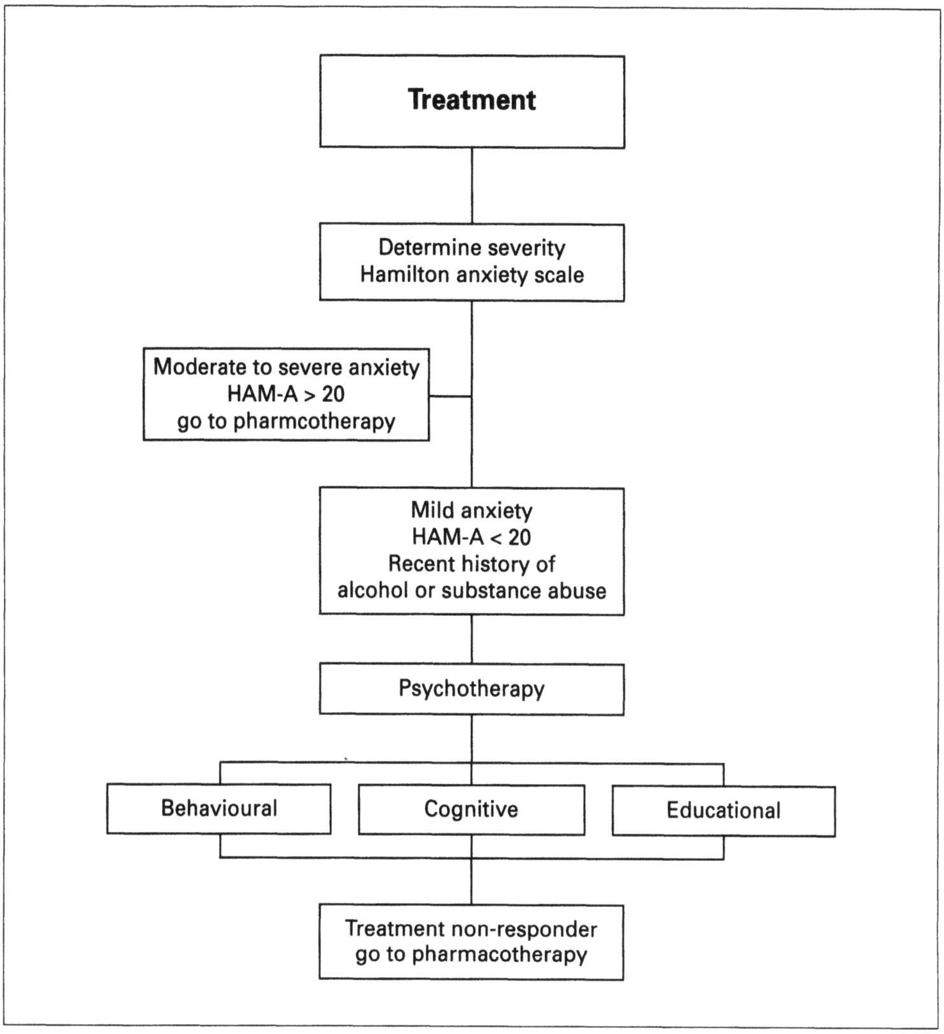

Figure 3.2
Treatment algorithm for generalised anxiety disorder initial treatment with psychotherapy

depressed patients (Rickels et al., 1993; Kahn et al., 1987; Laws et al., 1990). Patients with more cognitive discomfort may respond better to antidepressants than to a BDZ and those with more somatic discomfort may respond better to a BDZ (Hoehn-Saric et al., 1988; Hollander & Cohen, 1994).

8 Methodology for clinical investigation

A search to identify clinical trials of a duration of over 2 months conducted in patients with GAD in order to identify any successful long-term treatment showed that only a limited number of long-term studies in well-defined homogeneous

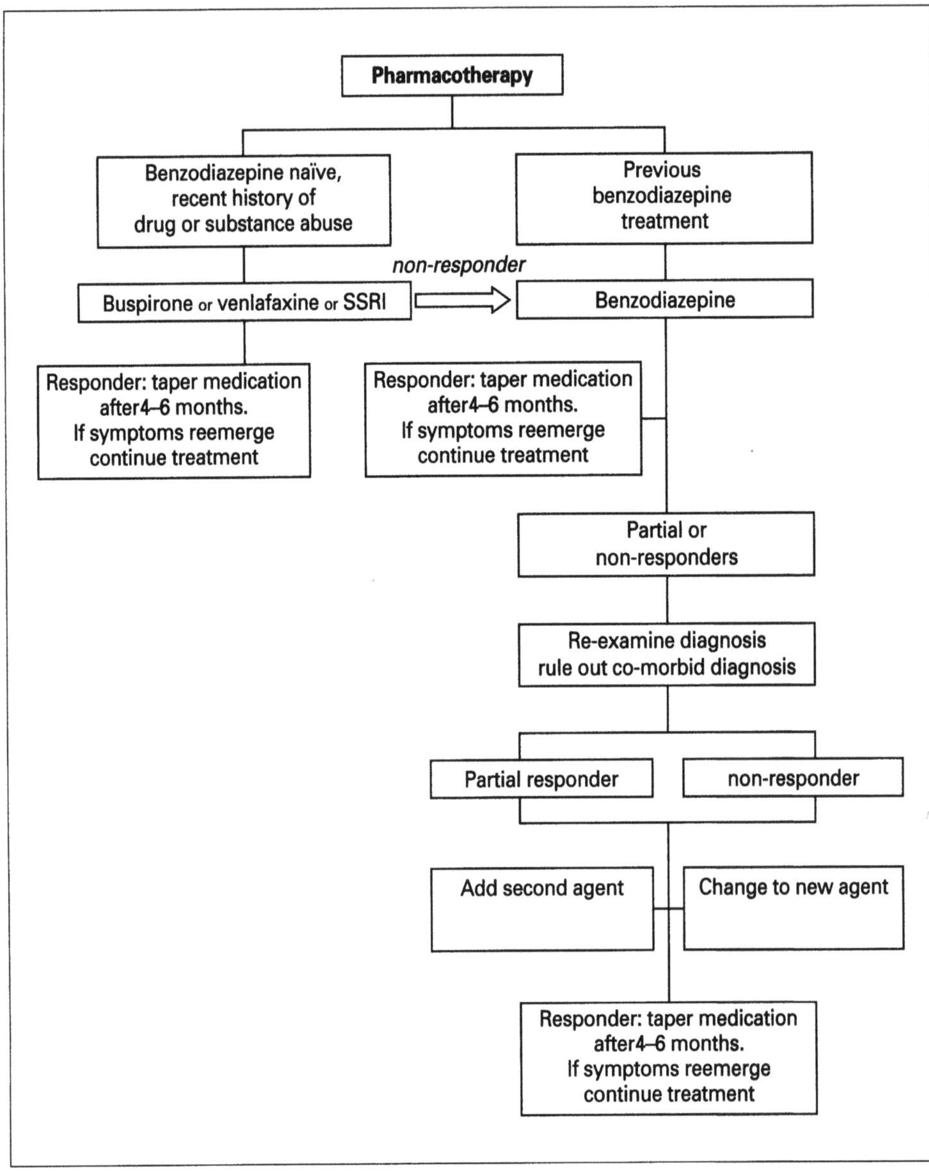

Figure 3.3
Treatment algorithm for generalised anxiety disorder pharmacotherapy

groups of GAD patients have been conducted (Mahe & Balogh, 2000). These studies presented various methodological issues that rendered the results inconclusive and no reference drug could be identified. Therefore, an adequate assessment of the long-term treatment effect of GAD remains to be conducted.

The Penn State Worry Questionnaire (PSWQ) was developed to measure in clinical studies aspects of clinically significant worry, the generality of worry over time and situations, the excessiveness of the experience and the uncontrollability of the process (Meyer et al., 1990; Molina & Borkovec, 1994). The PSWQ consists of one scale and had proven to possess high internal consistency (Van Rijsoort et al., 1999). The PSWQ is the most widely used measure of clinically significant worry and has proven to be reliable as well as valid in nonclinical and clinical samples. Moreover, the PSWQ has clear criterion validity (Molina & Borkovec, 1994).

9 Discussion

The lack of evidence of diagnostic reliability, high comorbidity and need for greater specificity of certain features of the disorder are all issues that require further investigation. It has been argued, for instance, that GAD may be better classified as a lifelong temperamental predisposition to worry, and thus an exaggeration of a normal personality disposition (Akiskal, 1998).

Although limited and conflicting, the neurophysiological and neuroimaging data provide some support for the involvement of the structures postulated by Gray in the mediation of generalised anxiety (Gray, 1988). However, further research utilising new emerging research techniques such as measurement of receptors in human brain tissue and state of the art neuroimaging studies is clearly needed to determine the biological correlates of GAD.

Treatment approaches for GAD are not widely well established, partly because of the confusion surrounding the definition of this disorder. Nevertheless, many treatment options, both pharmacological and psychological therapies are available for GAD patients. Buspirone and certain antidepressants, including the dual noradrenergic-serotonergic reuptake inhibitor venlafaxine, represent first-line therapy for GAD. Because GAD is a chronic condition, long-term treatment is often required. Most anxious patients experience a relapse after short-term treatment, while those treated for more than 6 months tend to exhibit a lower relapse rate than those treated for a shorter interval (Rickels & Schweizer, 1990; Rickels et al., 1980). Full remissions are in general less likely to occur in patients with poor relationships and personality disorders (Yonkers et al., 2000). These patients may be offered more intensive and possibly multi-modal therapy including psychological treatments.

References

Abelson JL, Glitz D, Cameron OG, Lee MA, Bronzo M & Curtis GC. Blunted growth hormone response to clonidine in patients with generalized anxiety disorder. Arch Gen Psychiatry 48 (2), 157–162, 1991

Akiskal HS. Toward a definition of generalized anxiety disorder as an anxious temperament type. Acta Psychiatr Scand 98 (393), 66–73, 1998

American Psychiatric Association. Diagnostic and statistical manual of mental disorders (4th ed.). Washington, DC, 1994

Ansseau M, Ollie JP, von Frenckell R, Jourdain G, Stehle B & Guillet P. Controlled comparison of the efficacy and safety of four doses of suriclone, diazepam, and placebo in generalized anxiety disorder. Psychopharmacology 104, 439–443, 1991

Avery DH, Osgood TB, Ishiki DM, Wilson LG, Kenny M & Dunner DL. The DST in psychiatric outpatients with generalized anxiety disorder, panic disorder, or primary affective disorder. Am J Psychiatry 142 (7), 844–848, 1985

Ballenger JC, McDonald S, Noyes R, Rickels K, Sussman N, Woods S, Patin J & Singer J. The first double-blind, placebo-controlled trial of a partial benzodiazepine agonist abecarnil (ZK 112-119) in generalized anxiety disorder. Psychopharmacol Bull 27 (2), 171–179, 1991

Barbee JG, Todorov AA, Kuczmierczyk AR, Mancuso DM, Schwab JJ, Maddock RJ, Hoehn-Saric R, Kelley LA & Davidson JRT. Explained and unexplained medical symptoms in generalized anxiety and panic disorder: Relationship to the somatoform disorders. Ann Clin Psychiatry 9 (3), 149–155, 1997

Barlow DH. Anxiety and its disorders: the nature and treatment of anxiety and panic. New York: Guildford, 1988

Barlow DH & Wincze J. DSM-IV and beyond: What is generalized anxiety disorder. Acta Psychiatr Scand 43, 722–730, 1998

Barlow DH, Rapee M & Brown TA. Behavioral treatment of generalized anxiety disorder. Behav Ther 23, 551–570, 1992

Barlow DH, Blanchard EB, Vermilyea JA, Vermilyea BB & Di Nardo PA. Generalized anxiety and generalized anxiety disorder: description and reconceptualization. Am J Psychiatry 143, 40–44, 1986

Beck JG, Stanley MA & Zebb BJ. Characteristics of generalized anxiety disorder in older adults: a descriptive study. Behav Res Ther 34, 225–234, 1996

Blazer D, George LK & Hughes D. Generalized anxiety disorder. In: LN Robins & DA Regier (eds): Psychiatric disorders in America: the Epidemiological Catchment Area Study. New York, NY: The Free Press, 180–203, 1991

Boehm C, Placchi M, Stallone F et al. A double-blind comparison of buspirone, clobazam, and placebo in patients with anxiety treated in a general practice setting. J Clin Psychopharmacol 10 (3), 38S–42S, 1990

Borkovec TD & Costello E. Efficacy of applied relaxation and cognitive-behavioral therapy in the treatment of generalized anxiety disorder. J Consult Clin Psychol 61, 611–619, 1993

Brawman-Mintzer O & Lydiard RB. Generalized anxiety disorder: issues in epidemiology. J Clin Psychiatry 57 (7), 3–8, 1996

Brawman-Mintzer O, Lydiard B, Crawford MM, Emmanuel N, Payeur R, Johnson M, Knapp RG & Ballenger JC. Somatic symptoms in generalized anxiety disorder with and without comorbid psychiatric disorders. Am J Psychiatry 151, 930–932, 1994

Brown TA, Barlow DH & Liebowitz MR. The empirical basis of generalized anxiety disorder. Am J Psychiatry 151, 1272–1280, 1994

Brown TA, Marten PA & Barlow DH. Discriminant validity of the symptoms constituting the DSM-III-R and DSM-IV associated symptoms criterion of generalized anxiety disorder. J Anxiety Disord 9, 317–328, 1995

Cameron OG, Smith CB, Lee MA, Hollingsworth PJ, Hill EM & Curtis GC. Adrenergic status in anxiety disorders: platelet alpha 2-adrenergic receptor binding, blood pressure, pulse, and plasma catecholamines in panic and generalized anxiety disorder patients and in normal subjects. Biol Psychiatry 28 (1), 3–20, 1990

Connor KM & Davidson JRT. Generalized anxiety disorder: neurobiological and pharmacological perspectives. Biol Psychiatry 44, 1286–1294, 1998

Cowley DS, Dager SR, McClellan J et al. Response to lactate infusion in generalized anxiety disorder. Biol Psychiatry 24, 409–414, 1988

Charney DS, Woods SW & Heninger GR. Noradrenergic function in generalized anxiety disorder: effects of yohimbine in healthy subjects and patients with generalized anxiety disorder. Psychiatry Res 27, 173–182, 1989

Davidson JRT, Dupont RL, Hedges D & Haskins JT. Efficacy, safety and tolerability of venlafaxine extended release and buspirone in outpatients with generalized anxiety disorder. J Clin Psychiatry 60, 528–535, 1999

DeMartinis N, Rynn M, Rickels K & Mandos L. Prior benzodiazepine use and buspirone response in the treatment of generalized anxiety disorder. J Clin Psychiatry 61 (2), 91–94, 2000

Di Nardo PA Moras K, Barlow DH, Rapee RM & Brown TA. Reliability of DSM-III-R and anxiety disorder categories: using the Anxiety Disorders Interview Schedule – Revised (ADIS-R). Arch Gen Psychiatry 148, 1512–1517, 1991

Di Nardo PA, Moras K, Barlow DH, Rapee RM & Brown TA. Reliability of DSM-III anxiety disorder categories. Arch Gen Psychiatry 50, 251–256, 1993

Dugas MJ, Gagnon F, Ladouceur R & Freeston MH. Generalized anxiety disorder: A preliminary test of a conceptual model. Behav Res Ther 36, 215–226, 1998

Durham RC & Allan T. Psychological treatment of generalized anxiety disorder. Br J Psychiatry 163, 19–26, 1993

Enkelman R. Alprazolam *versus* buspirone in the treatment of outpatients with generalized anxiety disorder. Psychopharmacology (Berl) 105, 428–432, 1991

Gelenberg AJ, Lydiard RB, Rudolph RL, Aguiar L, Haskins JT & Salinas E. Efficacy of venlafaxine extended release capsules in nondepressed outpatients with Generalized Anxiety Disorder. JAMA 283, 3082–3088, 2000

Gorman JM, Fyer MR, Goetz R, Askanazi J, Liebowitz MR, Fyer AJ, Kinney J & Klein DF. Ventilatory physiology of patients with panic disorder. [erratum appears in Arch Gen Psychiatry 48 (2), 181, 1991]. Arch Gen Psychiatry 45 (1), 31–39, 1988

Gray JA. The neuropsychological basis of anxiety. In: CG Last & M Hersen (eds): Handbook of anxiety sisorders. New York, NY: Pergamon Press, 10–37, 1988

Hackett D, Haudiquet V & Salinas E. A dose-response, 6 month evaluation of venlafaxine extended-release in outpatients with generalized anxiety disorder (abstract). The Summer Meeting of the British Association for Psychopharmacology July 25. J Psychopharmacol 13 (3), A44, 1999

Hamilton M. The assessment of anxiety by rating. Brit J Psychiatry Spec 32, 50–55, 1959

Hardt JV & Kamiya J. Anxiety change through electroencephalographic alpha feedback seen only in high anxiety subjects. Science 201, 79–81, 1978

Haskins T, Aguiar L, Pallay A & Rudolph R. Double-blind, placebo-controlled study of once daily venlafaxine XR (V-XR) in outpatients with generalized anxiety disorder. Presented at the annual meeting, Anxiety Disorders Association of America, San Diego, CA, March, 1999

Haskins T, Rudolph R, Pallay A et al. Double-blind, placebo-controlled study of once-daily venlafaxine XR in outpatients with generalized anxiety (GAD) [poster]. Presented at the 36th annual meeting of the American College of Neuropsychopharmacology, Dec 8–12, Waikoloa, Hawaii, 1997

Hedges DW, Reimherr FW, Strong RE, Halls CH & Rust C. An open trial of nefazodone in adult patients with generalized anxiety disorder. Psychopharmacol Bull 32 (4), 671–676, 1996.

Hegel MT, Ravaris C, Lewis C & Ahles TA. Combined cognitive-behavioral and time-limited alprazolam treatment of panic disorder. Behav Ther 25, 183–195, 1994

Hoehn-Saric R, McLeod DR & Zimmerli WD. Differential effects of alprazolam and imipramine in generalized anxiety: somatic vs psychic symptoms. J Clin Psychiatry 49, 293–301, 1988

Hoehn-Saric R, McLeod DR & Zimmerli WD. Symptoms and treatment responses of generalized anxiety disorder patients with high *versus* low levels of cardiovascular complaints. Am J Psychiatry 146, 854–859, 1989

Hoehn-Saric R. Psychic and somatic anxiety: worries, somatic symptoms and physiological changes. Acta Psychiatr Scand 98 (393), 32–38, 1998

Hollander E & Cohen LJ. The assessment and treatment of refractory anxiety. J Clin Psychiatry 55, 27–31, 1994

Hollister LE, Muller-Oerlinghausen B, Rickels K & Shader RL. Clinical uses of benzodiazepines. J Clin Psychiatry 13, 1–147, 1993

Kahn RJ, McNair DM & Frankenthaler LM. Tricyclic treatment of generalized anxiety disorder. J Affect Disord 13, 145–151, 1987

Katz RJ, Landau PS, Lott M et al. Serotonergic (5-HT2) mediation of anxiety-therapeutic effects of serazepine in generalized anxiety disorder. Biol Psychiatry 34, 41–44, 1993

Kendler KS, Neale MC, Kessler RC, Heath AC & Eaves LJ. Generalized anxiety disorder in women. A population-based twin study [see comments]. Arch Gen Psychiatry 49 (4), 267–272, 1992a

Kendler KS, Neale MC, Kessler RC, Heath AC & Eaves LJ. Major depression and generalized anxiety disorder. Same genes, (partly) different environments? Arch Gen Psychiatry 49 (9), 716–722, 1992b

Kessler RC, McGonagle KA, Zhao S, Nelson CB, Hughes M, Eshleman S, Wittchen HU & Kendler KS. Lifetime and 12-month prevalence of DSM-III-R psychiatric disorders in the United States. Results from the National Comorbidity Survey. Arch Gen Psychiatry 51 (1), 8–19, 1994

Ladouceur R, Blais F, Freeston MH & Dugas MJ. Problem solving and problem orientation in Generalized Anxiety Disorder. J Anxiety Disord 12, 139–152, 1998

Ladouceur R, Dugas MJ, Freeston MH, Rhéaume J, Blais F, Boisvert J-M, Gagnon F & Thobodeau N. Specificity of generalized anxiety disorder symptoms and processes. Behav Ther 30, 191–207, 1999

Ladouceur R, Talbot F & Dugas MJ. Behavioral expressions of intolerance of uncertainty in worry: Experimental findings. Behav Modif 21, 355–371, 1997

Ladouceur R, Dugas MJ, Freeston MH, Léger E, Provencher MD, Gagnon F, Thibodeau N & Boisvert J-M. Effectiveness of a new treatment for GAD: Evaluation in a group com-

parison design. Paper presented at the Annual Convention of the Association for advancement of behavior therapy, Miami Beach, FL, November, 1997
Laws D, Ashford JJ & Antee JA. A multicenter double-blind comparative trial of fluvoxamine *versus* lorazepam in mixed anxiety and depression treated in general practice. Acta Psychiatr Scand 81, 185–189, 1990
Lecrubier Y, Puech AT, Azcona A, Bailey PE & Letaste X. A randomized double-blind placebo-controlled study of tropisetron in the treatment of outpatients with generalized anxiety disorder. Psychopharmacology 112, 129–133, 1993
Lindesay J, Briggs K, Murphy E. The Guy's/Age Concern Survey: prevalence rates of cognitive impairment, depression and anxiety in an urban elderly community. Br J Psychiatry 155, 317–329, 1989
Luborsky L. Principles of psychoanalytic psychotherapy. New York, NY: Basic Books, Inc, 1984
Lydiard RB, Brawman-Mintzer O & Ballenger JC. Recent developments in the psychopharmacology of anxiety disorders. J Consult Clin Psychol 64, 660–668, 1996
Mahe V & Balogh. Long-term pharmacological treatment of generalized anxiety disorder. Int Clin Psychopharmacol 15, 99–105, 2000
Maier W, Gänsicke MW, Freyberger HJ, Linz M, Heun R & Lecrubier Y. Generalized anxiety disorder (ICD-10) in primary care from a cross-cultural perspective: a valid diagnostic entity. Acta Psychiatr Scand 101, 29–36, 2000
Marten PA, Brown TA, Barlow DH, Borkovex TD, Shear MK & Lydiard RB. Evaluation of the ratings comprising the associated symptoms criterion of DSM-III-R generalized anxiety disorder. J Ment Dis 181, 676–682, 1993
Maydeu-Olivares A & D'zurilla TJ. A factor analysis of the social Problem-Solving Inventory using polychoric correlations. Eur J Psychol Assessment 11, 98–107, 1996
McLeod DR, Hoehn-Saric R & Stefan RL. Somatic symptoms of anxiety: Comparison of self-report and physiological measures. Biol Psychiatry 21, 301–310, 1986
Meyer TJ, Miller ML, Metzger RL & Borkovec TD. Development and validation of the Penn State Worry Questionnaire. Behav Res Ther 28, 487–495, 1990
Molina S & Borkovec TD. The Penn State Worry Questionnaire: psychometric properties and associated characteristics. In: GCL Davey & F Tallis (eds): Worrying. Perspectives on theory, assessment and treatment, New York: Wiley, 265–283, 1994
O'Hanlon JF, Robbe HW, Vermeeren A, van Leeuwen C & Danjou PE. Venlafaxine's effects on healthy volunteers' driving, psychomotor, and vigilance performance during 15-day fixed and incremental dosing regimens. J Clin Psychopharmacol 18 (3), 212–221, 1998
Pollack MH, Zaninelli R, Goddard A, McCafferty JP, Bellew KM, Burnham DB & Iyengar MK. Paroxetine in the treatment of generalized anxiety disorder: Results of a placebo-controlled, flexible-dosage trial. J Clin Psychiatry 62, 350–357, 2001
Rice KM, Blanchard EB, Purcell M. Biofeedback treatments of generalized anxiety disorder: preliminary results. Biofeedback & Self Regulation 18, 93–105, 1993
Rickels K, Weisman K, Norstad N, Singer M, Stoltz D, Brown A & Danton J. Buspirone and diazepam in anxiety: a controlled study. J Clin Psychiatry 43 (12 Pt 2), 81–86, 1982
Rickels K, DeMartinis N, Garcia-Espana F, Greenblatt DJ, Mandos LA & Rynn M. Imipramine and buspirone in treatment of patients with generalized anxiety disorder

who are discontinuing long-term benzodiazepine therapy. Am J Psychiatry 157, 1973–1979, 2000

Rickels K, Downing R, Schweizer E & Hassman H. Antidepressants for the treatment of generalized anxiety disorder: a placebo-controlled comparison of imipramine, trazodone and diazepam. Arch Gen Psychiatry 50, 884–895, 1993

Rickels K, Schweizer E, Csanalosi , Case WG & Chung H. Long-term treatment of anxiety and risk of withdrawal. Arch Gen Psychiatry 45, 444–450, 1988

Rickels K, Case WG & Diamond L. Relapse after short-term drug therapy in neurotic outpatients. Int Pharmacopsychiatry 15, 186–192, 1980

Rickels K, Schweizer E, Case WG & Greenblatt DJ. Long-term therapeutic use of benzodiazepines. I. Effects of abrupt discontinuation. Arch Gen Psychiatry 47, 899–907, 1990

Rickels K & Schweizer E. The clinical course and long-term management of generalized anxiety disorder. J Clin Psychopharmacol 10 (Suppl), 101S–110S, 1990

Robins LN, Helzer JE, Weissman MM, Orvaschel H, Gruenberg E, Burke JD & Regier DA. Lifetime prevalence of specific psychiatric disorders in three sites. Arch Gen Psychiatry 41 (10), 949–958, 1984

Rocca P, Fonzo V, Scotta M, Zanalda E & Ravizza L. Paroxetine efficacy in the treatment of generalized anxiety disorder. Acta Psychiatrica Scand 95 (5), 444–450, 1997

Schwartz GE, Davidson FJ & Coleman DJ. Patterning of cognitive and somatic processes in the self-regulation of anxiety: effects of medication *versus* exercise. Psychosom Med 40, 321–328, 1978

Schweizer E, Rickels K, Case WG & Greenblatt DJ. Long-term therapeutic use of benzodiazepines. II. Effects of gradual taper. Arch Gen Psychiatry 47, 908–915, 1990

Schweizer E, Rickels K & Lucki I. Resistance to the antianxiety effect of buspirone in patients with a history of benzodiazepine use. N Engl J Med 313, 719–720, 1986

Sevy S, Papadimitriou GN, Surmont DW, Goldman S &Mendlewicz J. Noradrenergic function in generalized anxiety disorder, major depressive disorder, and healthy subjects. Biol Psychiatry 25 (2), 141–152, 1989

Shader RI & Greenblatt DJ. Use of benzodiazepines in anxiety disorders. N Engl J Med 328, 1398–1405, 1993

Stanley MA, Beck JG & Glassco JD. Treatment of generalized anxiety in older adults: A preliminary comparison of cognitive-behavioral and supportive approaches. Behav Ther 27, 565–581, 1996

Starcevic V, Fallon S & Uhlenhuth EH. The frequency and severity of generalized anxiety disorder symptoms: Toward a less cumbersome conceptualization. J Nerv Ment Dis 182, 80–84, 1994

Sussman N. Treatment of anxiety with buspirone. Psychiatr Ann 17, 114–120, 1987

Thayer JF, Friedman BH & Borkovec TD. Autonomic characteristics of generalized anxiety disorder and worry. Biol Psychiatry 39, 255–266, 1996

Tiihonen J, Kuikka J, Rasanen P, Lepola U, Koponen H, Liuska A, Lehmusvaara A, Vainio P, Koponen M, Bergstrom K et al. Cerebral benzodiazepine receptor binding and distribution in generalized anxiety disorder: A fractal analysis. Mol Psychiatry 2 (6), 463–471, 1997

Tiller JW, Biddle N, Maguire KP & Davies BM. The dexamethasone suppression test and plasma dexamethasone in generalized anxiety disorder. Biol Psychiatry 23 (3), 261–270, 1988

Tyrer PJ & Lader MH. Response to propranolol and diazepam in somatic and psychic anxiety. Br Med J 2, 14–16, 1974

Van Rijsoort SN, Emmelkamp PMG & Vervaeke G. The Penn State Worry Questionnaire and the Worry Domains Questionnaire: structure, reliability and validity in a Dutch population. Clin Psychol Psychother 6, 297–307, 1999

Wacker HR, Mullejans R, Klein KH et al. Identification of cases of anxiety according to ICD-10 and DSM-III-R using the Composite International Diagnosis Interview (CIDI). Int J Meth Psychiatric Res 2, 91–100, 1992

Walley EJ, Beebe DK & Clark JL. Management of common anxiety disorders. Am Fam Phys 50, 1745–1753, 1994

Wells A & Carter K. Preliminary tests of a cognitive model of generalized anxiety disorder. Behav Res Ther 37, 585–594, 1999

Wingerson D, Nguyen C & Roy-Byrne PP. Clomipramine treatment for generalized anxiety disorder. J Clin Psychopharmacol 12, 214–215. Letter, 1992

Wittchen H-U, Zhao S, Kessler RC & Eaton WW. DSM-III-R generalized anxiety disorder in the National Comorbidity Survey. Arch Gen Psychiatry 51 (5), 355–364, 1994

Wittchen HU, Zhao S, Kessler RC & Eaton WW. DSM-II-R. Generalized anxiety disorder in the National Comorbidity survey. Arch Gen Psychiatry 51, 355–364, 1994

Woodman CL, Noyes R, Black DW, Schlosser S & Yagla SJ. A 5-year follow-up study of generalized anxiety disorder. J Nerv Ment Dis 187, 3–9, 1999

Wu JC, Buchsbaum MS, Hershey TG, Hazlett E, Sicotte N & Johnson JC. PET in generalized anxiety disorder. Biol Psychiatry 29 (12), 1181–1199, 1991

Yonkers KA, Dyck IR, Warshaw M & Keller MB. Factors predicting the clinical course of generalised anxiety disorder. Br J Psychiatry 176, 544–549, 2000

Yonkers KA, Warshaw MG, Massion AO & Keller MB. Phenomenology and course of generalized anxiety disorder. Br J Psychiatry 168, 308–313, 1996

Chapter 4
Social phobia

1. Introduction

Social phobia (SP, also sometimes called social anxiety disorder) is common, impairing and responsive to treatment (Kessler et al., 1994, Schneier et al., 1994). It has also been termed "the neglected anxiety disorder" because it is often missed as a diagnosis (Liebowitz, 1999). A study showed that on subsequent administration of the SP section of the MINI questionnaire to patients who had presented with other psychiatric diagnoses, but had not been diagnosed by their physician as having SP, almost 25% met screening criteria for SP (Den Boer & Dunner, 1999). Therefore, physician recognition of SP remains suboptimal. Individuals with SP are 4 times more likely than the general population to develop other anxiety and mood disorders. They are also more likely to abuse alcohol and other substances. Social phobia is the most prevalent anxiety disorder and third most common psychiatric disorder in the US. However, this psychopathology is often underdiagnosed and a survey in Europe indicated that a diagnosis of phobia was made by general practitioners in only 24.2% of social phobics (Weiller et al., 1996). A recent, large-scale epidemiological study in the US showed that the 12-month prevalence rate of SP was 7.9% (6.6% for men, 9.1% for women) and 13.3% (11.1% for men, 15.5% for women) (Kessler et al., 1994). Another study which examined the prevalence of SP in the Swedish general population reported that the prevalence of this disorder was estimated at 15.6% but this prevalence rate varied between 1.9 and 20.4% across the different levels of distress and impairment that were used to define cases (Furmark et al., 1999). SP is characterised by early onset and generally appears between 13 and 20 years of age. It generally follows a chronic unremitting course. However, SP can be detected in children as young as 8 years of age and it occurs more commonly in the general population than any other anxiety disorder (Beidel & Turner, 1998). Patients suffering from this psychopathology are less likely ever to marry, and more likely to divorce, than matched controls without the disorder. They are more likely to be unemployed. SP, at least in its more severe forms, tends to be a chronic disorder without spontaneous remissions.

The essential features of SP in both the DSM-IV and ICD-10 criteria are displayed in Table 4.1. However, there are few differences between the two classification systems. In the ICD-10, public speaking to a large audience is not considered a phobic condition, as it is in DSM-IV, because ICD-10 specifies that the fear of scrutiny should be related to small groups of individuals (as opposed to crowds). Also, the DSM-IV specifies that the disorder places a socio-economic burden on the patient in terms of impairment of academic or occupational functioning, whereas ICD-10 does not. The ICD-10 recognises the importance of specific physical symp-

Table 4.1: Diagnostic criteria for social anxiety disorder according to DSM-IV and ICD-10

DSM-IV

A. A marked and persistent fear of one or more social or performance situations in which the person is exposed to unfamiliar people or to possible scrutiny by others. The individual fears that he or she will act in a way (or show anxiety symptoms) that will be humiliating or embarrassing.
B. Exposure to the feared social situation almost invariably provokes anxiety, which may take the form of a situationally bound or situationally predisposed panic attack.
C. The person recognises that the fear is excessive or unreasonable.
D. The feared social or performance situations are avoided or else are endured with intense anxiety or distress.
E. The avoidance, anxious anticipation, or distress in the feared social or performance situation(s) interferes significantly with the person's normal routine, occupational (academic) functioning, or social activities or relationships, or there is marked distress about having the phobia.
F. In individuals under age 18 years, the duration is at least 6 months.
G. The fear of avoidance is not due to the direct physiological effects of a substance (e.g. a drug of abuse, a medication) or a general medical condition and is not better accounted for by another mental disorder (e.g. panic disorder with or without agoraphobia, separation anxiety disorder, body dysmorphic disorder, a pervasive developmental disorder, or schizoid personality disorder).
H. If a general medical condition or another mental disorder is present, the fear is not of stuttering, trembling in Parkinson's disease, or exhibiting abnormal eating behaviour in anorexia nervosa or bulimia nervosa.
   Specify if
   Generalised: if the fears include most social situations (e.g. initiating or maintaining conversations, participating in small groups, dating, speaking to authority figures, attending parties).

toms, such as blushing, tremor, nausea, or urgency of micturition, while DSM-IV refers only to phobia symptoms that may take the form of a panic attack. To differentiate normal shyness from SP, both classification systems refer to the intensity of the experience in terms of distress it may cause and the recognition that the fear is excessive or unreasonable. The diagnostic criteria may also affect the prevalence rates found in epidemiologic surveys. In a study of 470 adults in the general population of Basel, Switzerland, using DSM-III-R and ICD-10 criteria, the lifetime prevalence of social anxiety in this sample was found to be higher according to DSM-III-R (16%) than ICD-10 (9.5%) due to the more stringent criteria of ICD-10 (Wacker et al. 1992).

DSM-IV but not ICD-10 incorporates the hypothetical distinction in SP by dividing the disorder into specific and generalised types. This typology is somewhat confused by the availability of the diagnostic category of avoidant personality disorder (as well as others) which very probably overlaps with that of generalised SP (Turn-

Table 4.1 (continued)

ICD-10
A. Either of the following must be present: Marked fear of being the focus of attention, or fear of behaving in a way that will be embarrassing or humiliating. Marked avoidance of being the focus of attention, or of situations in which there is a fear of behaving in an embarrassing or humiliating way. These fears are manifested in social situations, such as eating or speaking in public, encountering known individuals in public, or entering or enduring small group situations (e.g. parties, meetings, classrooms).
B. At least two symptoms of anxiety in the feared situation must have been manifest at some time since the onset of the disorder, together with at least one of the following symptoms: Blushing or shaking Fear of vomiting Urgency or fear of micturition or defecation.
C. Significant emotional distress is caused by the symptoms or by the avoidance, and the individual recognises that these are excessive or unreasonable.
D. Symptoms are restricted to, or predominate in the feared situations or contemplation of the feared situations.
E. Most commonly used exclusion clause. The symptoms listed in criteria A and B are not the results of delusions, hallucinations or other disorders, such as organic mental disorders, schizophrenia and related disorders, mood (affective) disorders or OCD, and are not secondary to cultural beliefs.

er, 1987). In theory, avoidant (anxious in ICD terms) personality disorder concerns problems in relating to people, whereas SP is characterised by difficulties in performing in public situations (Millon & Martinez, 1995). Clinically, however, the separation is far from obvious, nor is it necessarily useful. Although some significant differences between subtypes and APD were observed in terms of their clinical features, what these amount to is uncertain (Stravynski et al., 1996; Mannuzza et al., 1995; Widiger, 1992). Moreover, they appear to matter little so far as response to treatment is concerned (Brown et al., 1995; Turner et al., 1996). Clinically, APD, specific SP and generalised SP are more likely to represent differences of degree (of severity) rather than of kind.

Typical precipitating situations that produce phobia in the individual who has SP include being introduced, meeting people in authority, initiating conversation with a member of the opposite sex, dating, using the telephone, receiving visitors, being watched while doing something such as writing or typing, and speaking in public.

Most patients with SP have three to five specific feared situations, but some patients fear almost all social situations. Others may fear only public speaking or some other specific social or performance activity, leading to the suggestion that subtypes of the disorder may exist. In severe cases, SP impairs the fundamental capacity for intimacy, work performance, and leisure activities. It is conducive to depression and alcohol abuse.

Exposure to the social or performance situation almost invariably provokes immediate anxiety and accompanying somatic symptoms. The most common of these include palpitations (79%), trembling (75%), sweating (74%), tense muscles (64%), a sinking feeling in the stomach (63%), dry mouth (61%), hot or cold sensations (57%), and headaches or pressure in the head (46%) (Amies et al., 1983). Although such symptoms are similar to those present in other anxiety disorders, individuals with SP are particularly concerned about manifestations that they believe may display their phobia obviously to others. Blushing is thus more frequently a cause of concern to them than it is to individuals with agoraphobia (symptom frequency, 51% vs. 21%) (Turner & Beidel, 1989).

Central to cognitive-behavioral models of SP are the negative expectations that patients bring to social situations (Clark & Wells, 1995; Mattick et al., 1995). These expectations typically include fears of poor social performance, negative evaluations from others and uncontrollable anxiety. The natural result of these negative expectations is increased anxious apprehension, so that the socially anxious patient enters social situations hoping that negative outcomes will not occur but vigilant to their impending emergence. There is evidence that individuals with SP tend to believe that the way they feel is the way in which they are perceived by others (McEwan & Devins, 1983). Negative expectations lead to apprehension and vigilance in social situations. The resulting failure-focused attention makes adequate social performance more difficult and helps ensure that negative social cues will be noticed. Cognitive theories of SP hypothesise that self-focused attention, anticipatory and post-event processing are distinct features that contribute to social anxiety (Mellings & Alden, 2000). Self-focused attention occurs during social events and highlights specific types of information. Post-event rumination occurs between social events and reactivates memory traces, which results in deeper processing of the information recalled. Anticipatory processing occurs prior to social events and evokes the negative memories and predictions that begin the anxious cycle. Thus, all three operations contribute to biased processing of social information and hence SP, although at different points in time and in different ways. A recent study confirmed that compared to controls, patients with generalised SP were more likely to interpret ambiguous social events in a negative fashion and to catastrophize in response to unambiguous, mildly negative events (Stopa & Clark, 2000). The clinical value of a cognitive-behavioral model of SP lies in its ability to elucidate targets for intervention which aims to eliminate the specific patterns that engender and maintain social anxiety. This approach aims to correct dysfunctional thoughts that create apprehension and anxiety, correct core amplifying cognitions, modify failure-focused attention, decrease avoidance and safety behaviours. It also helps to evaluate performance and outcome situations.

Despite all the understanding of the physiological and cognitive mechanisms involved in SP, its underrecognition poses a serious obstacle to the delivery of effective treatments to patients who can benefit from them. Primary care clinicians may not be familiar with the diagnostic concept of SP. Although symptoms of SP may be excessive and disabling, individuals may consider themselves to be "shy" and believe this to be normal. Even if symptoms of SP are acknowledged to be a problem, they are commonly believed to constitute an aspect of personality that requires adjustment and coping, rather than medical treatment. Therefore this chapter is an attempt to classify the aetiology of SP outlining the potentials for treatment as revealed by current progress in psychopharmacology research.

2 Diagnosis and comorbidity

2.1 Subtypes

Although ICD-10 does not make reference to different forms of phobia, DSM-IV suggests the designation of a generalised subtype if the individual suffers from pervasive fear of most social situations. Three distinct subtypes of social anxiety have been identified: generalised social anxiety, in which the individual fears a multitude of social and performance situations; nongeneralised social anxiety, in which only two or three situations are feared; and public-speaking phobia, sometimes referred to as discrete or specific social anxiety. The generalised form of SP is the most severe and disabling subtype, highly familial and associated with a high level of comorbidity (Ballenger et al., 1998). It generally requires more intensive treatment. The latter two groups are often lumped together and referred to as suffering from either discrete or specific SP. There has been some recommendation that the public speaking-only group be treated as a separate group (Stein et al., 1996). Concerning SP in children, it has also been proposed that the condition of selective (formerly elective) mutism is probably a severe form of childhood SP, although other factors may also contribute to this condition (Ballenger et al., 1998).

The prevalence rates for SP vary according to whether ICD or DSM diagnostic criteria were used to define the disorder with lower lifetime rates reported in studies using ICD-10 criteria. The two classification systems differ in their recognition of public speaking anxiety and symptoms. In ICD-10, fear of speaking in small groups is recognised as SP, but public speaking anxiety is considered to be a normal anxiety. Similarly, the patients must experience blushing, fear of vomiting, or fear of urinary incontinence in a social situation to meet ICD-10 diagnostic criteria, whereas the presence of these symptoms is not mandatory in the DSM-IV classification. DSM-IV stipulates that if a patient's fears pervade most social situations, the patient should be diagnosed as having generalised SP. Patients with generalised SP appear different from those with discrete SP in a number of ways. They suffer from more functional disability and they have more comorbidity. The comparison of the characteristics of patients with generalised SP and public-speaking phobia suggests that those who had generalised social anxiety were younger, less well educated, and less likely to be employed than patients with public-speaking phobia (Heimberg et al., 1990). A recent study (a survey of 8,098 respondents in the age range of 15–54 years) further differentiated between SP subtypes and marked the distinction between SP characterised by pure speaking fears and that characterised by other social fears (Kessler et al., 1998). It was concluded that SP characterised by pure speaking fears was less persistent. It associated with less impairment and comorbidity with other psychiatric disturbances than was SP characterised by other social fears. On the other hand, individuals who have SP with multiple fears, including nonspeaking fears, appear to have the most impairment. They should be the main focus of prevention and intervention efforts.

Subtypes of SP may have different mean ages at onset. The generalised subtype may appear earlier, with patients having a mean age at onset of 11 years, in contrast to a mean age of 17 years for patients with the specific subtype (Mannuzza et al., 1995). It has also been reported that onset of SP prior to 11 years of age predicts nonrecovery in adulthood (Davidson et al., 1993).

Patients with SP showed a reduction in work productivity of around 12% compared with control subjects (Wittchen & Beloch, 1996). In addition, 11% of patients with social anxiety were unemployed (compared with 3% of controls); 8% reported taking time off work because of their condition, amounting to an average of 12 h in the previous week; and 23% reported substantially impaired working performance due to their SP symptoms.

2.2 Differential diagnosis

The clinical presentation of SP includes a wide range of somatic symptoms typical of anxiety reactions: palpitations, trembling/shaking, blushing, and sweating are identified in that order by both adults and children. Distinguishing between PD with agoraphobia and SP is sometimes difficult. Individuals with either of these conditions may experience panic attacks or avoid social conditions. The reasons for avoiding social situations, as well as the underlying conditions, may help to distinguish between the two diagnoses (Ball et al., 1995). In SP, fears pertain to situations in which scrutiny by others occurs; the focus is on possible public embarrassment, humiliation, or negative evaluation. In differentiating SP from agoraphobia, the type of shop feared by the patient may be a useful guide to the clinician. Patients suffering from SP fear buying goods in a small shop, where they will have to ask for what they want, whereas patients with panic agoraphobia fear supermarkets or shopping malls, where the crowded nature of the setting, not the possibility of social interaction, drives the anxiety. Whereas the SP patients feel anxious in a supermarket queue because of a fear of having to talk to the checkout clerk, the anxiety in the patients with agoraphobia is related to feeling trapped in the queue. In PD, patients are worried about the occurrence of a panic attack (at least two unexpected attacks must have occurred for the disorder to be diagnosed), while agoraphobic avoidance concerns situations in which escape or help may not be readily available. The core fear of individuals with agoraphobia is being trapped in situations where they cannot envision a way to escape, for example, getting trapped on the freeway, at a shopping mall, or in the checkout line in a supermarket (Judd, 1994). Patients with agoraphobia frequently benefit from contact with a familiar person in efforts to overcome this disorder, while individuals with SP generally eschew contact with others. Patients with agoraphobia and SP also differ with respect to the types of somatic symptoms they identify. Individuals with agoraphobia are more likely to report problems with limb weakness, feeling dizzy, breathing problems, fear of passing out and tinnitus whereas individuals with SP are more likely to complain of blushing and muscle twitches (Amies et al., 1983). In many instances, SP is found concurrently with PD, with or without agoraphobia. Between 17 and 50% of patients with SP have a comorbid lifetime diagnosis of PD (Schneier et al., 1992; Sanderson et al., 1990).

A study suggests that out of 50 SP patients, 90% had personality disorders, including APD (84%), dependent personality disorder (74%), borderline personality disorder (20%), obsessive compulsive personality disorder (20%), and schizotypal personality disorder (14%) (Alnaes & Torgersen, 1988). In the majority of cases, the onset of SP precedes the onset of the second psychiatric disorder by many years (Schneier et al., 1992). It will be important to determine whether the early identification and treatment of SP might prevent the development of a significant percentage of these comorbid disorders.

It is common for individuals with SP to develop a pattern of avoidant behaviour to protect themselves from these anxiety-provoking situations. Unfortunately, social avoidance frequently exacerbates problems with educational, occupational, and social functioning. It increases the individual's levels of distress.

There is a great deal of overlap between generalised SP and APD. The essential feature of APD is a pervasive pattern of social inhibition, feelings of inadequacy, and hypersensitivity to negative evaluation that begins by early adulthood and is present in a variety of contexts. In a study which compared a group of patients diagnosed with DSM-III SP to patients with APD on a battery of self-report psychological measures and psychophysiological, cognitive, and behavioural responses, it was noted that the patients with APD reported higher levels of phobia in a wider range of social situations, more somatic symptoms of phobia, and more obsessional symptoms (Turner et al., 1986). They also had a greater likelihood of past and/or current symptoms of depression and tended to have greater social-skill deficits. Therefore, SP and APD can be conceptualised as lying on a spectrum, with APD representing a more severe and pervasive form of SP (Holt et al., 1992). This hypothesis is supported by studies demonstrating that avoidant personality symptoms improve after treatment with medication usually effective for SPs (Versiani et al., 1992; Deltito & Stam, 1989). However, supporting the distinctiveness of APD are reports that some patients with the diagnosis of APD do not meet criteria for SP (Herbert et al., 1992).

A study reported that concurrent depression or dysthymia was diagnosed in 20% of SP patients at presentation (Stein et al., 1990). Depression often develops as a consequence of SP, with up to 80% of patients experiencing mood changes after initial development of social fears and avoidance (Turner et al., 1991).

Although the specifics of diagnostic subtyping are an issue of debate in the development of DSM-IV, it has become clear that some subtyping distinctions have clinical utility (Heimberg et al., 1993). Generalised social phobics appear more likely to receive a comorbid diagnosis of APD than other social phobics, although the degree of overlap between the two diagnoses is unclear. The generalised subtype was more frequently diagnosed among a group of social phobics with a previous history of alcoholism (Schneier et al., 1989). Generalised social phobics may fare less well in cognitive-behavioral group therapy than other social phobics and the subtypes may also respond differently to pharmacological intervention (Levin et al., 1989).

2.3 Comorbidity

It has been estimated that 70–80% of patients with SP have at least one other psychiatric disorder (Lecrubier & Weiller, 1997; Merikangas & Angst, 1995; Schneier et al., 1992). In a survey of primary care patients in France, 69% of all SP patients had other lifetime psychiatric disorders (Schneier et al., 1992). The most common comorbid conditions were simple phobia (59%), agoraphobia (44.9%), alcohol abuse (18.8%), major depression (16.6%), drug abuse (13%), dysthymia (12.5%), OCD (11.1%), bipolar disorder (4.7%), PD (4.7%) and somatization (1.9%). In approximately 80% of cases, SP precedes comorbid alcohol problems (Chambless et al., 1987). A matched-control study that supported these earlier findings showed that individuals with SP consume significantly more alcoholic drinks and are 2.5 times more likely to have a diagnosis of alcohol abuse or dependence than unaffected people (Wittchen et al., 1999). In addition, SP greatly increases the risk of being a heavy smoker or developing nicotine dependence (Wittchen et al., 1999).

An observation from a sample of 2096 consecutive primary care patients also suggests that the most comorbid condition was depressive disorder, which affected 70% of patients with SP of early onset (at less than 15 years of age), while the highest association was with agoraphobia (Lecrubier & Weiller, 1997). No association was observed with generalised anxiety. However, in patients with comorbid SP and depressive episode as a lifetime diagnosis, the onset of SP preceded the depression by more than 1 year in 76% of patients. Comorbidity with depression also had a strong influence on the general practitioner's diagnosis since in the comorbid group, 76% were recognised as cases but only 11% were identified as having an anxiety disorder; priority was given to the depressive symptomatology. It has been estimated that patients with SP are two to three times more likely to develop either major depression or dysthymia than a matched control group (Kessler et al., 1999). This relationship becomes stronger with the number of social fears, rather than the type of fear. Patients with comorbid depression usually have more severe symptoms, a lower opinion of their overall health, and an increased history of suicide attempts (Lecrubier & Weiller, 1997).

In addition, there is overlap of SP with other disorders such as autism, body dysmorphic disorder (a preoccupation with an imagined defect or defects in appearance that causes significant distress or impairment in social, occupational or other functioning), Asperger's syndrome (a pervasive developmental disorder characterised by an inability to understand how to interact socially) and schizotypal personality disorders. It has been suggested that a screening question based on three social situations or symptoms would have discriminatory value for the detection of SP in primary care (Ballenger et al., 1998). Screening questions such as: "are you markedly embarrassed and/or do you blush and tremble when asked to do things in public, like speak or eat or sign a check" may be helpful diagnostic guidance questions.

Interest in the comorbidity of SP with eating disorders has been considerable because of the frequent clinical observations that those with eating disorders are more likely also to suffer from SP. In a study including 63 consecutively presenting patients with a DSM-IV diagnosis of an eating disorder, more than 50% of the patients met the criteria for phobia even when a correction was made for body image (Godart et al., 2000). In these patients, the onset of SP occurred before the onset of eating disorders even if the latter started early in life.

Comorbidity in SP gives rise to greater disability and distress. The presence of comorbidity increases the likelihood of suicide attempts from 1% for "pure" SP to 15.7% in patients with comorbidity (Schneier et al., 1992). Some studies have emphasised the risk of suicide in SP (Schneier et al., 1992; Degonda & Angst, 1993). Although suicide attempts were noted more often in social phobics with comorbid depression, suicidal ideation was observed more frequently in SP without depression as well (Weiller et al., 1996).

2.4 Epidemiology

Epidemiological and clinical surveys in the past decade have put the lifetime prevalence of SP at between 9.5 and 16% in Western countries, depending on whether DSM-III-R, DSM-IV or ICD-10 criteria have been used (Ballenger et al., 1998; Magee et al., 1996; Weiller et al., 1996). Epidemiological studies, including those conducted in European countries such as Switzerland, Italy, Holland, France and Germany support the view that SP is among the most prevalent of the anxiety disorders in the general population (Angst & Dobler-Mikola, 1995; Bijl et al;, 1998; Lépine & Lellouch, 1995; Wittchen et al., 2000). Similar to the findings of epidemiological studies outside Europe, there are at first sight considerable variances in prevalence findings. Estimates vary from fairly low (Munich, 2.5%, Zurich, 3.2%, Florence, 1%) to considerably high (7.3%–16%) in other studies (Angst & Dobler-Mikola, 1995; Faravelli et al., 1989; Lépine & Pélissolo, 1999; Wacker et al;, 1992; Wittchen et al., 1992; 1998). A recent epidemiological study which aimed to use clinical methods in a community sample in Italy showed that sex ratio in SP was 2:1 (women : men) (Faravelli et al., 2000). The most common fear was speaking in public (89.4%), followed by entering a room occupied by others (63.1%) and meeting with strangers (47.3%). 86.9% of patients complained of more than one fear.

Women with social anxiety disorder may have an increased risk for developing agoraphobia (Lecrubier & Weller, 1997).

2.5 Natural history

SP, if untreated, is believed to be a chronic and unremitting disease (Hazen & Stein, 1995). A recent study in respondents with a lifetime diagnosis of SP who were interviewed using a semistructured interview schedule based on DSM-IV criteria supports the notion of SP as being a long-term disorder (the average duration of SP was 29 years in the sample studied) with a continuous pattern course (Chartier et al., 1998). Once SP started, it either continued for a lifetime or remitted without subsequent recurrence. However, unlike the findings of a previous study that found that the vast majority of patients remained ill, many individuals in the study of Chartier et al. (1998) do seem to remit (Reich et al., 1994). Therefore the picture may not be as bleak as one could conclude having looked only at one clinical sample. Factors perceived by respondents to precipitate SP were family and school environment, onset of adolescence, low self-esteem, temperament and poverty while factors which were perceived to improve symptoms were building self-esteem, exposure, determination, maturity and counselling. Factors such as avoidance, exposure to negative attention and comorbid disorders were perceived to worsen the symptoms.

2.6 Childhood and adolescence *versus* adult social phobia

The severity of SP in children was only recently recognised. Teachers do not often recognise the disorder because a child with SP is quiet and often does not cause trouble. However, when SP is severe, children may refuse to participate in class activities such as reading aloud and writing on the blackboard. As with adults, numerous problems are related to social anxiety among youth, including difficulty forming friendships, peer-neglect, lower social competence and alcohol abuse (LaGreca et al., 1988; Rubin et al., 1990). Severity of SP has been closely correlated with severity of selective mutism (Black & Uhde, 1995; Dummit et al., 1997). Family environment may play an important role in the maintenance of the disorder and therefore must be considered in relation to the overall clinical management of a child with SP. Remarkable similarity also exists between the types of common social situations feared by children and adults with SP. Public speaking, whether it is a presentation at school or at work, was the most commonly feared social situation.

When SP occurs during adolescence, further complications arise. Depression and social isolation are commonly associated with SP (Last et al., 1987). In order to gain some degree of control over their fears, many adolescents often use alcohol or other drugs. Of 73 adolescents hospitalised for alcohol abuse, 40% met the criteria for an anxiety disorder, the most common of which was SP (21%) (Clark et al., 1996). These disorders were not as common in adolescents in the community.

One specific form of SP that occurs in children is selective mutism (a consistent failure to speak in specific social situations despite speaking in others). It has been argued that this disorder is probably a form of SP and nearly 100% of children with selective mutism also meet criteria for SP (Dummit et al., 1997). Additionally, 70% have a first-degree family member with a history of SP (Black & Uhde, 1995).

Biological research on childhood SP holds the hope of clarifying factors that influence relationships between specific childhood and adult anxiety disorders. In particular, activity in an amygdala-based circuit may relate to the course of childhood social fears (Williams et al., 1996; Phillips & LeDoux, 1992; Daleiden & Vasey, 1997). As such, children with social fears most at risk for SP in adulthood are hypothesised to exhibit a unique amygdala response to facial cues, relative to children with few social fears that do not progress to SP.

The Social Anxiety Scale for Adolescents (SAS-A) was recently developed to assess social anxiety in adolescents (LaGreca & Lopez, 1998). The scale was developed to tap two major components of social anxiety identified in the adult literature. Fear of negative evaluation is a more cognitive feature, while social avoidance and distress concerns a behavioural pattern of anxiety in social situations.

3 Pathophysiology

3.1 Genetic

Family studies have shown that SP runs in families (Stein et al. 1998). Twin studies estimate that 30% of the variance in SP may be explained by genetic factors (Kendler et al., 1992). The concordance rate for SP in first degree relatives of individuals with pure SP was 16% as compared with 5% in the relatives of normal volunteers (Fyer et al., 1993). In a small study investigating monozygotic and dizygotic twins with SP, it was demonstrated that there was a higher concordance rate for specific social fears in the monozygotic twins (49%) as compared to the dizygotic twins (30%) (Torgersen, 1979). In a large study of female twins, it was reported that the concordance rate for SP was 44.4% for monozygotic twins and only 15.3% for dizygotic twins (Kendler et al., 1993). They concluded that, after controlling for environmental influences, genetic factors accounted for 30% of the liability for SP. Thus, these studies suggest that genetic factors may contribute to a significant loading for SP. Some data also suggest that the generalised subtype of SP may have a greater inheritable risk than the specific subtype. SP was present in 16% of relatives of patients with the generalised subtype, compared with only 6% of relatives of either patients with the specific subtype or normal controls (Mannuzza et al., 1995). Another study confirmed that first-degree relatives of probands with generalised SP showed a greatly increased incidence of generalised SP (26.4% compared to 2.7% in the relatives of control individuals) (Stein et al., 1998).

Recently, a functional polymorphism in the human serotonin transporter gene (SLC6A4*C) has been identified (Lesch et al., 1996). It was found to be linked to an anxiety-related personality trait, neuroticism, particularly anticipatory worry and fear of uncertainty. The relationship of SLC6A4*C to anxiety was replicated by sibpair linkage analysis in a recent study (Mazzanti et al. 1998). However, this report did not confirm the evidence for significant association between SCL6A4*C and anxiety which may suggest that this locus may not be directly affecting anxiety but is linked to another still unidentified functional variant. Nevertheless, the relationship of this polymorphism to SP remains yet to be investigated and clarified.

Several studies conducted in women with social anxiety disorder have provided evidence that genetic factors are important in the development of the generalised subtype (Stein, 1997; Hutchings & Dutton, 1997). In fact, relatives of patients with generalised social anxiety disorder have an increased risk, perhaps as much as 10-fold, of developing the generalised subtype (Stein et al., 1998). In contrast, relatives of patients with non-generalised social anxiety disorder are not more likely to have social anxiety disorder (Stein et al., 1998). They have an increased risk of having a relative with PD, but not family members with social anxiety disorder (Fyer et al., 1996). These findings suggest that comorbid conditions may be more likely in women with social anxiety disorder and that generalised social anxiety disorder, at least in women, may be mediated by genetic factors.

3.2 Neurophysiology

It has been hypothesised that patients with generalised SP may have central serotonergic dysregulation. A study designed to investigate abnormalities in the 5-HT function in SP *via* pharmacological challenges with the partial 5-HT agonist m-chlorophenylpiperazine (*m*-CPP) reported that social phobics had a greater cortisol response (peak change $\pm$ SD = 9.07 $\pm$ 7.50) than normal control subjects (5.89 $\pm$ 5.93) and OCD patients (7.04 $\pm$ 7.35) (Hollander et al., 1998). Female social phobics had a significant trend toward augmented cortisol response to *m*-CPP (9.06 $\pm$ 8.85) in comparison to female normal control subjects (3.96 $\pm$ 4.18) but did not differ from OCD control patients (6.70 $\pm$ 8.30). Prolactin response in the social phobics was normal. Therefore, this study may indicate preliminary evidence for 5-HT dysfunction in social phobics, particularly in female patients. However, it may also suggest a heightened HPA response rather than 5-HT dysfunction.

Dopamine dysregulation is also suspected in patients with generalised SP (Liebowitz et al., 1987). In a study designed to evaluate the density of dopamine reuptake sites in patients with SP, patients with this disorder were observed to exhibit lower striatal dopamine reuptake site densities compared with healthy subjects (Tiihonen et al., 1997). A study using PET technology demonstrated that dopamine D_2-receptor binding to the putamen (as measured with the radioligand [^{11}C] raclopride) was significantly associated with particular personality traits that may be relevant to SP (Farde et al., 1997). Specifically, it was reported that D_2-receptor density strongly correlated with the Karolinska Scale of Personality "detachment" scale ($r = -0.68$, $p < 0.001$, a significant correlation after Bonferroni correction for all comparisons). The detachment scale includes behaviours with tendency to avoid giving and taking confidences and to avoid involvement with other people. Whether or not detachment is actually a characteristic of individuals with generalised SP needs to be clarified by future research.

Surprisingly, the noradrenergic system has been little studied in SP despite the fact that anxiety attacks in social situations are commonly a feature of this disorder and despite the fact that SP is not infrequently comorbid with PD (Kessler et al., 1998).

Several studies have demonstrated an up-regulation of PBRs during acute stress and a down-regulation with chronic stress (Drugan et al., 1993; Weizman et al., 1994). PBRs are structurally different from central BDZ receptors since they are not associated with the GABA receptor/chloride ion channel complex. They are located on mitochondrial and plasma membranes of tissues throughout the body. PBR density changes may be associated with stress and anxiety states. A recent study showed that generalised SP patients had a significantly lower PBR B_{max} than control subjects (2764 ± 1242 vs. 4327 ± 1850 fmol/mg protein, $p = 0.00001$) (Johnson et al., 1998). The authors suggest that factors associated with this down-regulation in PBRs are likely to be linked pathophysiologically to a subset of chronic anxiety states rather than to nonspecific stress. This PBR abnormality has been observed with some anxiety disorders such as PD and GAD but not in OCD or major depressive disorder.

3.3 Neuroimaging

A study of conditioned anticipatory anxiety in healthy volunteers has demonstrated characteristic changes in blood flow in response to anxiety and this work has now been extended to patients with SP (Bell et al., 1999; Price & Friston, 1997). Two studies using magnetic resonance spectroscopy (MRS) have found abnormal choline metabolite levels in patients with SP (Davidson et al., 1993; Tupler et al., 1997). This may represent an abnormality in cell membrane composition or function in the disorder, though this remains to be replicated. Another recent study using brain SPECT technology with a specific ligand for the dopamine transporter site reported markedly reduced binding to the basal ganglia of patients with generalised SP (Tiihonen et al., 1997). Given the high rates of SP in Parkinson's disease, a condition known to be associated with abnormal brain dopaminergic function (anxiety disorders, particularly generalised anxiety, panic and SP occur in up to 40% of patients with Parkinson's disease and it seems that this pathology may not be a reaction to the illness but may rather be linked to specific neurobiologic processes accompanying this disease), this finding is intriguing and warrants further research for better understanding (Stein et al., 1990, Richard et al.,1996). It may be anticipated that studies using such brain investigation technology may add to our understanding of the role of particular neural systems in the mediation of anxiety and SP.

3.4 Environment

Family environment can have positive effects on the development of a child's social skills and parents can influence social approach by their verbal or non-verbal behaviours. Some children become less inhibited if their parents make a concerted effort to place them in social situations. However, if a child avoids encountering social situations, opportunities to learn social skills will be limited. Many studies have sought to assess the association of SP with childhood environmental factors. The identification of a temperamental construct known as behavioural inhibition to the unfamiliar (BIU) and its stability over time has prompted further research to attempt to establish its relationship to the later emergence of anxiety disorders and the utility of early intervention strategies (Kagan et al., 1988).

Certain biases in the cognitive processing of social cues help to maintain SP. Considerable effort is being directed towards understanding these processes. Cognitive theories of SP suggest that individuals with generalised SP tend to interpret ambiguous social events as negative even when a positive interpretation is readily available (Amin et al. 1998). It is also reported that the perceptions of patients with generalised SP differ from the perceptions of individuals with OCD and controls. The consequences of a negative interpretation bias for social scenarios can be particularly debilitating, leaving the individual concerned with a high vulnerability for neuropsychological impairment. Preference for negative interpretation of social scenarios appears to be specific for social anxiety and its maintenance (Amin et al., 1998). Importance of cognitive factors should be considered in psychological treatment studies, except that proof of the importance of addressing these factors in treatment has been rather elusive.

3.5 Gender and cultural differences

Specific phobias also appear to be more prevalent among women than men. In a recent survey, more women than men had animal (snakes, spiders) and situational phobias (lightning, closed spaces, darkness, heights), but no gender differences were found in the prevalence of mutilation phobias (injections, dentists, injuries) (Fredrikson et al., 1996). A recent study designed to investigate gender differences in SP reported that no differences were found on history of SP, SP subtype, or comorbidity of additional anxiety disorders, mood disorders, or APD (Turk et al., 1998). However, women exhibited more severe social fears as indexed by several assessment instruments. Some differences between men and women also emerged in their report of severity of fear in specific situations. Women reported significantly greater fear than men while talking to authority, acting/performing/giving a talk in front of an audience, working while being observed, entering a room when others are already seated, being the centre of attention, speaking up at a meeting, expressing disagreement to individuals they do not know well and giving a party. More women than men reported fear of going to a party, and more men than women reported fear of urinating in a public restroom. Gender differences in the presentation and management of SP may be influenced by fluctuations in levels of endogenous or exogenous reproductive hormones (Weinstock, 1999). Both oestrogen and progesterone may affect neurotransmitter systems implicated in the aetiology of mood and anxiety disorders. Preclinical studies suggest that oestrogen increases the density of dopamine receptors when applied to striatal neurons in the rat and has been shown to inhibit monoamine oxidase activity (Di Paolo, 1994; Häfner et al., 1993; Chakravorty & Halbreich, 1997). There are also complex interactions between oestrogen and serotonin systems. Estradiol administration in female rats causes acute increases in 5-HT_{2A} receptor density in the cerebral cortex and nucleus accumbens (Fink et al., 1996). Progesterone metabolites have been shown to act on GABA receptors in a manner similar to BDZs and barbiturates (Kroboth & McAuley, 1997; Majewska, 1986; 1992).

Some cultural differences appear to exist and in some other countries, the prevalence rate of SP is lower (e.g. Canada, 1.7%; Puerto Rico, 1% and Korea, 0.5%) (Weissman et al., 1996). Considering the impact of a second language on SP, a study conducted in South Africa pointed out that for many individuals who may be forced to speak in a second, third or even fourth language, it is not unlikely that this precipitates symptoms of SP (Stein et al., 1998). However, this putative phenomenon has not been well studied and surely deserves more attention in other countries.

Taijin-kyofu-sho (TKS) is thought to be a common, culture-bound disorder of SP in Japan and Korea. Recent data suggest that this disorder may not be as culture-bound as previously thought (Clarvit et al., 1996). This type of SP is noted most frequently in Asian countries and also responds well to treatment (Liebowitz, 1999). SP and TKS share common features, such as anxiety over being observed and social avoidance. The "offensive type" of TKS is characterised by fear of hurting the feelings of others by the expression of certain shortcomings within oneself. Offending others may occur in several ways such as embarrassing others by blushing, causing offence by emitting bodily odours or irritating others by shakiness of the voice. Thus, patients with offensive-type SP erroneously believe that their presence or body odour makes others uncomfortable, leading to social avoidance. Current research does not support a new diagnostic category or the expansion of criteria for SP to include the offensive type of TKS. However, SP should be considered in the differential diagnosis of patients with the offensive type of TKS.

4 Treatments

Current research has clearly indicated the need for treatment of this disorder (Montgomery, 1997). The introduction of effective medication and the spread of awareness that effective and specific treatment is available are therefore significant developments.

4.1 Psychological

Two general strategies are anxiety reduction and improvement in interpersonal functioning. The main anxiety reduction techniques are exposure and cognitive restructuring, and the main tool for improving social functioning is social skills training (Reilly et al., 1999).

Behavorial therapy exposure involves systematic and prolonged contact with the anxiety-evoking social setting or stimulus until a significant reduction in anxiety is achieved. An advantage of cognitive behaviour group therapy is that it is a short-term and symptom-focused intervention strategy. It is usually conducted in 12 to 15 sessions, each lasting 2.5 h. The group is led by two therapists, preferably one woman and one man, since either or both sexes may need to be represented in the different exposure situations. The group usually comprises 6 patients balanced as much as possible for sex, types of fears, and degree of impairment in the feared situation. Success of the intervention hinges upon careful assessment, which includes the identification of physical symptoms and anxiety-provoking cues. Exposure simulations in cognitive behaviour group therapy are based on the person's core fear in a particular situation as shown in Table 4.2.

Cognitive restructuring (a generic term for different models of cognitive modification) is a major component of cognitive behaviour group therapy (Shear & Beidel, 1998). It identifies systematic errors in thinking as inferred from the narrative of the patient. In therapy, both these and the underlying organising cognitive structures are challenged. Between sessions the patient is asked to identify his or her self-defeating thoughts as they arise in social situations and to challenge them using techniques taught during sessions. Cognitive restructuring may be used either as a technique or as an organising principle of therapy. Patients gain confidence from group exposure sessions with the therapist present, but homework is an important element of cognitive behaviour group therapy with much emphasis placed on daily practice. Patients are encouraged to do 30 minutes of cognitive preparation before an *in vivo* exposure by imagining the situation, identifying accompanying negative automatic thoughts, disputing these thoughts, deriving rational responses, and then setting goals for exposure.

In a series of studies and a meta-analysis of 42 treatment-outcome studies, the largest effect sizes were always seen in the groups that involved some form of exposure (Heimberg et al, 1990; Butler et al., 1984; Newman et al., 1994; Taylor, 1996). In these studies, the exposure was sometimes gradual, sometimes intensive, sometimes *in vivo* (done in real life), and sometimes imaginal. Although exposure is clearly important, the mechanism by which it works is not known. Habituation, initially thought to be the explanation, is a biological process by which repeatedly confronting a conditioned fear stimulus without a negative consequence leads to a reduction in reactivity to the stimulus. Often, when phobic individuals are exposed to an anxiety-provoking cue, their anxiety increases initially and then decreases if they are maintained in that situation for a period of time. Habituation implies a physiological process. In contrast, the assumption underlying cognitive therapies is that anxiety reduction may also occur through changing the individual's interpretation of a situation with disconfirming information.

Other procedures used in conjunction with exposure for the treatment of SP have not been shown to affect outcome to any significant degree, but they may nevertheless play a role in the treatment process (Mersch, 1995; Mattick & Peter, 1988; Scholing & Emmelkamp, 1993; Taylor et al, 1997; Mattick et al., 1989). Anxiety management training helps the individual to feel more comfortable in stressful situations and facilitates exposure. Anxiety management strategies include relaxation exercises, breathing, attention focusing and social effectiveness therapy (SET). SET uses an average of 28 treatment sessions over a period of about 16 weeks. A key

Table 4.2: Cognitive behaviour group therapy: Examples of common exposure simulations

Initiating conversation with a member of the opposite sex
Public speaking
Writing or using a keyboard in front of others
Eating or drinking in front of others
Working or playing with others watching
Assertion and interactions with authority figures
Job interviews
Joining ongoing conversation
Giving or receiving compliments
Making mistakes
Revealing personal information
Expressing opinions
Feeling trapped in a social situation

component of SET is social skills training that involves developing new strategies (sequences of behaviour) for coping with difficulties within the phobic situation or in various social settings by means of a sequence of modelling, role play with feedback between sessions. Lack of social skills can increase anxiety in social interactions and social skills training can therefore be helpful, particularly for the generalised subtype of SP. Both cognitive restructuring and social skills training may involve a fair degree of exposure during therapy in the clinic. A recent study supports the effectiveness of cognitive-behavioral interventions in routine care (Hunt & Andrews, 1998).

The exposure sessions of SET are based on individualised fears, especially focusing on the core fear. Initially, the exposure sessions use an imaginal format. Typically, *in vivo* or imaginal exposure sessions average 90 min. In SET, the therapist accompanies the patient during the first 12 weeks of *in vivo* exposure. The final four weeks of SET are devoted to independent programmed practice which is a way of turning over the treatment to the patients themselves and having them start to take responsibility for continuing the exposure. The patients are encouraged to find ways to put themselves in social situations, such as calling meetings at work and giving short presentations.

A study reported that SP patients with any diagnosis of personality disorder responded less well to a cognitive treatment (Turner, 1987). In several controlled studies, exposure treatment alone has been demonstrated to be more effective than a psychological placebo (Albano et al., 1995; Newman et al., 1994). In a double-blind comparison with a pill placebo, or atenolol, exposure was more effective than placebo, whereas atenolol was not (Turner et al., 1994). Efficacy has also been demonstrated for cognitive-behavioral combinations compared with psychological placebos (waiting list or credible non-specific treatment) (Heimberg et al., 1990; Turner et al., 1994).

4.2 Pharmacological

Treatment options which have been reported to result in improvement include monoamine oxidase inhibitors (MAOIs), reversible monoamine oxidase inhibitors (RIMAs), SSRIs and BDZ interventions. Pharmacological treatments which have shown some efficacy include the MAOI phenelzine, the SSRIs and the BDZ clonazepam (Bisserbe et al., 1994; Liebowitz et al., 1992; Van Vliet et al., 1994) (see Table 4.3). Although phenelzine has shown some efficacy for SP, its clinical use is complicated by adverse effects, including the risk of hypertensive reaction from ingestion of sympathomimetic amines. The tricyclic antidepressants do not appear to be effective for the treatment of SP (Simpson et al., 1998). As for BDZs, sedative effects and withdrawal problems make these drugs unsuitable for long-term use. Considering comorbid conditions, BDZs should not be prescribed at all in patients with alcohol dependence.

Moclobemide, a RIMA, may have efficacy in the treatment of SP, but absence of significant differences in most primary outcome measures suggests that its clinical effect is small (Schneier et al., 1998). However, it should also be emphasised that 23% of patients with severe or very severe SP treated with moclobemide for 8 weeks were rated as much or very much improved (compared to 0% for placebo) although numbers were too small to reach statistical significance. On the other hand, moderate or marked severely ill patients had response rates of 13% for moclobemide *versus* 25% for placebo. Another study suggested that higher doses of moclobemide (e.g. 600 mg) might be associated with a better response (Nutt & Montgomery, 1996). On the Liebowitz SP scale, there was a significant linear regression with the dose for weeks 8 and 12. However, current trends suggest that although the reversible inhibitors of monoamine oxidase A have fewer dietary restrictions compared with the MAOIs, these drugs may not be promising in the treatment of SP (Liebowitz, 1999).

Beta-blockers are often prescribed for professional performers to control normal performance-related anxiety and reduce autonomic symptoms such as tachycardia, tremor and sweating (James et al., 1977). However, placebo-controlled studies of atenolol have not shown efficacy in the treatment of generalised social anxiety disorder (Liebowitz et al., 1992; Falloon et al., 1981; Turner et al., 1994).

In clinical practice, selection of appropriate pharmacotherapy usually involves consideration of relevant comorbid conditions. SSRIs, as broad-spectrum compounds, may be used for the management of patients with SP that occurs comorbidly with PD, depression, PTSD and OCD (Isaac, 1999). In a 14-center study in the United States and Canada, paroxetine (20-50 mg daily) was compared with placebo during 11 weeks in 183 patients with SP (Stein et al., 1998). Active treatment reduced the anxiety score by 39% (placebo 17%), with 55% (placebo 24%) of paroxetine-treated rated very much or much improved by the clinician.

In a recent randomised double-blind placebo-controlled study, the effects of paroxetine (20–50 mg daily) in previously undiagnosed and untreated patients with social anxiety disorder were studied for 3 months (Allgulander, 1999). The primary outcome measures were the mean change from baseline in the Liebowitz Social Anxiety Scale (LSAS) total score and the proportion of responders on the clinician-rated global impression of improvement. In the intent to treat analysis, the categorical model of clinical global improvement showed a significant difference between the treatment groups beginning after 4 weeks. The proportion of responders on paroxetine was 70.5% and on placebo 8.3%. All scores for self-rated anxiety and avoidance behaviour showed differences between the treatments. The difference in LSAS score was significant from week 6.

Venlafaxine, an inhibitor reuptake of both serotonergic and noradrenergic properties, is also potentially effective (Kelsey, 1995).

Since relapse is common in patients who discontinue medications, long-term maintenance therapy and clinical trials may be necessary. A recent study that evaluated the efficacy, tolerability and effects on quality of life of sertraline, an SSRI, in the prevention of relapse of generalised SP, showed that in the intent to treat end-point analyses, 1 (4%) of 25 patients in the sertraline-continuation group and 9 (36%) of 25 patients in the placebo-switch group had relapsed at study end-point (Walker et al., 2000). The initial 20-week study was placebo-controlled and 15 responders to placebo also continued to receive double-blind placebo treatment in the continuation study. Eighty eight percent of patients in the sertraline-continuation group and only 40% of patients in the placebo-switch and placebo-responder groups completed the study.

Full therapeutic benefits may require weeks or months of continued therapy as patients test the anxiolytic effects of treatment by exposing themselves to fearful situations over time. It appears that most patients with SP maintain benefits for years during continued therapy (Pollack, 1999). However, relapse rates are high following drug discontinuation. For instance, 62% of patients who responded to paroxetine experienced relapse when pharmacotherapy was discontinued (Stein et al., 1996). At least 1 year of pharmacological treatment is recommended in order to avoid relapse and permit patients to enjoy the benefit of their treatment (Westenberg, 1999). Indications for long-term pharmacotherapy include patients with persistent ongoing significant symptoms, the presence of comorbidity, the presence of early onset with severe avoidant personality and a prior history of relapse.

4.3 Comparison, combination of drug *versus* cognitive-behavioural therapy

As both psychological and pharmacological treatments have been shown to be beneficial, some studies have sought to compare them singly or in combination (Falloon et al., 1981; Gelernter et al., 1991; Clark & Agras, 1991). In general, the combination of psychological treatments and medication has been rather disappointing due to the lack of strict experimental control with both approaches as the results need to be considered in the light of a potential response to placebo by socially phobic patients with both approaches. One of the difficulties in comparing the drug and psychological treatment literature is the almost invariable choice of different outcome measures in the two types of study. Trials of pharmacological agents usually choose the LSAS and CGI scale as the primary outcome measures. Effect sizes are

Table 4.3: Some treatments showing efficacy in social phobia.

Drugs	Study design	Results	References
MAOI			
Moclobemide	8-week double-blind study in 77 patients randomly assigned to moclobemide or placebo. Outcome was assessed by clinical global impressions from independent clinicians and self-ratings.	No significant effects of moclobemide on most primary outcome measure. ITT sample response rates at week 8 were 17.5% for the moclobemide group and 13.5% for placebo.	Schneier et al., 1998
Phenelzine	12-week double blind study in 133 patients who received CBGT, educational-supportive group therapy or phenelzine therapy (15–90 mg/day) or pill placebo. Outcome measures include LSAS & ADIS-R.	After 12 weeks, both phenelzine therapy and CBGT were associated with marked positive response. Although patients receiving phenelzine were rated less symptomatic than other patients were on most measures, both were more efficacious than the control conditions.	Heimberg et al., 1998
Brofaromine	10-week double-blind placebo-controlled study in 102 outpatients with social phobia with brofaromine (n = 52, 50–150 mg/day). Primary outcome measure was change from baseline to endpoint on the LSAS.	Brofaromine produced a significantly greater change from baseline in LSAS scores compared with placebo. Results showed a significant treatment effect with brofaromine producing greater changes from baseline LSAS scores compared to placebo ($p < 0.016$).	Pande et al., 1999
SSRIs			
Paroxetine	3-month double-blind study in 96 patients with generalised social phobia randomised for treatment with paroxetine (20-50 mg daily) or placebo.	In the ITT analysis, the proportion of responders on paroxetine was 70.5% and on placebo 8.3%. All scores for self-rated anxietyand avoidance behaviour showed differences between the treatments. The difference in LSAS score was significant from week 6.	Allgulander, 1999
	12-week placebo-controlled trial of paroxetine which analysed subgroups of patients classified as suffering from severe (LSAS total score ≥82, n = 85) or moderate (LSAS total score 52–81, n = 78) social phobia.	In the LSAS total score, the paroxetine-placebo difference was greater in patients in the severe subgroup (20, $P < 0.001$) than those in the moderate subgroup (13.7, $P < 0.001$). In the CGI improvement scores, the paroxetine-placebo difference was greater in the severe subgroup (34.2%, $P < 0.001$) than in the moderate subgroup (29.1%, $P < 0.02$).	Montgomery, 1998

Table 4.3 (continued)

Drugs	Study design	Results	References
Paroxetine (continued)	12-week double-blind trial. In 187 patients with generalised social phobia. Outcome measures were number of responders on the CGI Improvement Item and mean change from baseline on the LSAS total score.	55% of patients who received paroxetine and 23.9% of those who received placebo were significantly improved at the end of treatment (odd ratio = 3.88). Mean change from baseline on the LSAS total score was better in the paroxetine group (–30.5 ± 2.68; 39.1% decrease) than in the placebo group (–14.5 ± 2.63; 17.4% decrease), a difference of 21.7% favouring paroxetine.	Stein et al., 1998
	12-week double-blind placebo-controlled flexible-dose trial in 93 social phobia patients. Primary response measures were the Global Improvement item on the CGI scale & mean change from baseline in the patient-rated LSAS total score.	There was a significant drug effect on both the CGI global improvement score (% of sample that responded to treatment are as follows: paroxetine: 70.5 % vs. placebo 47.8%, $p = 0.031$) and the LSAS at 12 week.	Stein et al., 1999
	12-week double-blind treatment in 290 patients assigned randomly to paroxetine (20–50 mg/day flexible dose) or placebo. Primary efficacy outcomes were the LSAS total score and the CDI scale global improvement item.	Paroxetine produced a significantly greater reduction in LSAS total score (mean change from baseline: –29.4 vs. –15.6, $p \leq 0.001$) and a greater proportion of responders (65.7% vs. 32.4%, $p \leq 0.001$) compared with placebo at the end of 12 week.	Baldwin et al., 1999
Citalopram	12-week open-label study of citalopram (40 mg daily) in 22 patients. Social phobia symptoms were rated using the LSAS & the CGI scales.	Citalopram appears ot be effective in the treatment of social phobia. A significant difference between week 0 & week 12 on LSAS (fear subscale, $p < 0.001$; avoidance subscale, $p < 0.001$ and CGI ($p < 0.001$) scales were noted.	Bouwer & Stein, 1998
Fluvoxamine	6-week open label trial in 15 social phobia patients. Rating scales used to assess efficacy were HAM-D, HAM-A, BSFS, FQ, & SPRAS.	Ten patients completed the 6-week treatment period of flexible dosing (50–150 mg/day). A significant decrease in all scales from baseline to week 7 at the conclusion of the active treatment period was noted.	De Vane et al., 1999
	12-week double blind, placebo controlled trial in 92 patients with social phobia. Primary response criterion was the CGI. Secondary response criteria were BSPC, SPI and LSAS.	By study end, 42.9% of the patients taking fluvoxamine and 22.9% of those taking placebo were deemed unequivocal responders ($p = 0.04$). Fluvoxamine was superior to placebo on all social phobia rating scales at week 8 and beyond.	Stein et al., 1999

Table 4.3 (continued)

Drugs	Study design	Results	References
Sertraline	20-week double blind, placebo controlled trial in 204 patients with generalised social phobia. Primary efficacy assessments were the percentage of patients rated much or very much improved on the CGI improvement item.	Seventy one (53%) of 134 patients receiving sertraline and 20 (29%) of 69 patients receiving placebo were much or very much improved at the end of treatment ($p \leq 0.01$) according to CGI improvement ratings. Sertraline is an effective treatment for patients with generalised social phobia.	Van Amer-ingen et al., 2001
Tricyclic			
Imipramine	8-week open trial of imipramine (50-300 mg/day) in 15 patients with social phobia. Primary outcome measure was LSAS.	There was a modest mean decrease in the LSAS score for the Intent-to-treat ($p = 0.05$) and the completer sample ($p = 0.11$). However, the results do not support the efficacy of imipramine as a treatment for social phobia.	Simpson et al., 1998
SNRI			
Venlafaxine	Open-label trial (chart review) of venlafaxine (mean dose of 146.5 mg/day; range: 56.25–300, sem = 17.8) in 9 patients. Questionnaires (FQ, SDS, BDI & DAI) and physician ratings were analysed.	Venlafaxine appeared to be an effective treatment for social phobia in 8 of 9 patients (patient-rated & physician-rated CGI). Significant improvement was noted in the FQ social phobia and SDS social/leisure subscales.	Kelsey, 1995
	15-week open flexible doses study of venlafaxine (mean dose range: 112.5–187.5 mg/day) in 12 non-responders patients (with or without con-comitant APD) to SSRIs. Data from questionnaires (LSAS, CGI & HAMD) were assessed.	Venlafaxine improves social phobia and/or APD symptoms as shown by significant decrease in LSAS scores (fear score: 56.8 at week 0 to 22.5 at week 15, $p < 0.0.5$; avoidant score: 57.25 at week 0 to 22.7 at week 15, $p < 0.05$).	Altamura et al, 1999
Other drugs			
AED Gabapentin	14-week double-blind trial of gabapentin (dosed flexibly between 900 and 3600 mg/day in 3 divided doses) in 64 patients with social phobia. Efficacy assessments included the LSAS, BSPS, SPIN, CGI and MMFQ.	Significant decreases in the symptoms of social phobia were observed among patients with gabapentin as compared to placebo as evaluated by clinician- and patient-rated scales. On the LSAS, patients on gabapentin exhibited decreases in fear total scores that were nearly three times that observed among those on placebo. LSAS total avoidance decreases were twice that noted among patients on placebo.	Pande et al., 1999

Table 4.3 (continued)

Drugs	Study design	Results	References
Antidepressant ($5\text{-}HT_{2A}$ antagonist)			
Nefazodone	12-week open-label trial of nefazodone 200–600 mg/day) in 23 social phobia patients. Measured scales included the LSAS, BSPS and social phobic disorders rating form.	Analysis of social anxiety, social phobic avoidance and social functioning showed a significant change at baseline. 69.9% of patients were considered responders & 30.4 were noted as non-responders.	Van Ameringen et al., 1997

MAOI: Monoamine oxidase inhibitors, SSRI: Selective serotonin reuptake inhibitors; ITT: Intent-to-treat; NS: Not significant; HAM-A: Hamilton rating for anxiety; HAM-D: Hamilton rating for depression; CBGT: Cognitive behavioural group therapy. BSFS: Brief social phobia Scale; MSPS: Marks-Sheehan Phobia Scale, FQ: Fear Questionnaire and SPRAS: Sheehan Patient Rated Anxiety Scale; SDS: Sheehan Disability Scale; BDI: Beck Depression Inventory; DAI: Beck Anxiety Inventory; sem: Standard error of the mean; APD: Avoidant Personality Disorder; AED: Antiepileptic drug; SPIN: Social phobia inventory, MMFQ: Marks-Mathews' Fear Questionnaire. SNRI: Serotonin Noradrenalin Reuptake Inhibitors; ADIS-R: Anxiety disorder interview schedule-revised.

rarely reported. Studies of psychological therapies are more likely to employ scales developed by the particular investigating group as well as one or more older SP measures, such as the Fear of Negative Evaluation Scale (FNES) and the Fear Questionnaire. The CGI is rarely used. Effect sizes are sometimes reported, but studies often suffer from small numbers and inadequate controls. Another important problem is the use and implementation of a placebo group in psychological as in pharmacological studies. A waiting list may not be the best control for treatment, as it does not simulate it and therefore may not be as evocative of the "placebo" response. Owing to such methodological pitfalls, a psychological control condition that parallels the pharmacological placebo may not be achievable. Nevertheless, further comparisons of treatment with control conditions that mimic treatment at least partially ought to be tried.

However, more recent data seem to indicate that the onset therapeutic benefit of pharmacological treatment may be more rapid but those of cognitive-behaviour therapy may be more sustained (Shear & Beidel, 1998; Liebowitz et al., 1999). In a study which assessed the effects of maintenance treatment and durability of gains after the discontinuation of treatment, responders to either phenelzine or cognitive-behavioral therapy from an acute trial comparing these two treatments as well as pill placebo and a psychotherapy control (educational supportive group therapy) were enrolled into a 6-month maintenance and a treatment-free follow-up phase. Patients receiving pill placebo or psychotherapy did not enter the long-term study. The results suggest that phenelzine and cognitive-behaviour therapy may differ in their long-term effects and that there was a greater relapse rate among patients with generalised SP with phenelzine. Another study which assessed the 6-months efficacy of three different therapeutic treatment (moclobemide, cognitive behavioural therapy and combination of both) in patients with generalised SP reported that a combination of cognitive behavioural therapy and pharmacotherapy may be the best effective therapeutic treatment regimen (Prasko et al., 1999). In this study, whereas moclobemide alone is the best therapy choice for the decrease of the overall anxiety in the first months of treatment, positive therapeutic benefit of the drug on avoidant behaviour is less pronounced. On the contrary, cognitive-behaviour therapy induces more beneficial effects on avoidant behaviour that it significantly decreased.

Given the evidence that cognitive-behavioral intervention may offer long-term maintenance of treatment gains, cognitive behaviour therapy emerges as a potential strategy to aid medication discontinuation in patients with SP. There is consistent evidence that brief cognitive behaviour therapy may aid patients to discontinue pharmacological treatments.

4.4 Algorithm for treatment

A number of general principles may be useful in developing effective treatment strategies for patients with SP. In clinical practice, selection of appropriate pharmacologal treatment usually involves consideration of relevant comorbid conditions.

SSRIs, as broad-spectrum medications can be used for the management of patients with SP that that occurs comorbidly with PD, depression, PTSD and OCD. In patients who require rapid onset of effect, use of BDZs and combined BDZ-antidepressant therapy may be considered. However, comorbid alcohol abuse is a relative contraindication for the use of BDZs. Effective dose levels should be targeted for initial treatment (e.g., paroxetine, 20 mg/day) but clinical experience suggests that doses may be increased for partial responders or for patients who do not respond to initial therapy. Patients who experience poor or partial response to initial therapy may benefit from other pharmacological treatments such as venlafaxine (75–300 mg/day) or nefazodone (300–500 mg/day). Full therapeutic benefits may require weeks or months of continued treatment as patients test the anxiolytic effects of treatment by exposing themselves to fearful situations over time. Most patients may maintain benefits for years during continued therapy. However, relapse rates are high following drug discontinuation. It is reasonable to maintain pharmacotherapy for at least 1 year once patients experience robust clinical response before considering treatment discontinuation.

Although the strategy of combining pharmacotherapy and cognitive behaviour therapy has not been subjected to a large number of robust studies, combination therapy may provide synergistic or additive benefits. Behavioural therapy in the form of self-exposure instructions with pharmacotherapy for all patients with SP may be considered. Formal cognitive behavioural therapy should be considered for patients who remain symptomatic despite these interventions. It is important to consider psychosocial problems when treating patients with SP. As the SP symptoms are controlled by the treatment, some patients may experience difficulties with confidence, self-esteem and interpersonal relationships. These patients may benefit from psychotherapeutic exploration and treatment.

5 Methodology of clinical investigations

5.1 Rating Scales

Three types of criteria should be considered when evaluating global improvement in social anxiety: objective (i.e. whether the symptoms and avoidance behaviour have disappeared or decreased), adaptive (i.e. whether the patient has achieved a level of functioning that permits complete expression of his or her potential) and subjective (i.e. whether there is a perception of well-being). In recent years, several measures of SP including questionnaires and interviews that vary in goals, length and complexity have been constructed to assess these various criteria for clinical improvement.

Self-assessment questionnaires have several advantages over interviews, including ease of administration and cost reduction. The lack of a requirement for trained interviewers is a major advantage in many settings. Five questionnaires for assessing SP have been developed and thoroughly studied (see Table 4.4).

5.2 Self-assessment questionnaires

The Social Phobia & Anxiety Inventory (SPAI) was developed as a SP measure which is reasonably distinct from general anxiety, depression, and general distress as well as agoraphobia. Indeed, in some studies, the SPAI has been shown to be only weakly associated with state and trait anxiety, depression, social desirability and agoraphobia. The SPAI was developed with the goal of creating a measure that reliably discriminates between symptoms of SP and symptoms of other anxiety disorders, especially agoraphobia. Thus, the agoraphobia scale was added in order to control for the overlap in anxiety symptoms. The SPAI assesses behavioural, physiological and cognitive symptoms associated with SP. It is comprised of two subscales, the 32-item SP scale and the 13-item agoraphobia scale. Each item is scored on a 7-point Likert scale from 1 (never) to 7 (always). The SP scale measures the frequency with which respondents avoid or escape social situations. The agoraphobia scale was added to assess the extent to which respondents experience fear of panic attacks, concern about being trapped, and other agoraphobic fears, reactions which can lead to distress in social situations but which are not related to a fear of negative evaluation specific to SP. In screening patients with the SPAI, a difference score above 60 should prompt an evaluation for SP, and a difference score above 80 should alert clinicians to the probable presence of SP. A cutoff score of 80 was found to yield a 29% false negative rate, suggesting that the SPAI is a reasonably accurate screening measure (Turner et al., 1989). Scores for adolescents with SP may be somewhat lower than those reported with adult samples (Clark et al., 1994). In an adolescent sample, the SPAI scale proved to be positively correlated with fear of criticism and anxiety in heterosexual interactions, and negatively correlated with assertiveness (Clark et al., 1994).

Studies of criterion-related validity indicated that SPAI distinguished between patients with SP, those with other anxiety disorders and nonanxious control individuals in adult and adolescent samples (Clark et al., 1994). The SPAI also demonstrated sensitivity to change with treatment (Davidson et al, 1991; Beidel et al., 1993). In a study in which patients with SP received 12 weeks of either behaviour therapy (flooding), atenolol, or placebo, the results suggested that the SPAI was more sensitive to change with treatment than with the FNES and social avoidance distress scale (SADS).

The Social Phobia Scale (SPS) and Social Interaction Anxiety Scale (SIAS) are companion scales with similar design. The SPS was developed to measure anxiety when anticipating being observed or actually being observed by other people (e.g. public speaking, writing, eating). The SIAS was designed to assess anxiety in social interactional situations, such as initiating and maintaining conversations with friends, strangers, or potential mates. The SPS and SIAS each include 20 items. Each item is rated on a 5-point Likert scale (0 = not at all characteristic of me; 4 = extremely characteristic or true of me). Research is accumulating to suggest that the SIAS and SPS are reliable and valid measures of social anxiety and phobia (Ries et al., 1998). An underlying assumption of these measures is that they tap two specific dimensions of social anxiety – interaction anxiety and performance/observation anxiety. However, it is unclear whether or not the situations feared by individuals with SP actually cluster into these two categories. A recent study which performed an exploratory factor analysis of the SIAS and the SPS suggests that the factors involved (interaction anxiety, anxiety about being observed by others and fear that others will notice anxiety symptoms) as measured by these scales all load on a single higher-order factor which is social anxiety (Safren et al., 1998). Social anxiety represents different aspects of a single higher-order factor. This finding provides support for the current conceptualisation of SP as subsuming individuals with fears in vastly different social interaction and performance situations. In several studies, the SIAS scores discriminated between patients with generalised SP and those with non-generalised SP as per DSM-III-R criteria, but this did not prove to be the case for the SPS (Heimberg et al., 1992, Holt et al., 1992). Failure of the SPS to differentiate between generalised and non-generalised SP is probably due to the fact that the majority of individuals with the generalised subtype also fear performance-type situations. The SIAS and SPS have shown to be sensitive to the effects of cognitive and behavioural treatments in clinical outcome studies (Mattick et al., 1989). Several lines of evidence converge to support the utility of the SPS and SIAS scales in studies of SP and social anxiety. They discriminate social phobics from community volunteers and they are significantly correlated with other self-report measures of social anxiety and SP (Heimberg et al., 1992). Furthermore, the SIAS was more strongly related to several measures of social interactional anxiety and self-statements in social situations. The SPS was more strongly related to measures of performance/observation fear. Both scales showed excellent sensitivity to the presence of SP. Social phobics scored higher on both the SIAS and the SPS than agoraphobic subjects.

The FNES and SADS, a related pair of measures, are the first and most widely used questionnaire measures of social anxiety (Watson & Friend, 1969). The FNES was designed to measure apprehension about others' evaluations, expectation of negative evaluation, avoidance of evaluative situations, and distress related to negative evaluations. The SADS was designed to measure social avoidance and subjective distress, with items reflecting physiological symptoms and impaired performance excluded. Several studies attest to the ability of the FNES and SADS to detect change with psychological as well as pharmacological treatment (Beidel et al., 1993; Davidson et al. 1991).

5.3 Clinician/computer-administered scales

Interview measures have several advantages over questionnaires. The trained interviewer can monitor respondents' understanding of questions. He can provide respondents with supplemental information regarding the intention of questions.

The LSAS is a clinician-administered, semi-structured interview designed to assess DSM SP through the evaluation of fear and avoidance in social situations (Liebowitz, 1987). The LSAS includes 24 items, 13 describing performance situations and 11 describing social interactional situations. The LSAS demonstrated

Table 4.4: Social phobia/social anxiety scales

Self-assessment questionnaires and interview measures	**Description**	**Advantages and disadvantages**	**References**
Self-assessment questionnaires			
Social Phobia & Anxiety Inventory (SPAI)	Developed to assess social phobia as defined by DSM-III. It is comprised of two subscales, the 32-item social phobia scale and the 13-item agoraphobia scale. Each item is scored on a 7-point Likert scale from 1 (never) to 7 (always).	Good content validity for the DSM construct of social phobia. Excellent psychometric properties, is sensitive to change with treatment, and has been validated in a range of clinical and community samples including adults and adolescents. The measure provides detailed information regarding the type and severity of social anxiety symptoms.	Turner et al., 1989, 1995 Leon et al., 1995
Social Phobia Scale (SPS) and Social Interaction Anxiety Scale (SIAS)	Companion scales with similar design. The SPS was developed to measure anxiety when anticipating being observed or actually being observed by other people (e.g. public speaking, writing, eating). The SIAS was designed to assess anxiety in social interactional situations, such as initiating and maintaining conversations with friends, strangers, or potential mates.	Both demonstrated good internal consistency, stability over time & good criterion-related validity. Unlike the SPAI, the SPS and the SIAS have the advantage of providing separate scores for performance-type social anxiety and interactional anxiety. The SPS and SIAS are shorter than the SPAI, though they provide somewhat less information.	Mattick & Clarke, 1989; in: Heimberg et al., 1992
Fear of Negative Evaluation Scale (FNES) and Social Avoidance and Distress Scale (SADS)	The FNES (30-item inventory) and SADS (28-item inventory), a related pair of measures are the most widely used questionnaire measures of social anxiety. FNES was designed to measure apprehension about others' evaluations, expectation of negative evaluation, avoidance of evaluative situations, and distress related to negative evaluations. SADS was designed to measure social avoidance and subjective distress.	The FNES and SADS have been shown to have good internal consistency, acceptable retest reliability, and good convergent validity. However, though both instruments proved to be sensitive to change with treatments, they may not provide optimal information on symptom change due to their dichotomous response format. Neither measure is suitable as a diagnostic tool for social phobia.	Watson & Friend, 1969

Table 4.4 (continued)

Self-assessment questionnaires and interview measures	**Description**	**Advantages and disadvantages**	**References**
Semi-structured Interviews			
Liebowitz Social Anxiety Scale (LSAS)	A clinician-administered, semi-structured interview designed to assess DSM social phobia through the evaluation of fear and avoidance in social situations. Each item is rated separately for fear (scale from 0–3, 0 = none; 3 = severe) and avoidance (scale from 0–3; 0 = never (0%); 3 = usually (67–100%).	Assesses both anxiety and avoidance in a broad range of social situations. It is easy to administer and appears to be a useful tool for developing a fear hierarchy and treatment progress. However, further development of the LSAS is needed to improve the construct validity.	Liebowitz, 1987
Brief Social Phobia Scale (BSPS)	A semi-structured interview for assessing severity and treatment response in social phobia as defined by DSM criteria. The BSPS appears to have adequate content validity in that it captures the most common situations feared by individuals with social phobia as well as typical somatic symptoms associated with social phobia.	Brief and easy to administer, suggesting that it may be used as an efficient instrument for evaluating socialanxiety symptoms and for monitoring patients' progress in treatment. However, the BSPS does not include definitions for severity ratings of individual items, which may make reliable application of the measure problematic for clinicians.	Davidson et al., 1991

sensitivity to change with pharmacological as well as cognitive-behavioral treatment for SP (Brown et al., 1995; Liebowitz et al., 1992). Because the LSAS has been used in several studies with large samples of SP patients and because it has been more thoroughly evaluated than the Brief Social Phobia Scale (BSPS), the use of the LSAS is recommended. It should probably be used as primary outcome variable in clinical studies. Administration of the LSAS is straightforward, and it appears to be a useful tool for constructing a fear hierarchy. Recently, a french version of this scale has been validated (Yao et al., 1999). This French version, which showed a good empirical and concurrent validity, presented a good sensitivity to change after cognitive behavioural therapy in social phobics. It is clear that efforts should be made to adapt and validate the rating scales for different languages and cultures.

A recent study which investigated the distribution characteristics, reliability, validity and treatment sensitivity of the LSAS in a large population of patients with SP (N = 382) reported that the LSAS and its subscales were normally distributed and demonstrated excellent internal consistency (Heimberg et al., 1999). The LSAS appears to be a reliable, valid and sensitive measure of the effects of pharmacological treatments of SP over time in a double-blind clinical study. However, some weaknesses of the LSAS were also underlined. The pattern of correlations of LSAS subscales with one another and with the other measures suggests that the fear subscales and the avoidance subscales may not be sufficiently distinct in clinical samples (Heimberg et al., 1999). The lack of differentiation between LSAS fear and avoidance raises the question of the usefulness of the assessment of overall total scores (addition of fear and avoidance scores). This study showed that there was little to gain in the addition of the two subscales of fear and avoidance since the correlation of the total score with either fear or avoidance totals was 0.98. Another study also showed that the analysis of a two-factor model with the LSAS fear and avoidance ratings did not provide an adequate fit to the data, suggesting the need to further investigate the underlying structure of this scale (Safren et al., 1999). Separate factor analyses of the fear and avoidance items yielded four similar factors (social interaction, public speaking, observation by others and eating/drinking in public). While social interaction anxiety and avoidance as normally measured by the LSAS appear to be unifactorial, performance/observation anxiety and avoidance appear to be multifactorial. Further research to better understand the LSAS psychometric properties is required.

The BSPS is a semi-structured interview for assessing severity and treatment response in SP as defined by DSM criteria (Davidson et al., 1991). It is recommended that the BSPS be used following the administration of an initial diagnostic interview, so that the interviewer is familiar with the patient's SP symptoms. It is further suggested that the BSPS be administered with the patient looking at a copy of the scale. The BSPS is brief and easy to administer, suggesting that it may be used as an efficient instrument for evaluating social anxiety symptoms and for monitoring patients' progress in treatment.

A study designed to assess the utility, reliability and validity of computer-administered rating scales for social anxiety in a clinical trial used a computer-administered versions of the LSAS and BSPS (Kobak et al., 1998). Correlations between the computer and original versions were high at baseline, and remained high throughout the study. Mean score differences between computer and original versions were not significant at baseline. No significant differences were found between computer and traditional versions on the amount of change detected from baseline to endpoint. The results support the use of these computer-assisted symptoms rating scales of social anxiety as a viable alternative to the clinician-administered versions.

5.4 Health outcome assessments

Individuals suffering from SP are less likely to marry or to stay married. They have problems in the initiation and maintenance of intimate relationships, a disability that seems to be specific to SP rather than other anxiety disorders (Lecrubier et al., 2000). In a clinical survey, 92% of subjects estimated that their SP had a detrimental effect on their ability to work (Turner & Beidel, 1989). Individuals with SP are twice as likely to complain of poor health as those without SP and to have an increased rate of chronic illness including peptic ulcer (Davidson et al., 1993). Studies that have used the Sheehan Disability Scale have reported similar levels of impairment in SP as in depression or PD (Nutt & Montgomery, 1996). The Sheehan Disability Scale is a useful independent measure of the impairment experienced by patients with SP. It is a patient-rated instrument that has been widely used in treatment studies of the anxiety disorders to detect clinically relevant treatment-related differences. The scale measures the dimensions of work, social life and leisure activities. It also assesses family life and home responsibilities.

No scale has been specifically designed to examine quality of life in patients with social anxiety disorder. However, a number of generic scales have been devised which include the World Health Organisation Quality of Life-100 (WHOQOL-100), the WHOQOL-BREF, the Quality of Life Inventory (QOLI), and the short Form 36 items (SF-36) and 12 items (SF-12) scales. The WHOQOL-100 has 100 items examining overall quality of life and general health in a number of domains, including physical health, psychological, level of independence, social relationships, and environment. The WHOQOL-BREF is shorter, with 26 items and only 4 domains (physical health, psychological, social relationships, and environment).

Quality of life and functional impairment in patients with social anxiety disorder have been assessed in a double-blind study comparing patients with social anxiety disorder without comorbidities and matched controls (Wittchen & Beloch, 1996). Greater impairment in quality of life, as determined using the SF-36, was found in the social anxiety disorder group, with 47.7% severely or significantly impaired, compared with only 4.5% in the matched-control group. A study also reported that patients showed significant improvement in QOLI scores after cognitive-behavioral group therapy for SP (Frisch et al., 1992).

5.5 Assessment of recovery

Assessment of global improvement over three domains (symptoms, functionality and well-being or overall severity of illness) is necessary in order to assess a return to health or normal state (Bobes et al., 1998). The two most common criteria used to measure improvement in clinical studies of SP are achieving a rating on the CGI-S of markedly or moderately improved and reaching a prespecified level of improvement on a symptom scale (Liebowitz et al., 1992; Gergel et al., 1997; Schneier et al., 1998). Several studies have rather chosen the LSAS (van Vliet et al., 1994; 1997; Slaap et al., 1996; Fahlen et al., 1995). However, no single rating is currently adequate to define recovery and it is best to combine different measurements to assess both global and specific improvements in clinical severity and disability.

6 Discussion

It is now recognised that SP is not a trivial condition but a disorder with serious implications for the individual and society because it carries a greater degree of impairment than many other chronic disorders. Various studies suggest that SP is a chronic condition, with an average duration of 20 years, and is unlikely to remit spontaneously (Wittchen & Beloch, 1996; Davidson et al., 1993). Epidemiological studies have shown that only one quarter of patients recover, with the likelihood of recovery greater in patients with a higher educational level, higher age at onset, and no comorbid psychiatric conditions (Davidson, 1993). It is hoped that the proportion of patients recovering will increase as more patients are given the opportunity to receive treatment. Early identification programs should be devised to spot, treat and control the disease. Timely early recognition and treatment may prevent both immediate and long-term detrimental outcomes and possibly the onset of comorbid conditions.

Despite the increased interest in SP, many questions remain regarding the nature and boundaries of this disorder. The threshold between normal social anxiety and SP is arbitrary and difficult to define. There is a wider variation in the manifestations of SP than is seen in panic/agoraphobia. DSM-IV recognises two subtypes, generalised and nongeneralised, which are not operationally defined. There is considerable interest in defining and validating subtypes and seeking to establish their clinical significance. It may also be possible that in many sufferers the disorder becomes part of their life, with the impairments being regarded as normal functioning. Studies will need to be large enough to meaningfully compare nongeneralised SP, generalised SP and generalised SP with comorbid APD subtypes. The relationship of APD to SP requires further study.

Underrecognition and undertreatment persist but may be improved by creation of greater awareness of the disorder among primary health care physicians and the general public. The frequent co-occurrence of both Axis I and II disorders together with SP makes for a more severe and more complicated syndrome. Since comorbidity affects the choice of treatment, as well as its efficacy, assessment and treatment planning should take such comorbidity into account. The need to also educate clinicians involved in primary care as well as their patients about the difference between normal anxiety (experienced, for example, during public speaking) and pathologic anxiety needs to be recognised. The physiological response in each situation is different; whereas normal anxiety reaches a peak during the initial minutes of a presentation, the sustained level of intense anxiety felt in social anxiety disorder can severely disrupt functional ability. Future research aimed at examining why SP develops in some patients and not in others is crucial.

The LSAS and SPAI are clearly the most comprehensive and best validated SP measure to date. It has been suggested that the use of SPAI is excellent for the specific measure of SP symptoms (Herbert et al., 1991). Its use for the purpose of differential diagnosis has also been highlighted (Turner et al., 1989). Use of the SIAS and SPS in addition to the SPAI seems redundant. However the SIAS and SPS may increase our options for the assessment of SP. These scales may also be of use in determination of subtype of SP and in the analysis of the types of situations feared by social phobic patients.

The use of functional neuroimaging techniques during the performance of disorder-relevant neuropsychologic tasks promises to elucidate the neural circuitry of social anxiety and to better understand the implicated neurotransmitters with neuroanatomic precision. It may be anticipated that behavioural and molecular genetic approaches will clarify some of the risk factors for the development of SP that will help the development of innovative individualised treatment approaches. The precise action of serotonin, and its effects on, or modulation by, other neurotransmitter systems such as dopamine, remains poorly understood and should be a rich field of further research.

SP impacts on the quality of life of the whole family group and not just on the individual with the condition. The avoidance of social contact by the patient can limit the extent to which other members of the family socialise. Over time, the stress and strain takes its toll on close family members. There are data indicating that relatives of patients with SP lose more work days in their lifetime than relatives of patients with PD, obsessive disorder, or major depression (Faravelli et al., 2000).

Effective treatments have been identified, but there is a great divide between the methodologies of psychological and pharmacological studies that need to be resolved. Longer term follow up of outcome in drug studies and more reporting of effect sizes, larger and better controlled psychological studies are required. It is also important to formulate definitions for response and remission in SP. A full remission from SP may be considered as almost complete symptoms across the three domains of SP, which is maintained for a period of at least 3 months (Ballenger et al., 1998). Longitudinal studies and appropriate measures of the relevant dimensions of outcome are required to assess the long-term outcomes of SP, responses to pharmacological treatment and the possibilities for improving patient's abilities. Obviously, treatment strategies for patients with SP should consider gender differences in response to pharmacotherapy, psychiatric comorbidity, oral contraceptive use, pregnancy status and the specific nature of symptoms in the individual patient.

References

Albano AM, DiBartolo PM, Heimberg RG & Barlow DG. Children and adolescents: assessment and treatment. In: RG Heimberg, MR Liebowitz, DA Hope & FR Schnerer (eds): Social phobia: Diagnosis, assessments and treatment. New York, NY: Guildford Press, 387–425, 1995

Angst J & Dobler-Mikola A. The Zurich Study: anxiety and phobia in young adults. Eur Arch Psychiatr Neurol Sci 235, 171–178, 1995

Allgulander C. Paroxetine in social anxiety disorder. A randomized placebo-controlled study. Acta Psychiatr Scand 99, 1–6, 1999

Alnaes R & Torgersen S. The relationship between DSM-III symptom disorders (Axis I) and personality disorders (Axis II) in an outpatient population. Acta Psychiatr Scand 78, 485–492, 1988

Altamura AC, Piolo R, Vitto M & Mannu P. Venlafaxine in social phobia: a study in selective serotonin reuptake inhibitor non-responders. Int Clin Psychopharmacol 14, 239–245, 1999

Amies PL, Gelder MG & Shaw PM. Social phobia: a comparative clinical study. Br J Psychiatry 142, 174–179, 1983

Amin N, Foa EB & Coles ME. Negative interpretation bias in social phobia. Behav Res Ther 36, 945–957, 1998

Baldwin D, Bobes J, Stein DJ, Scharwächter I & Faure M. Paroxetine in social phobia/Social anxiety disorder. Br J Psychiatry 175, 120–126, 1999

Ball SG, Otto MW, Pollack MH, Uccello R & Rosenbaum JF. Differentiating social phobia and panic disorder: a test of core beliefs. Cogn Ther Res 19, 473–481, 1995

Ballenger JC, Davidson JRT, Lecrubier Y, Nutt DJ, Bobes J, Beidel DC, Ono Y & Westenberg HGM. Consensus statement on social anxiety disorder from the International Consensus Group on depression and anxiety. J Clin Psychiatry 59 (17), 54–60, 1998

Beidel DC, Turner SM & Cooley MR. Assessing reliable and clinically significant change in social phobia: Validity of the Social Phobia and Anxiety Inventory. Behav Res Therapy 31, 331–337, 1993

Beidel DC & Turner SM. Shy children, phobic adults. The nature and treatment of social phobia. Washington DC. American Psychological Association, 1998

Bell CJ, Malizia AL & Nutt DJ. The neurobiology of social phobia. Eur Arch Psychiatry Clin Neurosci 249 (Suppl), S11–S18, 1999

Bijl RV, Ravelli A & VanZessen G. Prevalence of psychiatric disorder in the general population: results of the Netherlands Mental Health Survey and Incidence Study (NEMESIS). Soc Psychiatr Epidemiol 33, 587–595, 1998

Bisserbe JC, Lépine J-P & the GRP Group. Moclobemide in social phobia: A pilot open study. Clin Neuropharmacol 17 (1), S88–S94, 1994

Black B & Uhde TW. Psychiatric characteristics of children with selective mutism: a pilot

study. J Am Acad Child Adolesc Psychiatry 34, 847–856, 1995
Bobes J. How is recovery from social anxiety disorder defined? J Clin Psychiatry 59 (17), 12–16, 1998
Bouwer C & Stein DJ. Use of the selective serotonin reuptake inhibitor citalopram in the treatment of generalized social phobia. J Affect Disord 49, 79–82, 1998
Brown EJ, Heimberg RG & Harlan RJ. Social phobia subtype and avoidant personality disorder: effect on severity of social phobia, impairment, and outcome of cognitive behavioral treatment. Behav Ther 26, 467–486, 1995
Butler G, Cullington A, Munby M, Amies P & Gelder M. Exposure and anxiety management in the treatment of social phobia. J Consult Clin Psychol 52 (4), 642–650, 1984
Chambless DL, Cherney J, Caputo GC & Rheinstein BJG. Anxiety disorders and alcoholism: a study with inpatient alcoholics. J Anxiety Disord 1, 29–40, 1987
Chartier MJ, Hazen AL & Stein MB. Lifetime patterns of social phobia: A retrospective study of the course of social phobia in a nonclinical population. Depress Anxiety 7, 113–121, 1998
Chakravorty SG & Halbreich U. The influence of estrogen on monoamine oxidase activity. Psychopharmacol Bull 33, 229–233, 1997
Clark DM & Wells A. A cognitive model of social phobia. In: RG Heimberg, MR Liebowitz, DA Hope et al (eds): Social phobia: Diagnosis, assessment, and treatment. New York, NY: Guildford Press, 69–93, 1995
Clark DB & Agras WS. The assessment and treatment of performance anxiety in musicians. Am J Psychiatry 148, 598–605, 1991
Clark DB, Bukstein OG, Smith MG, Kaczynski NA, Mezzich AC & Donovan JE. Identifying anxiety disorders in adolescents hospitalized for alcohol abuse or dependence. Psychiatr Serv 46 (6), 618–620, 1995
Clark DB, Turner S, Beidel D, Donovan J, Kirisci L & Jacob RG. Reliability and validity of the social phobia and anxiety inventory for adolescents. Psychol Assess 6, 135–140, 1994
Clarvit SR, Schneier FR & Liebowitz MR. The offensive subtype of Taijin-Kyofu-Sho in New York City: The phenomenology and treatment of a social anxiety disorder. J Clin Psychiatry 57, 523–527, 1996
Daleiden EL & Vasey MW. An information-processing perspective on childhood anxiety. Clin Psychol Rev 17, 407–429, 1997
Davidson JR, Hughes DL, George LK & Blazer DG. The epidemiology of social phobia: findings from the Duke Epidemiological Catchment Area Study. Psychol Med 23 (3), 709–718, 1993
Davidson JR, Krishnan KR, Charles HC, Boyko O, Potts NL, Ford SM & Patterson L. Magnetic resonance spectroscopy in social phobia: preliminary findings. J Clin Psychiatry 54 Suppl, 19–25, 1993
Davidson JRT, Potts NLS, Richichi EA, Ford SM, Krishnan KRR, Smith RD & Wilson W. The brief social phobia scale. J Clin Psychiatry 52, 48–51, 1991
Degonda M & Angst J. The Zurich study. XX. Social phobia and agoraphobia. European Arch Psychiatry Clin Neurosci 243, 95–102, 1993
Deltito JA & Stam M. Psychopharmacological treatment of avoidant personality disorder. Compr Psychiatry 30, 498–504, 1989

Den Boer JA & Dunner DL. Physician attitudes concerning diagnosis and treatment of social anxiety disorder in Europe and North America. Int J Psychiatry Clin Practice 3 (3), S13–S19, 1999

DeVane CL, Ware MR, Emmanuel NP, Brawman-Mintzer O, Morton WA, Villarreal G & Lydiard RB. Evaluation of the efficacy, safety and physiological effects of fluvoxamine in social phobia. Int Clin Psychopharmacol 14, 345–351, 1999

Di Paolo T. Modulation of brain dopamine transmission by sex steroids. Rev Neurosci 5, 27–42, 1994

Drugan RC, Paul SM, Crawley JN. Decreased forebrain [35S]TBPS binding and increased [3H]muscimol binding in rats that do not develop stress-induced behavioral depression. Brain Res 631, 270–276, 1993

Dummit ES III, Klein RG, Tancer NK, Asche B, Martin J & Fairbanks JA. Systematic assessment of 50 children with selective mutism. J Am Acad Child Adolesc Psychiatry 36 (5), 653–660, 1997

Fahlen T, Nilsson HL, Borg K, Humble M & Pauli U. Social phobia: the clinical efficacy and tolerability of the monoamine oxidase -A and serotonin uptake inhibitor brofaromine. A double-blind placebo-controlled study. Acta Psychiatr Scand 92(5), 351–358, 1995

Falloon I, Lloyd G-G & Harpin R-E. The treatment of social phobia: real-life rehearsal with non-professional therapists. J Nerv Ment Dis 169, 180–184, 1981

Faravelli C, Guerrini Degl'Innocenti B & Giardinelli L. Epidemiology of anxiety disorders in Florence. Acta Psychiatr Scand 79, 308–312, 1989

Faravelli C, Zucchi T, Viviani B, Salmoria R, Perone A, Paionni A, Scarpato A, Vigliaturo D, Rosi S, D'Adamo D et al. Epidemiology of social phobia: a clinical approach. Eur Psychiatry 15, 17–24, 2000

Faravelli C, Zucchi T, Viviani B, Salmoria R & Perone A. Epidemiology of social phobia: a clinical approach. Eur Psychiatry 15, 17–24, 2000

Farde L, Gustavsson JP & Jönsson E. D2 dopamine receptors and personality traits. Nature 385, 590, 1997

Fredrikson M, Annas P, Fischer H & Wik G. Gender and age differences in the prevalence of specific fears and phobias. Behav Res Ther 34, 33–39, 1996

Fink G, Sumner BE, Rosie R, Grace O & Quinn JP. Estrogen control of central neurotransmission: effect on mood, mental state, and memory. Cell Mol Neurobiol 16(3), 325–344, 1996

Frisch MB, Cornell J, Villanueva M & Retzlaff PJ. Clinical validation of the quality of life inventory: a measure of life satisfaction for use in treatment planning and outcome assessment. Psychol Assess 4, 92–101, 1992

Furmark T, Tillfors M, Everz PO, Marteinsdottir I, Gefvert O & Fredrikson M. Social phobia in the general population: prevalence and sociodemographic profile. Soc Psychiatry Psychiatr Epidemiol 34, 416–424, 1999

Fyer AJ, Mannuzza S, Chapman TF, Lipsitz J, Martin LY & Klein DF. Panic disorder and social phobia: effects of comorbidity on familial transmission. Anxiety 2 (4), 173–178, 1996

Fyer A, Mannuzza S, Chapman T, Liebowitz M & Klein D. A direct interview family study of social phobia. Arch Gen Psychiatry 50, 286–293, 1993

Gelernter CS, Uhde TW, Cimbolic P, Arnkoff DB, Vittone BJ, Tancer ME & Bartko JJ. Cog-

nitive-behavioral and pharmacological treatments of social phobia. A controlled study. Arch Gen Psychiatry 48 (10), 938–945, 1991
Gergel I, Pitts C, Oakes R & Kumar R. Significant improvement in symptoms of social phobia after paroxetine treatment. Biol Psychiatry 42, 26S, 1997
Godart NT, Flament MF, Lecrubier Y & Jeammet P. Anxiety disorders in anorexia nervosa: Co-morbidity and chronology of appearance. Eur Psychiatry 15, 38–45, 2000
Häfner H, Riecher-Rössler A, An Der Heiden W, Maurer K, Faktenheuer B & Loffler W. Generating and testing a causal explanation of the gender difference in age at first onset of schizophrenia. Psychol Med 23, 925–940,1993
Hazen AL & Stein MB. Clinical phenomenology and comorbidity. In: MB Stein (ed): Social phobia: clinical and research perspectives. Washington, DC: American Psychiatric Press, 1995
Heimberg RG, Dodge CS, Hope DA, Kennedy CR, Zollo LJ & Becker RE. Cognitive behavioral group treatment for social phobia: Comparison with a credible placebo control. Cogn Ther Res 14 (1), 1–23, 1990
Heimberg RG, Holt CS, Schneier FR, Spitzer RL & Liebowitz MR. The issue of subtypes in the diagnosis of social phobia. J Anxiety Disord 7 (3), 249–269, 1993
Heimberg RG, Liebowitz MR, Hope DA, Schneier FR, Holt CS, Welkowitz LA, Juster HR, Campeas R, Bruch MA, Cloitre M et al. Cognitive behavioral group vs. therapy for social phobia. 12 week outcome. Arch Gen Psychiatry 55, 1133–1141, 1998
Heimberg RG, Mueller GP, Holt CS, Hope DA & Liebowitz MR. Assessment of anxiety in social interaction and being observed by others: The social interaction and anxiety scale and the social phobia scale. Behav Ther 23, 53–73, 1992
Heimberg RG, Hope DA, Dodge CS & Becker RE. DSM-III-R Subtypes of social phobia: Comparison of generalized social phobics and public speaking phobics. J Nerv Ment Dis 178 (3), 172–179, 1990
Heimberg RG, Horner KJ, Juster HR, Safren SA, Brown EJ, Schneier FR & Liebowitz MR. Psychometric properties of the Liebowitz social anxiety scale. Psychol Med 29, 199–212, 1999
Herbert JD, Bellack AS & Hope DA. Concurrent validity of the Social Phobia and Anxiety Inventory. J Psychopathol Behav Assess 13, 357–368, 1991
Herbert JD, Hope DA & Bellack AS. Validity of the distinction between generalized social phobia and avoidant personality disorder. J Abnorm Psychol 101, 332–339, 1992
Hollander E, Kwon J, Weiller F, Cohen L, Stein DJ, DeCaria C, Liebowitz M & Simeon D. Serotonergic function in social phobia: comparison to normal control and obsessive-compulsive disorder subjects. Psychiatry Res 79, 213–217, 1998
Holt CS, Heimberg RG & Hope DA. Avoidant personality disorder and the generalized subtype of social phobia. J Abnorm Psychol 101, 318–325, 1992
Hunt C & Andrews G. Long-term outcome of panic disorder and social phobia. J Anxiety Disord 12 (4), 395–406, 1998
Hutchings PS, Dutton MA. Symptom severity and diagnoses related to sexual assault history. J Anxiety Disord 11, 607–618, 1997
Isaac M. Where are we going with SSRIs? Eur Neuropsychopharmacol 9 (3), S101–S106, 1999

James IM, Griffith DN & Pearson RM et al. Effect of oxprenolol on stage-fright in musicians. Lancet ii, 952–954, 1977

Johnson MR, Marazziti D, Brawman-Mintzer, Emmanuel NP, Ware MR, Morton A, Rossi A, Cassano GB & Lydiard BR. Abnormal peripheral benzodiazepines receptor density associated with generalized social phobia. Biol Psychiatry 43, 306–309, 1998

Judd L. Social phobia: A clinical overview. J Clin Psychiatry 55 (6), 5–9, 1994

Kagan J, Reznick SJ & Snidman N. Biological bases of childhood shyness. Science 240, 167–171, 1988

Kelsey JE. Venlafaxine in social phobia. Psychopharmacol Bull 31, 767–771, 1995

Kendler KS, Neale MC, Kessler RC, Heath RC & Eves LJ. The genetic epidemiology of phobias in women. The interrelationship of agoraphobia, social phobia, situational phobia and simple phobia. Arch Gen Psychiatry 49, 273–281, 1992

Kendler R, Neale M, Kessler R, Heath A & Eaves L. Major depression and phobias: The genetic and environmental sources of comorbidity. Psychol Med 23 (2), 361–371, 1993

Kessler RC, Stang P, Wittchen HU, Stein M & Walters EE. Lifetime comorbidities between social phobia and mood disorders in the US National Comorbidity Survey. Psychol Med 29, 555–567, 1999

Kessler RC, McGonagle KA, Zhao S, Nelson CB, Hughes M, Eshleman S, Wittchen H-U & Kendler KS. Lifetime and 12-month prevalence of DSM-III-R psychiatric disorders in the United States: Results from the National Comorbidity Survey. Arch Gen Psychiatry 51 (1), 8–19, 1994.

Kessler RC, Stein MB & Berglund P. Social phobia subtypes in the National Comorbidity Survey. Am J Psychiatry 155, 613–619, 1998

Kobak KA, Schaettle SC, Greist JH, Jefferson JW, Katzelnick DJ & Dottl SL. Computer-administered rating scales for social anxiety in a clinical drug trial. Depress Anxiety 7, 97–104, 1998

Kroboth PD & McAuley J. Progesterone: does it affect response to drug? Psychopharmacol Bull 33, 297–301, 1997

LaGreca AM, Dandes SK, Wick P, Shaw K & Stone WL. Development of the Social Anxiety Scale for Children: Reliability and concurrent validity. J Clin Child Psychol 17, 84–91, 1988

La Greca AM & Lopez N. Social anxiety among adolescents: Linkages with peer relations and friendships. J Abnorm Child Psychol 26 (2), 83–94, 1998

Last CG, Strauss CC & Francis G. Comorbidity among childhood anxiety disorders. J Nerv Ment Dis 175, 726–730, 1987

Lecrubier Y, Wittchen HU, Faravelli C, Bobes J, Patel A & Knapp M. A European perspective on social anxiety disorder. Eur Psychiatry 15, 5–16, 2000

Lecrubier Y & Weiller E. Comorbidities in social phobia. Int Clin Psychopharmacol 12 (6), S17–S21, 1997

Leon AC, Murzuk PM, Portera L. More reliable outcome measures can reduce sample size requirements. Arch Gen Psychiatry 52, 867–871, 1995

Lesch PK, Bengel D, Heils S, Sabol SZ, Greenberg BG, Petri S, Benjamin J, Müller CR, Hamer DH & Murphy DL. Association of anxiety-related traits with a polymorphism in the serotonin transporter gene regulatory region. Science 274, 1527–1531, 1996

Liebowitz MR. Update on the diagnosis and treatment of social anxiety disorder. J Clin Psychiatry 60 (Suppl. 18), 22–26, 1996

Liebowitz MR. Social phobia. Modern problems. Pharmacopsych 22, 141–173, 1987

Liebowitz MR, Campeas R & Hollander E. Possible dopaminergic dysregulation in social phobia and atypical depression (Letter). Psychiatr Res 22, 89–90, 1987

Liebowitz JM, Schneier F, Campeas R, Hollander E, Hatterer J, Fyer A, Gorman JM, Papp L, Davies S, Gully R & Klein DF. Phenelzine vs. atenolol in social phobia. A placebo-controlled comparison. Arch Gen Psychiatry 49, 290–300, 1992

Lépine JP & Pélissolo A. Epidemiology and comorbidity of social anxiety disorder. In: HGM Westenberg & JA den Boer (eds): Focus on psychiatry. Social anxiety disorder. Amsterdam: Synthesis Publishers, 29–43, 1999

Lépine JP & Lellouch J. Diagnosis and epidemiology of agoraphobia and social phobia. Clin Neuropharmacol 18, S15–S26, 1995

Levin AP, Schneier FR & Liebowitz MR. Social phobia: Biology and pharmacology. Clin Psychol Rev 9, 129–140, 1989

Liebowitz MR, Heimberg RG, Schneier FR, Hope DA, Davies S, Holt CS, Goetz D, Juster HR, Lin S-H, Bruch MA et al. Cognitive-behavioral group therapy *versus* phenelzine in social phobia: Long term outcome. Depress Anxiety 10 (3), 89–98, 1999

Magee WJ, Eaton WW, Wittchen HU, McGoagle KA & Kessler RC. Agoraphobia, simple phobia and social phobia in the National Comorbidity Survey. Arch Gen Psychiatry 53, 159–168, 1996

Majewska M. Neurosteroids: endogenous bimodal modulators of the GABA-A receptor mechanism of action and physiological significance. Prog Neurobiol 38, 379–395, 1992

Majewska MD, Harrison NL, Schwartz RD, Barker JL & Paul SM. Steroid hormone metabolites are barbiturate-like modulators of the GABA receptor. Science 232 (4753), 1004–1007, 1986

Mannuzza S, Schneier FR, Chapman TF, Liebowitz MR, Klein DF & Fyer AJ. Generalized social phobia. Reliability and validity. Arch Gen Psychiatry 52 (3), 230–237, 1995

Mattick RP & Peter L. Treatment of severe social phobia: effects of guided exposure with or without cognitive restructuring. J Consult Clin Psychol 56, 251–260, 1988

Mattick RP, Page A & Lampe L. Cognitive and behavioral aspects. In: MB Stein (ed): Social phobia: clinical and research perspectives. Washington, DC: American Psychiatric Press, 189–227, 1995

Mattick RP, Peters L & Clarke JC. Exposure and cognitive restructuring for social phobia: controlled study. Behav Ther 20, 3–23, 1989

Mazzanti CM, Lappalainen J, Long JC, Bengel D, Naukkarinen H, Eggert M, Virkkunnen M, Linnoila M & Goldman D. Role of the serotonin transporter promoter polymorphism in anxiety-related traits. Arch Gen Psychiatry 55, 936–940, 1998

McEwan KL & Devins GM. Is increased arousal in social anxiety noticed by others? J Abnorm Psychol 92, 417–421, 1983

Mellings TMB & Alden LE. Cognitive processes in social anxiety: the effects of self-focus, rumination and anticipatory processing. Behav Res Ther 38, 243–257, 2000

Merikangas KR & Angst J. Comorbidity and social phobia: evidence from clinical, epidemiologic, and genetic studies. Eur Arch Psychiatry Clin Neurosci 244, 297–303, 1995

Mersch PPA. The treatment of social phobia: the differential effectiveness of exposure *in vivo* and an integration of exposure *in vivo*, rational emotive therapy and social skills training. Behav Res Ther 33, 259–269, 1995

Millon T & Martinez A. Avoidant personality disorder: In: WJ Livesley (ed): The DSM-IV personality disorders. New York: Guildford Press, 218–233, 1995

Montgomery SA. Implications of the severity of social phobia. J Affect Disord 50, S17–S22, 1998

Montgomery SA. Social phobia: the need for treatment. Int Clin Psychopharmacol 12 (Suppl 6), S3–S9, 1997

Newman MG, Hofmann SG, Trabert W, Roth WT & Taylor CB. Does behavioral treatment of social phobia lead to cognitive changes? Behav Ther 25, 503–517, 1994

Nutt D & Montgomery SA. Moclobemide in the treatment of social phobia. Int Clin Psychopharmacol 11 (Suppl 3), 77–82, 1996

Pande AC, Davidson JR, Jefferson JW, Janney CA, Katzelnick DJ, Weisler RH, Greist JH & Sutherland SM. Treatment of social phobia with gabapentin: A placebo-controlled study. J Clin Psychopharmacol 19 (4), 341–348, 1999

Phillips RG & LeDoux JE. Differential contribution of amygdala and hippocampus to cued and contextual fear conditioning. Behav Neurosci 106, 274–285, 1992

Pollack MH. Social anxiety disorder: Designing a pharmacologic treatment strategy. J Clin Psychiatry 60 (Suppl 9), 20–26, 1999

Prasko J, Kosova J, Paskova B, Praskova H, Klaschka J, Seifertova D & Sipek J. Pharmacotherapy and/or cognitive-behavioral therapy in the treatment of social phobia – Controlled study. Psychiatrie 3 (1), 13–18, 1999

Price CJ & Friston KJ. Cognitive conjunction: a new approach to brain activation experiments. Neuroimaging 261–270, 1997

Reich J, Goldenberg I, Nasile R, Goisman R & Keller M. A prospective follow-along study of the course of social phobia. Psychiatry Res 54, 249–258, 1994

Reilly CE, Sokol L & Butler AC. A cognitive approach to understanding and treating anxiety. Hum Psychopharmacol Clin Exp 14, S16–S21, 1999

Richard IH, Schiffer RB & Kurlan R. Anxiety and Parkinson's disease. J Neuropsychiatry Clin Neurosci 8 (4), 383–392, 1996

Ries BJ, McNeil DW, Boone ML, Turk CL, Carter LE & Heimberg RG. Assessment of contemporary social phobia verbal report instruments. Behav Res Ther 36, 983–994, 1998

Rubin KH, LeMare LJ & Lollis S. Social withdrawal in childhood: Developmental pathways to peer rejection. In: SR Asher & JD Coie (eds): Peer rejection in childhood. New York: Cambridge University Press, 1990

Safren SA, Turk CL & Heimberg RG. Factor structure of the social interaction anxiety scale and the social phobia scale. Behav Res Ther 36, 443–453, 1998

Safren SA, Heimberg RG, Horner KJ, Juster HR, Schneier FR & Liebowitz MR. Factor structure of social fears: The Liebowitz social anxiety scale. J Anxiety Disord 13 (3), 253–270, 1999

Sanderson WC, Di Nardo PA, Rapee RM & Barlow DH. Syndrome comorbidity in patients diagnosed with a DSM-III-R anxiety disorder. J Abnorm Psychol 99, 308–312, 1990

Schneier FR, Johnson J, Hornig CD, Liebowitz MR & Weissman MM. Social phobia: Comorbidity and morbidity in an epidemiologic sample. Arch Gen Psychiatry 49, 282–288, 1992

Schneier FR, Heckelman LR, Garfinkel R, Campeas R, Fallon BA, Gitow A, Street L, Del Bene D & Liebowitz MR. Functional impairment in social phobia. J Clin Psychiatry 55 (8), 322–331, 1994
Schneier FR, Martin LY, Liebowitz MR, Gorman JM & Fyer AJ. Alcohol abuse in social phobia. J Anxiety Disord 3, 15–23, 1989
Schneier FR, Goetz D, Campeas R, Fallon B, Marshall R & Liebowitz MR. Placebo-controlled trial of moclobemide in social phobia. Br J Psychiatry 172, 70–77, 1998
Scholing A & Emmelkamp PMG. Exposure with and without cognitive therapy for generalized social phobia: effects of individual and group treatment. Behav Res Ther 31, 667–681, 1993
Shear MK & Beidel. Psychotherapy in the overall management strategy for social anxiety disorder. J Clin Psychiatry 59 (Suppl 17), 39–44, 1998
Simpson HB, Schneier FR, Campeas RB, Marshall RD, Fallon BA, Davies S, Klein DF & Liebowitz MR. Imipramine in the treatment of social phobia. J Clin Psychopharmacol 18 (2), 132–135, 1998
Slaap BR, van Vliet IM, Westenberg HG & Den Boer JA. Responders and non-responders to drug treatment in social phobia: differences at baseline and prediction of response. J Affect Disord 39 (1), 13–19, 1996
Stein DJ, Van der Linden G & Schmidt A. Social phobia when using a second language. South African Med J 88 (1), 61, 1998
Stein DJ, Berk M, Els C, Emsley RA, Gittelson L, Wilson D, Oakes R & Hunter B. A double-blind placebo controlled trial of paroxetine in the management of social phobia (social anxiety disorder) in the South Africa. South African Med J 89, 402–406, 1999
Stein MB. Phenomenology and epidemiology of social phobia. Int Clin Psychopharmacol 12 (Suppl) S23–S26, 1997
Stein MB, Chartier MJ, Hazen AL, Kozak MV, Tancer ME, Lander S, Furer P, Chubaty D & Walker JR. A direct-interview family study of generalized social phobia. Am J Psychiatry 155 (1), 90–97, 1998
Stein MB, Fyer AJ, Davidson JRT, Pollack MH & Wiita B. Fluvoxamine treatment of social phobia (social anxiety disorder): A double-blind, placebo-controlled study. Am J Psychiatry 156, 756–760, 1999
Stein MB, Walker JR & Forde DR. Public speaking fears in a community sample: prevalence, impact on functioning, and diagnostic classification. Arch Gen Psychiatry 53, 169–174, 1996
Stein MB, Liebowitz MR, Lydiard B, Pitts CD, Bushnell W & Gergel I. Paroxetine treatment of generalized social phobia (social anxiety disorder). A randomized controlled trial. JAMA 280, 708–713, 1998
Stein MB, Tancer ME, Gelernter CS, Vittone BJ & Uhde TW. Major depression in patients with social phobia. Am J Psychiatry 147, 637–639, 1990
Stein MB, Heuser IJ, Juncos JL & Uhde TW. Anxiety disorders in patients with Parkinson's disease. Am J Psychiatry 147, 217–220, 1990
Stein MB, Chartier MJ, Hazen AL, Kroft CD, Chale RA, Cote D & Walker JR. Paroxetine in the treatment of generalized social phobia: open-label treatment and double-blind, placebo-controlled discontinuation. J Clin Psychopharmacol 16, 218–222, 1996
Stein MB, Chartier MJ, Hazen AL, Kozak M, Tancer ME, Lander S, Furer P, Chubaty D &

Walker J. A family study of generalized social phobia. Am J Psychiatry 155, 90–97, 1998

Stopa L & Clark DM. Social phobia and interpretation of social events. Behav Res Ther 38, 273–283, 2000

Stravynski A, Lelliott P, McNamee G et al. A typology of social phobia based on content of patients' complaints. 26th Congress of the European Association for Behaviour and Cognitive Therapy, Budapest, 2–5 October, 1996

Taylor S, Woody S, Koch WJ, McLean P, Paterson RJ & Anderson KW. Cognitive restructuring in the treatment of social phobia. Efficacy and mode of action. Behav Modif 21 (4), 487–511, 1997

Taylor S. Meta-analysis of cognitive-behavioral treatments for social phobia. J Behav Ther Exp Psychiatry, 27, 1–9, 1996

Tiihonen J, Kuikka J, Bergstrom K, Lepola U, Koponen H & Leinonen E. Dopamine reuptake site densities in patients with social phobia. Am J Psychiatry 154 (2), 239–242, 1997

Torgersen S. The nature and origin of common phobic fears. Br J Psychiatry 134, 343–351, 1979

Tupler LA, Davidson JRT, Smith RD, Lazeyras F, Charles HC & Krisnan KR. A repeat proton magnetic resonance spectroscopy study in social phobia. Biol Psychiatry 42, 419–424, 1997

Turner SM, Beidel DC, Wolff PL, Spaulding S & Jacob RG. Clinical features affecting treatment outcome in social phobia. Behav Res The 34 (10), 795–804, 1996

Turner RM. The effects of personality disorder diagnosis on the outcome of social anxiety symptom reduction. J Pers Disord 1, 136–143, 1987

Turner AM, Beidel DC, Wolff PL et al. Clinical features affecting treatment outcome in social phobia. Behav Res Ther 34, 795–804, 1996

Turner SM & Beidel DC. Social phobia: clinical syndrome, diagnosis, and comorbidity. Clin Psychol Rev 9, 3–18, 1989

Turner SM, Beidel DC & Jacob RG. Social phobia: a comparison of behaviour therapy and atenolol. J Consult Clin Psychol 62, 350–358, 1994

Turner SM, Beidel DC & Dancu CV. Social phobia and anxiety Inventory Manual. North Tonawanda NY: MHS, 1995

Turner SM, Beidel DC, Dancu CV & Keys DJ. Psychopathology of social phobia and comparison to avoidant personality disorder. J Abnorm Psychol 95, 389–394, 1986

Turner SM, Beidel DC, Borden JW, Stanley MA & Jacob RG. Social phobia: Axis I and II correlates. J Abnorm Psychol 100, 102–106, 1991

Turk C, Heimberg R, Orsillo SM, Holt CS, Gitow A, Street LL, Schneier FR & Liebowitz MR. An investigation of gender differences in social phobia. J Anxiety Disord 12 (3), 209–223, 1998

Van Ameringen M, Mancini C & Oakman JM. Nefazodone in social phobia. J Clin Psychiatry 60 (2), 96–100, 1999

Van Ameringen MA, Lane RM, Walker JR, Bowen RC, Chokka PR, Goldner EM, Johnston DG, Lavallee Y-J, Nanday S, Pecknold JC et al. Sertraline treatment of Generalized Social Phobia: A 20 week, double-blind, placebo-controlled study. Am J Psychiatry 158, 275–281, 2001

Van Vliet IM, den Boer JA & Westenberg HGM. Psychopharmacological treatment of social phobia. Clinical and biochemical effects of brofaromine, a selective MAO-A inhibitor. Eur Neuropsychopharmacol 2, 21–29, 1992

van Vliet IM, den Boer JA, Westenberg HG & Pian KL. Clinical effects of buspirone in social phobia: a double-blind placebo-controlled study. J Clin Psychiatry 58 (4), 164–168, 1997

Van Vliet IM, den Boer JA & Westenberg HGM. Psychopharmacological treatment of social phobia: a double blind placebo controlled study with fluvoxamine. Psychopharmacol (Berl) 115, 128–134, 1994

Versiani M, Nardi AE, Mundim FD, Alves AB, Liebowitz MR & Amrein R. Pharmacotherapy of social phobia: a controlled study with moclobemide and phenelzine. Br J Psychiatry 161, 353–360, 1992

Wacker HR, Müllejans R, Klein KH & Battegay R. Identification of cases of anxiety disorders and affective disorders in the community according to ICD-10 and DSM-IIIR by using the Composite International Diagnostic Interview (CIDI). Int J Meth Psychiatric Res 2, 91–100, 1992

Walker JR, Van Ameringen MA, Swinson R, Bowen R, Chokka PR, Goldner E, Johnston DC, Lavallie YJ, Nandy S, Pecknold JC, Hadrava V & Lane RM. Prevention of relapse in generalized social phobia: Results of a 24-week study in responders to 20 weeks of sertraline treatment. J Clin Psychopharmacol 20 (5), 636–640, 2000

Watson D & Friend R. Measurement of social-evaluative anxiety. J Cons Clin Psychol 33, 448–457, 1969

Weiller E, Bisserbe J-C, Boyer P, Lepine J-P & Lecrubier Y. Social phobia in general health care. An unrecognised undertreated disabling disorder. Br J Psychiatry 168, 169–174, 1996

Weinstock LS. Gender differences in the presentation and management of social anxiety disorder. J Clin Psychiatry 60 (Suppl 9), 9–13, 1999

Weissman MM, Bland RC, Canino GJ, Greenwald S, Lee CK, Newman SC, Rubio-Stipec M & Wickramaratne PJ. The cross-national epidemiology of social phobia: a preliminary report. Int Clin Psychopharmacol. 11 (Suppl 3), 9–14, 1996

Weiller E, Bisserbe J-C, Boyer P, Lepine J-P & Lecrubier Y. Social phobia in general health care: an unrecognised undertreated disabling disorder. Br J Psychiatry 168, 169–174, 1996

Weizman R, Laor N, Karp L, Dagan E, Reiss A, Dar DE, Wolmer L & Gavish M. Alteration of platelet benzodiazepine receptors by stress of war. Am J Psychiatry 151 (5), 766–767, 1994

Westenberg HGM. Facing the challenge of social anxiety disorder. Eur Neuropsychopharmacol 9 (Suppl 3), S93–S99, 1999

Widiger TA. Generalized social phobia *versus* avoidant personality disorder: a commentary on three studies. J Abnorm Psychol 101, 340–343, 1992

Williams JMG, Mathews A & MacLeod C. The emotional Stroop task and psychopathology. Psychol Bull 120, 3–24, 1996

Wittchen HU, Ahmoi Essau C, von Zerssen D, Krieg J-C & Zaudig M. Lifetime and six-month prevalence of mental disorders in the Munich follow-up study. Eur Arch Psychiatry Neurosci, 241–258, 1992

Wittchen HU, Nelson CB & Lachner G. Prevalence of mental disorders and psychosocial impairments in adolescents and young adults. Psychol Med 28, 109–126, 1998

Wittchen HU, Nelson CB & Kessler RC. Social fears and DSM-IV social phobia: prevalence, risk factors and comorbidity. Psychol Med 29, 309–329, 1999

Wittchen HU, Feutsch M, Sonntag H, Muller N & Liebowitz M. Disability and quality of life in pure and comorbid social phobia: findings from a controlled study. Eur Psychiatry 15, 46–58, 2000

Wittchen HU & Beloch E. The impact of social phobia on quality of life. Int Clin Psychopharmacol 11 (Suppl 3), 15–23, 1996

Yao SN, Note I, Fanget F, Albuisson E, Bouvard M, Jalenques I & Cottraux J. Social anxiety in social phobics: Validation of Liebowitz's social anxiety scale – French version. Encephale 25 (5), 429–435, 1999

Chapter 5
Panic disorder

1 Introduction

Patients with PD experience recurrent episodes of panic, characterised by an intense feeling of impending doom or apprehension. These effects may be accompanied by several physical manifestations of anxiety (see Tab. 5.1). A three-part phenomenological model for PD has been formulated (Klein, 1981). The acute panic attack is the keystone of this model, characterised by sudden and spontaneous, crescendo-like onset of autonomic symptoms and a subjective sense of dread. These attacks last between 10 and 30 min in most instances, and then the patient returns to baseline functioning. The second feature is anticipatory anxiety. The patient begins to worry that an attack will occur again. Rather than returning to baseline after each attack, the patient now exists in a more chronic state of anxiety, always anticipating the onset of an attack. Finally, a subset of patients with PD develops phobic avoidance. In many of these patients, incapacitating agoraphobia supervenes, as they fear leaving the security of home in case a panic attack occurs. The question of whether panic attacks play a fundamental role in the development of agoraphobia remains controversial (Klein et al., 1983; Basoglu et al., 1994). Nevertheless, most patients with agoraphobia had panic attacks before becoming phobic (DeNardo et al., 1983; Noyes et al., 1986; Uhde et al., 1985).

PD, which is twice as common among women as among men, is an anxiety disorder whose defining feature is recurrent panic attacks. It is a chronic disorder, with fluctuations in panic frequency and intensity over time, accompanied by variations in phobic avoidance. Panic attacks are highly prevalent in the community. A recent world-wide epidemiologic survey demonstrated that 12% of primary care patients experience at least one panic attack during their lifetimes and 3.5% have a history of PD (Lecrubier and Üstün, 1998). Prompt recognition and treatment of panic attacks is important because sufferers are at particular risk of developing other psychiatric conditions such as agoraphobia, anxiety and depression (Ballenger, 1998).

A recent study showed that among women, PD is frequently associated with comorbid agoraphobia and that these Axis I disorders seems to develop on an underlying anxious-fearful personality (Barzega et al., 2001). The presence of an anxious trait may explain other characteristics of PD in women, in particular the more chronic course of illness. Among men PD is more commonly associated with a more severe personality psychopathology.

Antipanic therapy is almost always chronic in nature. Many antipanic agents are also antidepressants, although not all antidepressant agents are effective against panic.

2 Diagnosis and aetiology

A panic attack is a discrete period of intense fear or discomfort during which some somatic symptoms of anxiety, such as dyspnea, chest pain, palpitations, dizziness, and choking, develop abruptly and reach a peak within 10 minutes. One of the most important symptom combinations is that of palpitations, sweating, shortness of breath and fear of dying. This combination of symptoms is often interpreted by patients as a heart attack, and it brings them to the emergency room. However, panic attacks can occur in situations of extreme stress in people who do not have PD and isolated attacks do not indicate a diagnosis of PD. According to the DSM-IV (see Tab. 1), PD may be diagnosed when there are recurrent, unexpected panic attacks and preoccupation with the panic attacks for at least 1 month, such as the person acknowledges persistent concern about future attacks, worries about the implications or consequences of attacks, or makes significant changes in behaviour to avoid attacks (APA, 1994). Frightened of the recurrence of panic, such patients do not want to be in places or situations where they believe they could be either physically or socially trapped, or alone and unable to get help. Patients with these symptoms generally exhibit an increased sensitivity to anxiogenic agents (adrenaline, isoprenaline, yohimbine, fenfluramine, sodium lactate, carbon dioxide, β-carbolines and caffeine).

Panic attacks can also be generated through a number of pharmacological stimulants, such as sodium lactate, carbon dioxide, yohimbine, *m*-CPP and most recently, the CCK tetrapeptide (CCK_4) (Albus et al., 1992; Keck et al., 1993). Recent studies have revealed that acute administration of CCK_4 or its synthetic analogue pentagastrin induces panic-like symptoms in patients with PD and healthy volunteers reliably and in a dose-dependent manner (Van Megen et al., 1994; 1996; Lines et al., 1995). The physiological and behavioural effects elicited by these compounds closely resemble the symptom profile during naturally occurring panic attacks. Furthermore, patients display an enhanced sensitivity to challenge with CCK_B receptor agonists like pentagastrin and CCK_4, as compared to healthy subjects (Van Mergen et al., 1994). Pre-treatment with the CCK_B antagonist L-365, 260 reduced the propensity of CCK_4 to induce panic attacks in PD patients as well as the number and intensity of anxiety symptoms in a dose-dependent fashion (Bradwejn et al., 1994). A study that investigated the effect of the SSRI fluvoxamine on CCK_4-induced panic attacks showed that treatment with fluvoxamine (150 mg daily) significantly decreased the sensitivity of PD patients for CCK_4 while placebo was without effect (Van Megen et al., 1997). Of the patients who responded to treatment, 83% no longer experienced a panic attack when rechallenged with CCK_4, whereas in the non-responder group this was only 28%. In the fluvoxamine group, the treatment response assessed by the HAM-A showed a statistically significant treatment effect. The results of this study strengthen the validity of the CCK_4 test as an experimental human model for panic attacks. It also yields evidence to support that both CCK_4 and 5-HT are implicated in the regulation of panic attacks.

The large number of physical symptoms reported by PD patients raises the possibility that there is a diagnostic overlap between it and somatization disorder

Table 5.1: DSM-IV criteria for panic attack (4 of the 13 criteria required for diagnosis)

1.	Palpitations, pounding heart, or accelerated heart rate
2.	Sweating
3.	Trembling or shaking
4.	Sensation of shortness of breath or smothering
5.	Feeling of choking
6.	Chest pain or discomfort
7.	Nausea or abdominal distress
8.	Dizziness, unsteadiness, light-headedness, or faintness
9.	Derealization (external environment does not appear real) or depersonalisation (self does not feel real)
10.	Fears of losing control or going crazy
11.	Fears of dying
12.	Presthesias
13.	Chills or hot flushes

(Katon, 1984; Katon et al., 1987). Two studies of panic patients found prevalence rates of somatization disorder varying from 25% by DSM-III criteria to 71% according to the Feighner criteria (King et al., 1986; Sheehan & Sheehan, 1982). Conversely, estimates of the prevalence of PD in patients with somatization disorder (or Briquet's Syndrome) range from 10 to 45% (Liskow et al., 1986; Swartz et al., 1986; Zoccolillo & Cloninger, 1986). Such findings have led to question the validity of the categorical distinction between somatization and other Axis I disorders, including panic (Orenstein, 1989).

The aetiology of PD remains unknown, although investigators have identified several contributory factors. First, there may be a genetic predisposition (Weissman, 1993; Kendler et al., 1995). Family members of patients with PD have a greater prevalence of the disorder than do relatives of controls without PD (Goldstein et al., 1994; Battaglia et al., 1995).

Developmental factors and temperament may play a role, including a history of separation anxiety with parents (King et al., 1994; Silove et al., 1995; Shear, 1996). Among some patients, there appears to be an association between PD and traumatic experiences. These include traumatic suffocation, family dysfunction, and sexual abuse, the last being more common among women (David et al., 1995; Stein et al., 1996; Moisan & Engels, 1995). In addition to the proposed causative factors for PD symptoms, other factors including psychosocial stressors, illness, drugs such as caffeine, marijuana and cocaine, and even severe weight loss may be involved (Charney et al., 1985).

Sleep panic attacks are frequent in patients with PD. It has been suggested that sleep panic attacks occurred in the transition phase between stage 2 and stage 3 sleep (Hauri et al., 1989). It appears that nocturnal panic attacks are unique, different from stage 4 sleep terrors, and different from dream anxiety attacks. In fact, patients with recurrent sleep panic had significantly more panic attacks per week than those without sleep panic (Agargün et al., 1996). In addition, the patients with recurrent sleep panic had more severe panic symptoms than others. The recurrent sleep panickers were more severely ill than the other panickers. Sleep panic attacks may affect clinical variables and modify the severity of illness in patients with PD. The prevalence of sleep panic may be as high as 62% and the prevalence of recurrent sleep panic as high as 40% (Agargün & Kara, 1997). Sleep panic seems to be in relation to the presence of major depression and to modify the severity of illness.

2.1 Comorbidity

Comorbidity between panic and depression is common: two-thirds of primary care patients with current PD also meet diagnostic criteria for depression (Lecrubier & Üstün, 1998). Panic-depression comorbidity leads to greater symptomatology, in terms of frequency and severity of panic attacks, work and social impairment, chronic illness and increased use of medical services.

Twenty-seven percent of the patients with PD, 18% with major depression and 11% with neither disorder had experienced, at some point in their life, alcohol problems meeting the DSM-III criteria for alcohol abuse (Weissman, 1991; Bandelow, 1999; Pollack & Marzol, 2000). PD, like major depression, is associated with the self-perception of poor physical and emotional health, increased risk of alcohol abuse and marital and financial problems, increased medication and emergency room use and suicide attempts (Weissman, 1991). These impairments are important to consider in the assessment of the risks and benefits of currently available short and long-term treatments of PD.

2.2 Epidemiology

PD has a prevalence of 1–2% and results in considerable morbidity and increased mortality (Weissman et al., 1997; Katerndahl & Realini, 1993; Katon, 1996). Epidemiological studies have found that PD is most common at the age from 30 to 44 years and panic attacks usually have their onset in young adulthood (Weissman, 1992; Timmerman, 1995). However, it is uncommon in late life and it rarely starts for the first time after the sixth decade of life (Regier et al., 1988; Flint, 1994). However, one study that examined anxiety disorders in elderly patients (ages 60 and older) reported that PD can begin in later life (Raj et al., 1993). Although some evidence suggests a bimodal age at onset of panic attacks, in general late onset panic attacks represents a less severe disorder associated with lower levels of comorbidity, less hypochondriasis and a greater number of positive coping behaviours (Katerndahl & Talamantes, 2000).

PD, as well as panic attacks, is twice as frequent in women compared with men (Andrade et al., 1996; Lydiard, 1996; Yonkers et al., 1998). PD appears to have some distinct features in women who report more individual panic-related symptoms (Dick et al., 1994, 1994a). Women also have an elevated risk of developing agoraphobia and other avoidance behaviours as a complication of PD (Andrade et al., 1996; Yonkers et al., 1998). Comorbid psychiatric disorders, such as GAD and simple phobia, also are more common in women with PD (Marshall, 1996; Wisner et al., 1996).

Women with PD also appear to be particularly vulnerable to somatization disorder as a comorbid condition (Yonkers et al., 1998; Marshall, 1996). In fact, some studies suggest that somatization disorder is 4 times more likely to occur in women with PD (Battaglia et al., 1995). Women with comorbid PD and somatization disorder are more likely to have relatives with antisocial personality disorder (Battaglia et al., 1995). Greater risk for comorbid disorders may also contribute to the greater functional impairment and more severe clinical course reported in women with PD in comparison with men with PD (Wisner et al., 1996; Hollifield et al., 1997).

Relapses are common after short-term treatment periods and maintenance treatment is often required since a substantial subgroup of patients suffer from persistent attacks and agoraphobia (Barlow, 1992). Depression appears to occur in a high percentage of patients with PD, which may be related to the uncontrollable nature of panic attacks. Suicidal ideation and suicide attempts are common in PD and often associated with lifetime diagnosis of major depressive disorder episodes and alcohol and other substance abuse (Weissman et al., 1989; Lepine et al., 1993). A recent study designed to clarify the linkage between panic-specific clinical and cognitive variables and suicide indicators in patients with PD seems to confirm this association between PD and suicide (Schmidt et al., 2001). A number of significant predictors for suicidal ideation (e.g., overall anxiety symptoms, level of anticipatory anxiety, avoidance of bodily sensations, attentional vigilance toward bodily perturbations and phrenophobia, i.e. fear of cognitive incapacitation was reported. Such relationship between panic attacks and suicide attempts has also been reported in adolescence (Pilowsky et al., 1999). In a study that controlled for demographic factors, major depression, the use of alcohol, and the use of illicit drugs in 13- to 14-year-old adolescents, it was observed that adolescents with panic attacks were three times more likely to have expressed suicidal ideation and approximately two times more likely to have made suicide attempts than adolescents without panic attacks. In a naturalistic 6-year study designed to study PD patients who developed major depression in the long-term, a sample of 55 patients initially treated with alprazolam or imipramine during a period of 9 weeks were followed up (Lepola et al., 1996). At the beginning of the study, patients with major depression were excluded. At the 3-year visit six patients had major depression. At the 6-year visit, nine patients had developed an episode of major depression, but five of them had no panic attacks. Five patients had mild, three had moderate and one patient had severe depression. This study shows that PD patients had prolonged anxiety symptoms lasting for years in many cases and indicating a long-term drug treatment.

3 Pathophysiology

The first episode of panic attacks occurs in many patients, especially women, upon either threatened or actual separation from or loss of a loved person. Such patients often have histories of childhood separation anxiety. A common precipitant for male patients is a life-threatening event or illness.

One of the most striking features of a patient's description of an acute attack is the physical nature of these symptoms. Unlike other forms of anxiety, in which affects like worry and tension predominate, patients with PD invariably begin describing the illness with reference to their hearts, lungs, gastrointestinal tracts and "nerves". A number of agents such as sodium lactate, carbon dioxide, yohimbine, caffeine, isoproterenol and NE have been shown to produce an anxiety attack in panic patients if given in the laboratory (Liebowitz et al., 1986; Gorman et al., 1988; Charney et al., 1984; Uhde et al., 1986; Rainey et al., 1984; Pyke & Greenberg, 1986). The three agents that have been most extensively studied are sodium lactate, carbon dioxide and yohimbine. It is most likely that each one of these has its primary effect on one or more brainstem loci that, when triggered, provoke the massive autonomic discharge characterising the panic attack.

One group of theories views the panic attack as an alarm reaction triggered by signs of impending suffocation. These theories followed from the observation of a close relationship between PD and respiratory abnormalities, including dyspnea, signs of abnormal ventilatory control and enhanced sensitivity to biological "suffocation indicators" such as CO_2, lactate, and doxopram (Klein, 1993). These theories are being extended to childhood anxiety disorders. Several groups note an association between various childhood anxiety disorders and smothering respiratory illness (Pine et al., 1994; 1998b; Mrazek, 1992). Moreover, preliminary evidence suggests the presence of similar abnormalities in ventilatory physiology among children with anxiety disorders and adults with PD (Pine et al., 1997). It has also been suggested that childhood separation anxiety disorder may predispose to PD through the effect of separation experiences on the respiratory and endorphin systems (Klein, 1993). Consistent with this hypothesis, it was shown that separation from a "safe person" moderates the anxiogenic response to CO_2 challenge in adult PD.

Fear of panic is a specific, focused anxiety that may be manifest in a variety of ways, such as preoccupation or worry about having a panic attack, the degree of expectation or prediction that a panic attack may occur, and a tendency to fear panic, the consequences of panic, or the bodily sensations associated with panic. It has now been established that a fear of the bodily sensations is a consistent characteristic of patients with PD, but there is a controversy over whether this is a cause or a consequence of panic, or both.

Anticipatory anxiety is a central symptom of PD and its measurement is essential. To fully understand the meaning of anticipatory anxiety, three separate constructs embedded in the idea of fear of panic may be described. The first one is the worried or apprehensive preoccupation with having a panic attack. The second construct is the specific expectation or prediction that a panic attack will occur and will be dangerous. Finally, the ongoing tendencies to fear and/or fear-related bodily sensations are noteworthy. Most current treatment studies include a daily rating of the degree of preoccupation, worry, or anxious anticipation about having a panic episode and this type of measure is essential. Anticipatory anxiety is variable enough to lead to a strong endorsement of the use of a daily self-report. Both the frequency (i.e. percent of the day spent worrying about having a panic attack) and the intensity of the anxiety should be recorded. A standard time frame for assessing anticipatory anxiety, matched to the panic time frame (i.e. 2 weeks) is highly useful. A measure of prediction or expectation of having a panic episode in the near future (e.g. in the next week) is useful as is a measure of prediction of panic severity. The expectation of panic could be measured with Likert scales incorporated into the daily diary. The patient should be asked to rate the likelihood of experiencing a panic episode in the next week (subjective probability of panic, panic expectancy) and to rate its expected aversiveness.

A measure of phobic symptoms is essential. Phobic fear and avoidance should be measured separately, since they occur with different frequency and respond differently to treatment. Assessment of phobic severity must always refer to fear avoidance when the patient is unaccompanied, i.e. alone. The most important consideration in rating phobic symptoms in PD patients is whether or not the phobia is panic related. In general, patients with PD tend to avoid situations or activities because they fear that the situation or activity will provoke a panic attack or because they are afraid of the consequences if an unexpected panic attack occurs. All studies of PD should include a self-report scale and a clinician's rating, encompassing both fear and avoidance.

3.1 Autonomic and central nervous system dysfunctions

PD has been conceptually linked with the sympathetic nervous system. Recently, increased cardiovascular mortality, including sudden death, has been reported in patients with PD and in men with high levels of phobic anxiety (Coryell et al., 1982; Weissman et al., 1990; Kawachi et al., 1994). These findings may provide indirect evidence of sympathetic involvement in PD because the cardiac sympathetic nerves have a critical role in the development of fatal ventricular arrhythmias (Esther, 1992). A recent study which tested nervous system function in patients with PD by using sensitive methods such as direct nerve recording (clinical microneurography) suggested that whereas muscle sympathetic activity, arterial plasma concentration of NE and the total and cardiac NE spillover rates to plasma were similar in patients and control subjects at rest, epinephrine spillover from the heart was elevated in patients with PD (Wilkinson et al., 1998). Responses to laboratory mental stress were almost identical in patient and control groups. Epinephrine is released from the heart at rest in patients with PD, possibly due to loading of cardiac neuronal stores by uptake from plasma during surges of epinephrine secretion in panic attacks. These findings support the idea that the core abnormalities in PD will not be found in the sympathetic nervous system itself, but instead in those central neurobiological systems that regulate sympathetic nervous system function. These data also suggest that the panic attack originates in the brain only secondarily if there is an excessive sympathetic nervous discharge.

PD has been associated with abnormalities of central serotonin or catecholamine neurotransmission (Paniccia & Rapaport, 1995; Sheehan et al., 1993). A role for serotonergic neuromodulation in the aetiology of PD has been suggested mainly by the observations that increased serotonergic neurotransmission increases anxiety even up to the level of panic attacks in patients with PD and that decreased serotonin uptake is present in patients with anxiety disorder (Kahn & Wetzler, 1991; Iny et al., 1994). This corresponds to the observation that in animal models an increase of serotonergic function is anxiogenic while a decrease of serotonergic function is anxiolytic (Chopin and Briley, 1987). It may therefore be hypothesised that increased serotonergic neurotransmission in PD is due to genetically determined decreased uptake. However, neuroendocrine challenge studies have not robustly supported the involvement of serotonin in PD. A study of the cortisol response to 5-hydroxytryptophan did not clearly differentiate panic patients from controls (van Vliet et al., 1996).

A challenge agent with recently discovered panicogenic properties is CCK_4. CCK_4 reliably induces somatic, sensorial and cognitive symptoms of panic attack in both PD patients and healthy subjects, with the patients being more sensitive to the action of the peptide. The panic symptoms are usually accompanied by an increase in anxiety and fear (Bradwejn et al., 1990, 1991, 1992; Jerabek et al., 1999).

There is a strong evidence of involvement of the BDZ site in PD. Inverse agonists are specifically panicogenic in man (Dorow et al., 1983). Agonists reduce anxiety and panic symptoms but are less effective in PD patients than in controls and antagonists provoke panic attacks in PD patients in a dose-dependent manner (Roy-Byrne et al., 1990; Nutt et al., 1990). These observations have led to theories that there may either be a "shift" in BDZ-$GABA_A$ receptor function in PD or that putative endogenous agonists are released which are not, however, sufficient in blocking the symptoms (Nutt et al., 1990).

The GABA system is another leading candidate for the central neurobiologic system regulating sympathetic nervous system function where an abnormality could explain the pathogenesis of PD. Among other evidence, GABA-ergic transmission is critical to the function of the brain areas involved in fear and anxiety (Charney et al., 1998; Nutt et al., 1990; Robertson et al., 1978; Rago et al., 1988).

PD has been consistently associated with a blunting of GH responses to challenges of clonidine (an α_2-adrenergic agonist) and GH releasing factor (Rapaport et al., 1989, Uhde et al., 1992). Neurohormonal factors may be involved in some cases (Boulenger et al., 1996; Abelson & Curtis, 1996; Birchall, 1994). Exogenous progesterone and triphasic oral contraceptives have been associated with the induction of panic attacks (Wagner & Berenson, 1994; Deci et al., 1992).

Sodium lactate infusion is reported to reliably provoke panic in patients with PD, but at least one third of patients and possibly more have no marked response (Pitts & McClure, 1967; Liebowitz et al., 1984). In general, racemic sodium lactate is a stronger panic inducer than either carbon dioxide or sodium bicarbonate (Klein, 1991). This difference in potency may be due to the fact that racemic lactate induces panic by two synergistic mechanisms: (1) conversion to carbon dioxide and (2) a direct, pharmacologic stimulation of a suffocation alarm.

The DST has been most widely studied as a marker for primary or endogenous major depression. The occurrence of nonsuppression in PD suggests biological features common to the two disorders. Among PD patients, nonsuppression was clearly associated with intolerance to BDZ withdrawal (Coryell et al., 1989). Nonsuppressors had more severe symptoms and a lower likelihood of placebo response (Corryell and Noyes, 1988). PD patients who had shown nonsuppression before or during an 8-week study of diazepam or alprazolam were much more likely than those who had consistently normal DST results to relapse during the gradual discontinuation of these drugs 6 months later. Since DST nonsuppression in PD apparently indicates a more persistent and chronically disabling condition, this liability to symptom persistence may be long-term and endure for years (Coryell et al., 1991).

Several interesting research and clinical observations can be explained with reference to a brainstem locus for acute panic. It is possible, for example, that the putative brainstem locus or loci are prone to peripheral excitation as well. Reference to brainstem loci of panic explains the sudden, unpredictable onset of the attack and the predominance of autonomic symptoms during the attack. Such a view may explain why any stimulus, including sudden fright, that creates an asynchrony between metabolic demand and physiological function, may be capable of causing a panic attack in a susceptible individual.

There is ample reason to suggest that anticipatory anxiety is a limbic lobe phenomenon which is believed to be the centre of many basic human emotions, including rage, arousal and fear. In a study which included patients with PD and volunteers who underwent sodium lactate infusion under a PET scanning, only those patients who went on to panic during the subsequent infusion showed an abnormal symmetry in blood flow through a specific limbic structure, the parahippocampal gyrus (Reiman et al., 1984; 1986). Because the abnormality was found in subjects about to have an attack, it probably represents the cortical events of anticipatory anxiety, although this needs to be confirmed. However, another study which tested the temporal cortex activation during experimentally induced anxiety (i.v. bolus injection of 50 μg CCK_4) in normal volunteers using PET and MRI technology reported cerebral blood flow (CBF) increases in the anterior cingulate gyrus, the claustrum-insular-amygdala region, and the cerebellar vermis (Benkelfat et al., 1995). This study suggests that muscular artefacts resulting in extracranial increases in CBF might have confounded previous results linking temporal lobe activation to anxiety states. It also argues to systematically coregister structural and functional images in brain imaging studies. Clinically, anticipatory anxiety can become a greater problem for the patient than panic attacks themselves. In many cases, even when the attacks spontaneously cease to occur, the patient still dreads having them. Such patients may experience high levels of anticipatory anxiety merely by thinking of a situation associated with having an attack, such as driving a car or going to the restaurant. At times, it appears that the level of anticipatory anxiety reaches a point that by itself triggers an actual attack. This may explain the finding that patients who panic during sodium lactate infusion had higher baseline levels of anxiety immediately before infusion than nonpanicking patients (Liebowitz et al., 1984).

3.2 Brain imaging

Several observations suggest that PD should be characterised by right frontal hyperactivation. The right hemisphere predominantly controls and processes autonomic changes and interoceptive perceptions, both important factors in the development and maintenance of PD (Ehlers & Breuer, 1992; Pauli et al., 1991). Most patients with PD are characterised by avoidance withdrawal behaviour, which seems to be controlled by right frontal brain regions (Rachman, 1988; Sutton & Davidson, 1997). A recent study which examined FBA in patients with PD supports the hypothesis that patients with PD are characterised by greater activation of a right frontal avoidance-withdrawal system in negatively valenced situations (Wiedemann et al., 1999). Whereas no FBA was found in the control participants, patients with PDs were characterised by an FBA with a relatively reduced right alpha power during rest and when confronted with anxiety-relevant stimuli (emergency situations).

In a study which employed fully quantitative [^{11}C]flumazenil PET, a global decrease in binding in BDZ-naïve, drug-free patients with PD who had no comorbid conditions and did not abuse alcohol was reported (Malizia et al., 1998). These changes were maximal in ventral basal ganglia, orbitofrontal and temporal cortex.

3.3 Respiratory function and carbon dioxide sensitivity

Hyperventilation is an important part of the pathogenesis of panic, but probably at least 50% of patients with PD show no evidence of chronic hyperventilation when evaluated at rest (Gorman et al., 1986).

A well-established finding is that patients with PD are sensitive to the panic-provoking effects of CO_2 inhalation (Gorman et al., 1994; Perna et al., 1994). This observation is central to many of the biological theories of PD pathophysiology. In fact, this characteristic has been so well replicated that CO_2 responsivity has been examined as a potential biologic risk factor for the disorder. First-degree family members of patients with PD are more likely than first-degree relatives of control subjects to experience panic attacks during 35% CO_2 inhalation (Perna et al., 1996). It was also found that PD patients who panic in response to 35% CO_2 inhalation are more likely to have a positive family history of PD than patients who are 35% CO_2-nonresponsive (Perna et al., 1996). These intriguing observations have led to the hypothesis of CO_2-responsiveness as a key biological characteristic that might be inherited in PD. Thus, CO_2 hypersensitivity has been suggested to be a "trait" marker of PD, representing an underlying vulnerability (Perna et al., 1995). This trait may be due to an inherently unstable autonomic nervous system or a "false suffocation alarm" (Papp et al., 1993; Klein, 1993). As such, respiratory measures in children, as in adults, are hypothesised to identify a familial form of anxiety that exhibits varying expressions across development. During childhood, it is associated with separation anxiety, whereas during adolescence, this form of anxiety is associated with spontaneous panic attacks that may eventually develop into PD (Pine et al. 1998a, 1998b).

A study demonstrated increased sensitivity to the 35% CO_2 during the early follicular, compared to the midluteal phase of the cycle in PD patients but not in normal controls (Perna et al., 1995). It was concluded that along with higher prevalence of PD in women, infrequent onset in the prepubertal and postmenopausal periods, and changes in panic vulnerability during pregnancy indicate a significant role of ovarian hormones in the clinical modulation of PD.

3.4 Genetic

Evidence for a genetic liability for PD has been obtained in twin as well as family studies (Torgersen, 1983; Maier et al., 1993; Battaglia et al., 1995). Studies of the diagnosis of PD (with or without agoraphobia) have also reached the same conclusion that this psychopathology is a familial phenotype (Crowe et al., 1983; Mendlewicz et al., 1993; Fyer et al., 1996). First-degree relatives of probands with PD have a three- to 21-fold higher lifetime risk of PD than relatives of unaffected probands. Analysis of pedigrees in several of these family studies have been consistent with the possibility that a single major locus contributes to the inheritance of PD, but polygenic inheritance has not been excluded (Crowe et al., 1983; Vieland et al., 1996). However, although genetically identical twins are more likely to both have PD than are twins who are no more genetically identical than ordinary brothers and sisters, there are many cases in which one identical twin has PD and the other does not. The conclusion may be that although genes are involved in causing PD, they cannot be the whole story. It seems clear that what is inherited is a susceptibility to panic rather than PD itself. Patients with PD very likely inherit a susceptibility to panic that has its basis in an unusually sensitive fear network, with the central nucleus of the amygdala playing a significant role.

3.5 Impact on cognitive processes

In a recent study designed to explore the relationship between PD and memory, anxiety and fear with verbal description of one or more fearful situations in the participants (30 patients with PD, 12 healthy volunteers, 12 with GAD and 12 with major depression) was induced and they were asked in a neutral manner what they felt if they thought of themselves in such situations (Berksun, 1999). The results of this study showed that none of the patients in the PD group could recall any acceptable fearful event or episode in their past. All but one person among healthy volunteers and all the patients with conditions other than PD could recall one or more fearful events or episodes in a period as brief as 30 s. A possible hypothesis embracing this observation is that the fear-relevant emotional-autonomic cluster in these patients is not cognitively linked to the fearful events or the scenarios of the past life memory traces. Thus, patients are unable to recall or produce any themes or scenarios other than the simple apprehension of a heart attack or a similar fear. Patients with PD have a defect in fear-relevant episodic memory, and their panic attacks arise from automaticity in recollecting fear-relevant emotional-automatic cluster. The cluster as a component of fear appears to have been dissociated from cognitive structure, episodic or informative memory trace, or from information structure.

In the use of structured interviews, there have been some discussions (Shear & Maser, 1994). The structured format and the time-consuming nature of these interviews have led to the practice of hiring junior individuals with little or no clinical experience to conduct these interviews. There was concern that such a practice could lead to significant error. It is recommended that an experienced clinician be involved in the final diagnostic decision.

4 Treatments

4.1 Psychological

The behavioural cognitive treatment of PD is based on Clark's model of the disorder (Clark, 1986). This states that patients experience panic because they persistently interpret a range of bodily sensations in a catastrophic way. The sensations that are misinterpreted are usually those that are involved in normal anxiety responses. The patient believes that these symptoms are indicative of immediate impending physical or mental disaster and this belief worsens the anxiety symptoms.

The behavioural cognitive treatment of PD consists of helping the patient to construct alternative non-threatening interpretations of the sensations, using cognitive restructuring and behavioural experiments.

Desensitisation and exposure may be the best remedy for phobic avoidance, but substantial numbers of patients do not respond to these treatments or to other forms of psychotherapy, including dynamic psychotherapy.

In younger adults, cognitive-behavioral therapy is considered more effective than supportive or psychodynamic therapy for panic. Thus far, there is no evidence to suspect that older adults respond differently. In a recent study, 15 older PD patients (ages 55–80) were treated with ten 90-minute sessions of individual cognitive-behavioral therapy, including diaphragmatic breathing, relaxation, cognitive techniques and interoceptive and *in vivo* situational exposure (Swales et al., 1996). The goal of interoceptive exposure is to reduce the fear of internal somatic states such as breathlessness, dizziness, or accelerated heart rate. Patients voluntarily bring on these states by hyperventilating, spinning in a chair, jogging in place, and so on until they are able to tolerate the associated physical sensations. Treatment gains in frequency and severity of panic attacks, behavioural avoidance, cognitive measures, decreased self-reported physiological arousal, depressive symptoms and role impairment were achieved and maintained at a 3-month follow-up.

4.2 Pharmacological

Several studies have demonstrated that medications, particularly those that affect serotonergic neurotransmission and cognitive behavioural therapy, are indeed robustly effective in patients with PD (Kent et al., 1998; Welkowitz et al., 1991; Papp et al, 1997). In general, drugs that have been shown to have efficacy in the treatment of PD are as follows: tricyclic antidepressants, SSRIs, BDZs and MAOIs (see Tab. 5.2). They cause a global reduction of panic and agoraphobia.

4.2.1 *Benzodiazepines*

It has been well established that the BDZs are effective in the treatment of PD. Brain imaging studies utilising radiolabeled BDZ receptor binding agents demonstrate reduced numbers of BDZ CNS receptors in PD. Although BDZs have been used for many years in the treatment of panic symptoms, they are not effective in comorbid depression and their use is limited by dependence problems and withdrawal reactions (Lenox et al., 1984; Hallfors & Saxe, 1993). Other disadvantages associated with BDZ use include side effects such as sedation and cognitive effects, and the need for multiple daily doses (Westenberg, 1996).

4.2.2 *Tricyclic antidepressants*

Tricyclic antidepressants have the advantage of a single daily dose, a low risk of dependence and withdrawal phenomena and efficacy against comorbid depression. Most of the studies have used imipramine or clomipramine (Zitrin et al., 1978; 1980; Sheehan et al., 1980; Kahn et al., 1987; Johnston et al., 1988). However, they have a delayed therapeutic onset of up to 4 weeks or more and induce a transient exacerbation of symptoms during the first week of treatment in approximately one third of patients (Pohl et al., 1988). In a study which assessed the efficacy of desipramine (DMI), it was shown that the number of patients having panic attacks at post-placebo showed a marginally significant reduction (pre-placebo: 10, post-placebo: 8, week 6, DMI: 3, $p < 0.06$) (Kalus et al., 1991). However, significant reduction from pre-placebo to week 6 was noted for somatic anxiety, psychic anxiety and phobic anxiety. This study raises concerns on an over-reliance on panic attack measures in relation to other PD symptomatology as the primary criterion for assessing both PD morbidity and treatment response.

It is now well established that imipramine increases anxiety, worsens somatic symptoms and precipitates panic attacks after the first dose and commonly leads to patients dropping out of treatment early (Cassano et al., 1988; Sheehan et al., 1980). The acute effect of imipramine is to exacerbate the symptoms of panic and

Table 5.2: Summaries of studies in the pharmacological treatment of panic disorder (PD). The Sheehan Panic and Anticipatory Anxiety Scale (PAAS), CBT: Cognitive behaviour therapy. SCL-90 was developed by Derogatis, 1977. Clinician Global Impression (CGI).

Drugs	Design	Results	References
SNRI			
Venlafaxine	Retrospective chart review of 9 patients in an open-label trial. Patients were given a standard screening questionnaire before their first visit: Fear Questionnaire (FQ), 13 of 14 items from Pilowsky's hypochondriasis scale, Sheehan Disability Scale (SDS), Beck Depression & Anxiety Inventory. Patients were diagnosed with SP by clinical interview using DSM-III-R. All patients had the generalised subtype of SP.	Mean final dose of venlafaxine was 146.5 mg/day (range: 56.25–300) given in a bid dosing schedule. Significant improvement was seen in the SP. The mean improvement in the FQ was 62.9% ($p < 0.02$) and 48% in the blood-injury phobia subscale ($p = 0.051$). The social/leisure subscale of the SDS improved by 55.5% ($p < 0.02$) and showed a trend toward improvement in the work subscale (47.8%, $p = 0.09$).	Kelsey, 1995
	8-week double blind, placebo controlled trial (1 site of a five-centre; 25 outpatients (20 men and 5 women; Age: 36.7 ± 11.2 yr.). 13 received venlafaxine and 12 received placebo. After 4–10 day single-blind placebo washout period, patients were randomised to either venlafaxine or placebo. Primary efficacy determinants were an 11-point CGI and the number of panic attacks as assessed by psychiatrists on a weekly basis.	Mean dose for patients receiving venlafaxine was 166 ± 39.2 mg qd. Significant differences in outcome between venlafaxine and placebo were evident at the endpoint visit for the CGI improvement score (placebo: 5.09 * 2.12, venlafaxine 7.08 ± 2.35). Although a slight decrease in panic attacks was noted after venlafaxine at endpoint (placebo: 1.73 ± 2.01, venlafaxine: 1.00 * 1.71), this did not reach significant level.	Pollack et al., 1996
	Open-label, fixed-flexible dose (mean daily dose = 47 mg/day) study in DSM-IV PD patients (n = 13, 10 women and 3 men; mean age: 34 ± 9.7; duration of illness: 7.88 ± 5.2 years) for 10 weeks duration. HAM-A was administered at weeks 1, 5 and 10. The CGI scales & SAFTEE-up event form were filled out weekly. Patients recorded panic attack at baseline and then weekly.	The mean panic attack frequency decreased from 4.15 ± 1.99 at baseline to 0 by week 10 ($p < 0.012$). Statistically significant decreases were noted from week 4 onwards ($p < 0.05$). An overall significant effect was noted from baseline to week 10 for CGI severity ($p < 0.0001$) and global improvement ($p < 0.001$). Significant changes were evident from week 4 forward for severity ($p < 0.001$). Scores on HAM-A progressively decreased over the 10-week trial (Baseline: 15.3 ± 3.6, week 5: 5.0 ± 3.9, week 10: 3.2 ± 1.6). Statistically significant decrease was evident by week 5 ($p < 0.001$) and by week 10 ($p < 0.0001$).	Papp et al., 1998

Table 5.2 (continued)

Drugs	Design	Results	References
MAOI			
Moclobemide	Randomised placebo-controlled trial. Patients were assigned to one of the 4 groups of treatment (N = 55, 1. Moclobemide + CBT, 2. Moclobemide + clinical management (psychological placebo), 3. Placebo + CBT or 4. Placebo + clinical management) for 8 weeks. The primary outcome variable was agoraphobic avoidance, assessed by the Fear Questionnaire agoraphobia subscale, ranging from 0–40. 2 other self-report measures were the Mobility Inventory & the disability scales were used. Patients kept a diary to monitor frequency, duration and intensity of panic attacks.	In the week prior to treatment, patients had an average of 4.34 (± 3.57) full attacks per week, with a mean duration of 6.32 (± 1.95) and a mean intensity of 6.32 (± 1.95) on a scale from 0–10. Both moclobemide + CBT and placebo + clinical management were superior to moclobemide + clinical management and placebo + clinical management with respect to the primary efficacy measure FQ agoraphobia at week 8.	Loerch et al., 1999
SSRI			
Sertraline	A double blind, parallel, placebo-controlled, fixed dose investigation with sertraline (50, 100 and 200 mg) or placebo (N = 178 out-patients with PD) for 12 weeks. A 2-week single-blind placebo lead-in period ensured an adequate number of panic attacks prior to randomisation upon which improvement could be compared. The PAAS provided the primary efficacy measure, the number of panics.	In the pooled sertraline treatment group, panic attacks were reduced 65% from baseline compared to a 39% reduction in the placebo group. Reductions among the sertraline dose groups favoured lower doses (71% and 83% for 50 mg and 100 mg respectively compared to 42% for 200 mg).	Londborg et al., 1999
	After 2 weeks of single-blind placebo, patients with PD, with or without agoraphobia, were randomly assigned to 10 weeks of double blind, flexible-dose treatment with either sertraline (50–200 mg/day) or placebo. The principal efficacy instrument was the PAAS scale from the number of panic attacks was obtained.	Sertraline-treated patients exhibited significantly greater improvement at end point than did patients with placebo for the primary outcome variable, panic attack frequency. Significant differences between groups were also evident for clinician and patient assessments of improvements as measured by the CGI impression ($p = 0.01$) and severity ($p = 0.009$) scales & PD severity scale ratings.	Pollack et al., 1998

Table 5.2 (continued)

Drugs	Design	Results	References
Citalopram	A double blind, placebo and clomipramine controlled parallel group 8-week study. 475 patients with PD, with or without agoraphobia, were randomised to treatment with either placebo, clomipramine 60 or 90 mg/day, or citalopram 10 or 15 mg/day, 20 or 30 mg/day, or 40 or 60 mg/day. Primary efficacy analysis was based upon the relative number of responding patients at week 8.	Treatment with citalopram at 20 or 30 mg, 40 or 60 mg and clomipramine were significantly superior to placebo as assessed by the number of patients free of panic attacks. All rating scales suggested that citalopram 20 or 30 mg was more effective than citalopram 40 or 60 mg	Wade et al., 1997
Fluoxetine	Patients who responded to acute fluoxetine treatment (a 2-week single blind placebo lead-in followed by a 10-week double blind acute therapy phase with three treatment arms of placebo or fluoxetine 10 mg or fluoxetine 20 mg) were randomised to 24 weeks of continued fluoxetine or placebo. Outcome measuresincluded an analysis of relapse (defined as worsening of CGI-Improvement score to ≥ 4 for 2 consecutive visits).	Fluoxetine responders randomised to continue on their acute-phase fluoxetine dose experienced statistically significant improve-ment in panic attack frequency and phobia rating scale score over 24 weeks of therapy, while those switched to placebo experienced worsening.	Michelson et al., 1999
Tricyclics			
Desipramine	A 6-week open trial of desipramine (50- 300 mg/day) pre-ceded by a 10 day placebo lead-in, in 15 patients with PD. Measures recorded were panic attack frequency (self-report patient diaries), somatic, psychic and phobic anxiety (SADS-Change items), global clinical impression (CGI scale) and depressive symptomatology (SCL-90).	Improvement resulted from a reduction in non-panic attack symptomatology. Significant improvement from pre-placebo to week 6 was noted for somatic anxiety, psychic anxiety and phobic anxiety. Longer duration of illness and residual psychic anxiety were associated with poorer response.	Kalus et al., 1991
5-HT1$_A$ agonists			
Gepirone	An uncontrolled 6-week study in 21 patients with concurrent DSM-III-R diagnosis of PD with agoraphobia and GAD. Scales used were the CGI, Sheehan Panic Attack, Marks and Gelder Phobia, HAM-A, HAM-D and Symptom checklist.	17 (70.6%) of patients had at least a 50% reduction in their panic attacks by week 6. Ten patients (59%) had 0 panic attacks by week 6. On the HAM-A scale, 65% had a 50% or greater reduction in total score, mostly beginning in week 1.	Pecknold et al., 1993

even to precipitate full-blown attacks. The most likely cause for this is that increased central and peripheral availability of NE leads to increased central arousal and anxiety and may also give rise to peripheral side effects such as tremor that are interpreted as panic symptoms. As a practical point, it would seem prudent to start patients on the smallest possible dose of imipramine (10 mg daily) and to increase this slowly and in small increments to minimise this problem. Thus, after chronic administration, stabilisation of NE activity would occur, with improvement in symptoms.

There have been several reports comparing treatment with imipramine alone and various behavioural or psychological therapies (Telch et al., 1985).

4.2.3 SSRIs

SSRIs are effective in reducing panic symptomatology and are better tolerated than BDZs, tricyclic antidepressants and MAOIs (Sheehan & Harnett-Sheehan, 1996; Westenberg, 1996). Because the amygdala is known to receive dense serotonergic input from the raphe nuclei, this may be a prime site for the anxiolytic action of the SSRIs, whereby an increase in 5-HT inhibits excitatory cortical and thalamic neurons (Gorman et al., 2000).

Fluvoxamine, paroxetine, sertraline and citalopram have been the most extensively studied of the SSRIs. The treatment response to SSRIs is associated with a characteristic initial, self-limited increase in anxiety, which peaks over the first week of treatment and thereafter subsides as the treatment effect emerges. Counselling patient about this adverse effect is important to prevent their premature withdrawal from treatment.

Paroxetine, the first SSRI licensed for the treatment of PD, was shown to have an efficacy equivalent to clomipramine in eliminating panic attacks and associated anxiety (Lecrubier et al., 1997). However, it had an earlier onset of action than clomipramine and was better tolerated. Since in the treatment of PD it is usual to start with low doses of SSRIs and build up the dose slowly, an initial dose of 10 mg of paroxetine is recommended, with titration up to the recommended daily dose of 40 mg (Dunner, 1998).

Sertraline has demonstrated efficacy in the treatment of PD in some placebo-controlled studies (Gorman & Wolkow, 1994). However, there are no comparative data against active treatments and its long-term effects in PD. A 10-weeks double-blind, flexible-dose study of sertraline in patients suffering from PD, with or without agoraphobia, showed that patients receiving sertraline exhibited significantly greater reductions in panic attack frequency and global severity of illness than did patients treated with placebo (Pollack et al., 1998). The initiation of treatment with a low starting dose of sertraline of 25 mg/day appears to be a useful strategy to minimise early treatment discontinuation secondary to adverse events.

Considering the efficacy of citalopram in PD, a study designed to establish and estimate its dose range in the acute treatment showed that its most advantageous benefit/risk ratio for the treatment of this disorder was associated with 20 or 30 mg/day (Wade et al., 1997). Response rates with the physician's assessment of Global Improvement Scale (CGI) and the Patient Global Improvement Scale (patCGI) was significantly greater with citalopram 20–30 mg (CGI 41%, patCGI 42%) and clomipramine (39%; 38%) than placebo (21%; 21%) at week 8. Anorgasmia appears to be the only dose-related adverse event, with patients reporting it more frequently as the dose of citalopram increased (placebo 0%, citalopram: 10–15 mg, 2%; 20–30 mg, 9%; 40–60 mg, 10%). Anorgasmia is also significantly higher in the clomipramine group when compared to placebo (placebo 0%; clomipramine 60–90 mg: 10%). A study designed to evaluate the efficacy and tolerability of citalopram in the long-term (1 year) treatment of adult outpatients with PD with or without agoraphobia showed that citalopram in the dosage range of 20 to 60 mg/day is effective, well tolerated and safe in the long-term treatment (Lepola et al., 1998). A recent study designed to compare citalopram and paroxetine in the treatment of PD showed them to have similar anti-panic properties (Perna et al., 2001).

In addition to their psychic effects, SSRIs may eliminate most of the troubling physical effects that occur during panic by affecting heart rate, blood pressure, breathing rate and glucocorticoid release, leading to a secondary decrease in anticipatory anxiety as a patient recognises that the seemingly life-threatening physical manifestations of panic have been blocked.

4.2.4 Other treatments

The 5-HT_{1A} agonists and brain CCK_B receptor antagonists have not proved clinically effective (Sheehan et al., 1993; Kramer et al., 1995). However, an uncontrolled open label 6-week study suggests that treatment with low-dose (12 mg) gepirone, a 5-HT_{1A} agonist, may induce some antipanic activity in a chronic, moderately to severely ill population with PD, agoraphobia and GAD (Pecknold et al., 1993). Of the patients, 58.8% had zero panic attacks by week 6. It was suggested that gepirone may be a more effective antipanic drug than buspirone, perhaps because gepirone is devoid of dopamine receptor affinity.

The 5-HT_3 antagonist ondansetron may be partly effective but the clinical relevance of these findings requires confirmation (Schneier et al., 1996).

Minor tranquilisers are helpful in treating the anticipatory anxiety of PD patients but do not block the panic attacks that are refractory to all classes of antipsychotic drugs that may even exacerbate the condition. In such cases, a combination of drug treatment to block panic attacks and behaviour therapy to overcome anticipatory anxiety and phobic avoidance should be more effective that either treatment administered alone.

4.2.5 Algorithm for treatment

The SSRIs may be the generally preferred pharmacological treatment in primary care of PDs. Although paroxetine is the only SSRI currently approved by the Food and Drug Administration to treat PD, other SSRIs commonly used such as sertraline and fluoxetine are also effective (Oehrberg et al., 1995; Gorman & Wolkow, 1994, Scheier et al., 1990). With regard to dosing, primary care physicians need to be advised to start low and go slow to avoid precipitating a panic attack (Altshuler, 1994).

Clinically, blockade of panic attacks with antipanic medications often does not relieve phobic avoidance. Psychotherapeutic approaches aimed at teaching the patient that nothing serious will actually occur during exposure to phobic stimuli may then be required. Such treatments are varied, ranging from simple explanation of this fact to more formal combinations of hierarchical *in vivo* desensitisation and cognitive restructuring. If the patient does not respond to an SSRI, then nefazodone, a 5-HT_2 antagonist that has been found to be particularly effective in the treatment of depression complicated by agitation and anxiety, may be used (Zajecka, 1996). However, though the SSRI appears to be the main first-line treatment prescribed by most specialists, current practice suggests some cultural differences in treatment particularly when these are administered by general practitioners (GPs).

In the United States, nearly all patients diagnosed with PD receive prescription drug therapy and SSRIs are regarded as first-line therapy. However, BDZs continue to be administered to patients although they are usually prescribed only for short-term (see Fig. 5.1). It is recognised that general practitioners tend to start their patients on an excessively high dose of SSRI therapy, a dose more commonly used to treat depression (which can cause increased anxiety) rather than starting them at the more appropriate level of approximately half of the standard antidepressant dose. Some specialists recommend treatment with cognitive behaviour therapy and pharmacological therapy to achieve the maximum response rate.

In France, although SSRIs are the standard of care, there tends to be a high preference for BDZ prescription by GPs. Interviewed specialists state that most of their patients referred from a GP are already receiving BDZs and that they find it difficult to withdraw patients from BDZs. Specialists express concern that GPs overprescribe BDZs. There may be a need to educate GPs regarding the detrimental side effects associated with BDZ use and withdrawal as well as the advantages of prescribing SSRIs. In general, psychiatrists prescribe SSRIs for more than 50% of patients for a period of six months. For patients older than age 50 who have been on tricyclic antidepressant therapy, physicians often recommend switching to an SSRI because of the anticholinergic side effects of the tricyclics.

In Germany, SSRIs are prescribed to the vast majority of patients (90% or more) while a small minority of them receive tricyclic antidepressants and MAOI. German physicians often prescribe herbal and plant-based pharmaceuticals for PD. This practice is unique to Germany. Physicians report that an average of 10% of patients are prescribed BDZs. However, this percentage includes those patients in whom short-term use is indicated. More than half of the patients receive cognitive behaviour therapy with pharmacological therapy. Experts maintain that when cognitive behaviour therapy is used in conjunction with pharmacological therapy, treatment is successful in about 80% of patients.

In Spain, many doctors choose to administer a BDZ in conjunction with a low-dose SSRI, then to gradually increase the dose of the SSRI while simultaneously tapering the patient off the BDZ. As a result, the patient may be taking only an SSRI or an SSRI with a minimally effective dose of a BDZ. If the SSRI fails, the physician

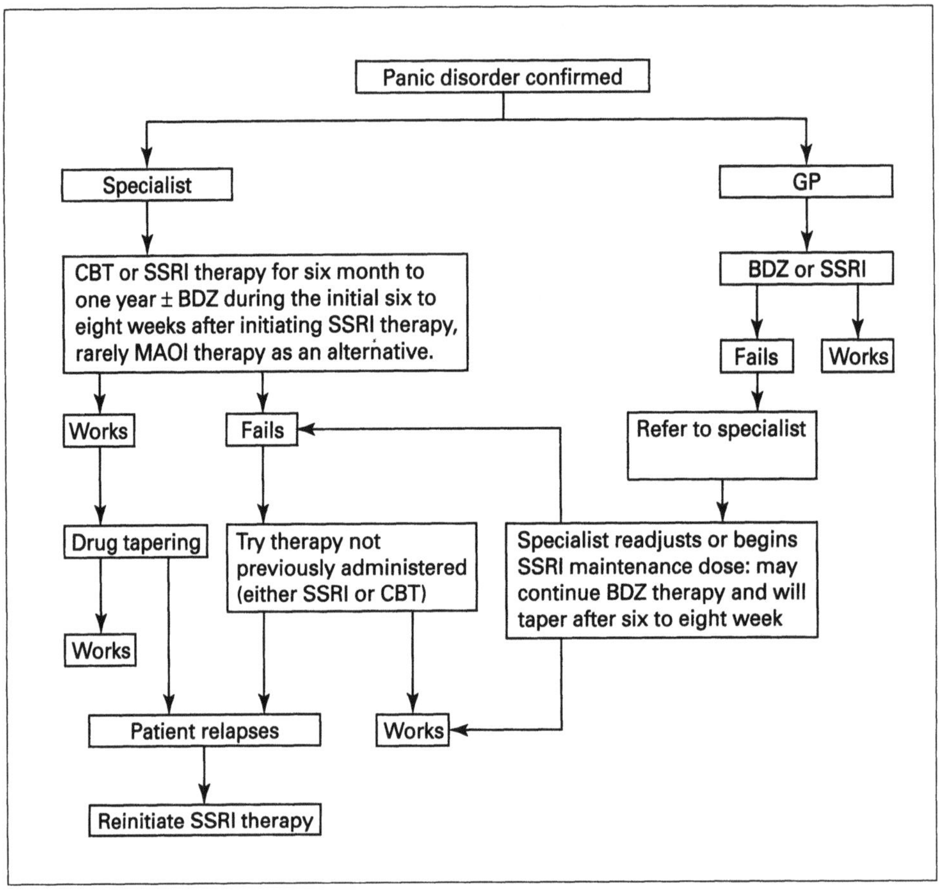

Figure 5.1
Current treatment procedure for panic disorder in the United States.

may choose to switch to a tricyclic or MAOI. Psychotherapy is not widely used in the management of PD in Spain.

In the United Kingdom, patients with PD are much less likely to receive specialist attention than patients in the other countries because GPs tend to be more conservative about referring patients. The SSRIs, particularly paroxetine, have become the preferred first-line treatment among GPs. However, unlike in the other countries, GPs in the United Kingdom continue to prescribe beta blockers as a non-addictive alternative to the BDZs. Specialists criticise the use of beta blockers for PD treatment because randomised, placebo-controlled trials failed to demonstrate that beta blockers are more effective than placebo. Specialists agree that patients receiving both cognitive behaviour therapy and prescription drug therapy show the most rapid improvement.

In Japan, BDZs are prescribed to nearly 100% of patients diagnosed with PD. In addition, unlike in Europe and the United States, tricyclic antidepressants are prescribed in approximately 50% of patients and beta blockers are prescribed in approximately 15% of patients either in conjunction with BDZs or rarely, alone. Doctors may use brief psychotherapy or patient education in addition to drug therapy.

5 Methodology for clinical investigation

The field has grappled with the problem of appropriate outcome measures for PD. Reduction of panic attack frequency has been widely utilised but has been unreliable as a single measure, and most investigators now use multidomain measures.

A daily, self-reported measure of panic attacks (sometimes referred to as a panic diary) is essential to all studies of PD. Limited symptom episodes, including autonomic surges, are monitored along with full panic episodes. The self-report should include such information as the time of day, the duration and severity of panic episodes, the severity of each of the individual symptoms, and an indication of whether the episode was unexpected situation bound or situation predisposed. There should also be a way to register the degree of the increment over the baseline anxiety. Accurate assessment of panic attacks requires a discussion with the patients to establish that they understand how to identify and monitor panic. A script with a graphic illustration of the type of onset and escalation of panic sensations may be helpful.

Panic frequency is highly variable. When an unstable signal is being measured, longer time frames are preferable. A minimum length of monitoring time for panic frequency should be 2 weeks, although 4 weeks is preferable (Shear & Maser, 1994). An entry criterion for panic frequency is important in studying where panic is the main target symptom. When an entry criterion for panic frequency was used, there was a lower placebo response rate for a requirement of two than for one panic episode per week. This may suggest that a requirement for panic attacks may select for severe illness, counteracting to some extent the problem of regression to the mean. However, it is conceivable that one may wish to study treatment of PD in patients with clinically significant anticipatory anxiety and/or phobic avoidance, even if current panics are infrequent. In this case, an entry criterion for panic frequency would not be used.

5.1 Psychometric scales

The Panic-Associated Symptom Scale (PASS) measures the severity of the core symptoms of PD (Deltito et al., 1991). It is not a diagnostic scale and does not include items such as insomnia, poor concentration, generalised anxiety and depressed mood. Considering the daily fluctuations in PD symptoms, the score is taken from an assessment of the previous week's symptoms.

The items are displayed in Table 5.3. The five core symptoms include situational attacks, limited symptoms attacks, anticipatory anxiety and phobia score. Situational is defined as occurring in or when just about to enter a situation known from past

Table 5.3.: PASS score

> 3 Symptoms panic attacks		**Score**		**Item code**
Situational (SiPA)	Number in last week =	0	0	
		1	1	PASS 1
		2–7	2	
		8+	3	
	Average intensity =	0–3	0	
		4–6	1	PASS 2
		7–9	2	
		10	3	
Spontaneous (SpPA)	Number in last week =	0	0	
		1	1	PASS 3
		2–7	2	
		8+	3	
	Average intensity =	0–3	0	
		4–6	1	PASS 4
		7–9	2	
		10	3	
Limited symptom attacks (LSA)	Number in last week =	0	0	
		1–8	1	PASS 5
		8+	2	
	Average intensity =	0–3	0	
		4–6	1	PASS 6
		7–10	2	
Anticipatory anxiety (AA)	Number in last week =	0	0	
		1–30	1	
		31–60	2	PASS 7
		61–90	3	
		91–100	4	
	Average intensitiy =	0–3	0	
		4–6	1	PASS 8
		7–9	2	
		10	3	
Phobia Score (PS)	Overall phobia score =	0	0	
		1–2	1	
		3–4	2	PASS 9
		5–6	3	
		7–8	4	
		9–10	5	

experience to be associated with panic attacks. All non-situational attacks are labelled spontaneous attacks, which therefore include attacks that might be triggered by cognitions or physical stimuli but do not occur in or just before entering phobic situations. Each type of attack has two components, frequency and intensity.

Panic attacks are distinct from most other symptoms in that they have an all-or-nothing quality and patients' distress levels vary from no panic attacks to any panic attacks at all. The PASS is intended to be a more valid measure than individual symptoms, such as panic attacks. Its comprehensiveness and higher correlations with disability and global improvement scores make it a useful clinical tool. Data from a large body of patients generally confirm the scoring ranges and balances of items with proof for concurrent validity and internal consistency (Deltito et al., 1990).

Data suggest that the presence of anxiety focused on bodily sensations may be predictive of posttreatment outcome in both medication and psychosocial treatments (Clark, 1995). There are several measures available to rate this dimension of anticipatory anxiety, including the Anxiety Sensitivity Inventory (ASI), the Agoraphobic Cognitions and the Body Sensations questionnaires, the Panic Appraisal Inventory and the Panic Belief Questionnaire (Reiss et al., 1986; Peterson & Reiss, 1992; Chambless et al., 1984; Greenberg, 1989). More recently, the Suffocation Fear Scale (SFS) has been devised (Taylor & Rachman, 1994). However, the most widely used measure of anxiety sensitivity is the ASI, a 16-item self-report measure that assesses fear of anxiety and beliefs about possible consequences of anxiety (e.g., "It scares me when I feel faint"). The ASI has been translated into many languages, including Spanish, German, French, Hebrew, Greek, Mandarin and Dutch. In particular, studies utilising the ASI have demonstrated that anxious responding to panicogenic challenges can be predicted by high scores on this measure (Rapee et al., 1992; McNally, 1994). Moreover, individuals with high ASI scores report more intense panic symptoms following voluntary hyperventilation when compared with low ASI participants (Asmundson et al., 1994) Thus, the ASI is commonly used in studies of PD as a self-reported index of fears of anxiety symptoms. On the other hand, the SFS was created to assess anxiety related to suffocation, which has been shown to be a central component of claustrophobic reactions (Booth & Rachman, 1992). The underlying rationale for the measure is that claustrophobic reactions can be accounted for by fears of suffocation and restriction. However, the results of a recent study suggest that the ASI may be a more useful tool than the SFS in predicting self-reported and respiratory responses to CO_2 challenges in PD patients (Shipherd et al., 2001).

A new measure of severity and impairment called the Panic Disorder Severity Scale (PDSS) using the Yale-Brown Obsessive Compulsive Scale (Y-BOCS) as a model has been developed (Shear et al., 1997; Goodman et al., 1989). The 7-item interview rates criterion symptoms separately on a 0 to 4 scale. Items include panic frequency, distress during panic, severity of anticipatory anxiety, agoraphobic fear/avoidance, fear/avoidance of physical sensations, and panic-related impairment in work and in social situations. The use of the PDSS as a single measure of key areas of PD symptomatology in clinical trials is recommended. However, since it is a new instrument, further research is required to validate its use in the long-term follow-up of patients and determine scores in a normal population and in a primary care setting.

The Comprehensive Panic Profile (CPP) is a comprehensive self-report instrument designed to assess seven aspects of panic symptomatology including panic frequency, panic severity, panic cognitions, fear of panic symptoms, avoidance, panic coping strategies, and confidence in panic strategies (Clum, 1990a; 1990b; 1995). Each of the seven sections of the CPP may be described as follows:

1. *Frequency of panic attacks*
   The frequency of panic attacks (FPA) questionnaire assesses the frequency of full- and limited-symptom panic attacks over a 2-week period in a retrospective fashion (Clum, 1995). This inventory lists the 13 DSM-IV symptoms of a panic attack and provides a description of both a full- and limited-symptom panic attack. The patient is required to estimate the number of full- and limited-symptom attacks in the last 2 weeks. This particular method of assessing panic attacks is commonly used in the treatment outcome literature (Gould et al., 1993; Barlow et al., 1989).
2. *Panic Attack Symptoms Questionnaire*
   The Panic Attack Symptoms Questionnaire (PASQ) is a 36-item questionnaire designed to assess (Clum et al., 1990) the severity of symptoms experienced during a typical recent panic attack. Participants are asked to endorse the presence and duration of a range of panic attack symptoms on a 5-point Likert scale. Higher scores on this inventory reflect more severe panic attacks. Prior research has supported the validity of using symptom duration as a measure of panic severity with good reliable consistency (Clum et al., 1990; Febbraro et al., 1999). The PASQ has also been shown to have adequate discriminant validity in distinguishing between patients with anxiety problems who panic *versus* those who do not (Clum et al., 1990).
3. *Panic Attack Cognitions Questionnaire*
   The Panic Attack Cognitions Questionnaire (PACQ) is a 25-item scale developed to measure negative cognitions associated with a typical panic attack (Clum et al., 1990). Patients are required to rate on a 4-point Likert scale their level of preoccupation with a series of negative thoughts that occur during panic attack. Higher scores represent a more serious problem with dysfunctional thoughts during a typical panic attack. It has been suggested that the PACQ reliably differentiates patients who panic from anxious persons who do not panic and has excellent internal consistency (Clum et al., 1990; Febbraro et al., 1999).
4. *Fear of Having a Panic Attack*
   The Fear of Having a Panic Attack (FHPA) is a 15-item scale designed to assess fear of experiencing panic-related symptoms at times other than during a panic attack. This questionnaire was based on the ASI but was modified to reflect better the notion of "fear of fear" with regard to worrying about the risk of experiencing additional panic attacks (Reiss et al., 1986; Chambless et al., 1984).
5. *Avoidance Questionnaire*
   The Avoidance Questionnaire (AQ) is a 22-item instrument based on the Motility Inventory for Agoraphobia and developed to assess level of agoraphobic avoidance (Chambless et al., 1985). Using a 5-point Likert scale, the AQ requires patients to rate their desire to escape or avoid certain situations that previous

research has shown to be problematic for individuals diagnosed with PD or PD with agoraphobia (Chambless et al., 1985).

6. *Coping Strategies Questionnaire*
The Coping Strategies Questionnaire (CSQ) is a 27-item questionnaire that uses a 5-point Likert scale to measure the frequency of the use of coping strategies to decrease or control the thoughts and feelings associated with panic attacks. Higher scores on the CSQ suggest the use of more coping strategies on a more frequent basis. The CSQ is a condensed version of the coping questionnaire that prior research has shown to have good discriminant validity (Borden et al., 1988). The CSQ was found to posses excellent internal consistency reliability (Febbraro et al., 1999).
7. *Confidence in Coping Strategies Questionnaire*
The confidence in coping strategies questionnaire (CCSQ) is a 10-item inventory designed to assess confidence in the ability to cope with problematic situations associated with panic attacks. Items are scored on a 9-point Likert scale. Higher scores denote higher degrees of confidence in one's ability to use effective techniques for coping with panic attacks. The CCSQ was shown to have good internal consistency (Febbraro et al., 1999).

5.2 Assessing response and remission

There is definition of treatment response in the DSM classification of PD. However, proposals for defining response and remission in PD were made (Ballenger et al., 1998). A response may be considered as a stable, clinically significant improvement (usually occurring after 4 to 8 weeks of treatment) such that the patient no longer has the full range of symptoms, but continues to show more than minimal symptoms. Almost complete resolution of symptoms across the five domains of PD maintained for a period of at least 3 months may be considered as full remission. To achieve such definition of remission may require at least 9 to 12 months of treatment intervention. The first 6 to 9 months may be necessary to observe the initial response and consolidation of that response. A further period of 3 months may be required to demonstrate stable and almost complete resolution of symptoms and thus meet the criterion for full remission.

6 Discussion

Because of the physical manifestations of panic attacks, which can mimic cardiorespiratory, gastrointestinal and otoneurologic illness, a high proportion of patients with PD initially present in the general medical setting (about 80%) (Simon & Vonkorff, 1991; Katerndahl & Realini, 1995). Over 70% of panic patients use primary care to obtain mental health services (Leon et al., 1997). Consequently, PD is over-represented in patient populations with chest pain and normal coronary arteries, palpitations, irritable bowel syndrome and unexplained vertigo and dizziness. Despite the increased use of health care services in panic patients, there is a high rate of physician nonrecognition of PD (61% in primary care) (Spitzer et al., 1994). Other studies have shown that even when anxiety is recognised in the primary care setting, treatment remains inadequate. Even in psychiatric settings, panic patients have markedly low rates of utilisation for both cognitive-behavioral therapy and adequate antidepressant treatment (Taylor et al., 1989; Goismann et al., 1993; Swinson et al., 1992; Yonkers et al., 1992). Hence, there is a need for improved treatment interventions for PD especially in primary care setting (Roy-Byrne et al., 1999).

Although panic attacks are an important component of the PD syndrome, their episodic nature makes them subject to substantial intrinsic variability. Hence the importance of considering multiple symptom domains when assessing outcome (Shear & Maser, 1994). Some efforts should be made to address the identification and definition of subthreshold panic symptoms. Individuals with subthreshold panic may be distressed and impaired and may respond to treatment known to be effective for PD. However, little is known about subthreshold phenomena to determine what the definition of a subthreshold PD should be. One of the puzzles in understanding PD is the frequent observation that even when patients report few or no panic attacks, they still exhibit avoidant behaviour. This has led to the widespread recommendation that clinical trials examining antipanic treatments should measure the effect of the putative treatment on more domains than just the reduction in frequency or severity of panic attacks (Shear & Masur, 1994). Agoraphobia is probably the most treatment-resistant symptom in PD. Although effective pharmacotherapy does significantly reduce agoraphobia avoidance, *in vivo* exposure is often used to decrease avoidance behaviours. There is no standard measure employed to improve agoraphobic avoidance, making comparisons across studies and treatments difficult. In a recent trial, 69% of patients became free of avoidance (Marchesi et al., 1977). Improvement in agoraphobic avoidance occurs with all the effective treatments, probably more or less equally, although this has not been rigorously studied. In general, there is too little information about the long-term course information of PD and long-term effects of treatment intervention. It may be essential to conduct a 12-month follow-up assessment after almost any treatment study. A follow-up assessment soon after the end of a treatment comparison is also recommended.

As it has been suggested, psychotherapy may work, in part, by strengthening the ability of cortical projections to assert reason over automatic behavioural and physical responses (LeDoux et al., 1996). Medications may be only partially helpful in reversing the incessantly gloomy predictions of patients with PD or in helping them rearrange relationships that are based on safety and dependency. Most studies suggest that classic BDZ receptor full agonists, the barbiturates and the 5-HT_{1A} receptor agonists, often are of limited utility in the treatment of PD. For instance, most studies point out that classic BDZ agonists require high and motor-impairing doses to alleviate panic attacks (Pollack & Rosenbaum, 1988). To truly make fair comparisons about therapeutic agents, we need a better understanding of their relative merits in the long run. Depending on the severity of the patient's symptoms that often correlate with how long a patient has had PD, psychotherapy may become invaluable. Obviously, both medication and psychotherapy can be effective treatments for PD which operate at different levels of the brain. A single measure of anxiety related to the prediction of panic may produce a conflation of two different phenomena: the expectation or prediction of having a panic attack and how bad it would be to have one. Treatments may affect these two dimensions differentially. For example, if panic attacks are suppressed with imipramine, the patient may predict or expect panic less but still dread it. Cognitive behaviour therapies may have the opposite effect: panic may still occur and still be predicted, while the dread of panic is markedly diminished.

The percentage of patients who become free of panic attacks is generally 50–80% of patients studied in acute trials lasting 6–8 weeks with multiple medications (Den Boer, 1998). In patients who are treated for longer periods, this percentage most often rises. It is generally true that the longer PD patients are treated, the more complete and comprehensive is their response. In the large cross-national trial, after 8–12 months of treatment, three fourths of patients were free of panic attacks (Cross National Collaborative Panic Study, 1993). In the recent large 12-month comparison of paroxetine and clomipramine, the respective panic-free rates were 85% and 72%, rising from an average of 55% at 3 months (Lecrubier & Judge, 1997). In general, efficacies of short-term treatments have been demonstrated, but high rates of recurrence and relapse justify the exploration of long-term treatment strategies as well. In order to prevent relapse in the discontinuation of treatment, it is suggested that it involve choosing the correct time in which the patient is stable and confident in his or her ability to manage anxiety. It should also involve family and patient eduction, followed by a slow taper of the medication over 2–6 months (Ballenger, 1992). Group behaviour therapy may be helpful in managing emergent symptoms and increasing the percentage of patients who successfully discontinue medications.

Several other studies have looked for possible predictors of non-response in PD. A comorbid depression, or even depressive symptoms, appears to be a robust predictor of non-response in long-term studies (Maier and Buller, 1988, Scheibe & Albus, 1996). These factors do not appear to be of great predictive value for short-term treatment effect (Black et al., 1994). Comorbid depression does not appear to be an obstacle for short-term treatment success with pharmacotherapy, but in the long term, it may make patients relapse. The observation of a history of major depression in patients with a lifetime PD and depressed patients who experience a panic attack at some time in their lives highlights the value of pharmacotherapy with a broad-spectrum agent that can treat the symptoms of comorbid psychiatric disorders effectively (Dunner, 1998). Clearly, the patient's quality of life needs to be taken into consideration in planning long-term treatment and also in evaluating the efficacy of its outcome. An integrated view of the issue of quality of life in patients with anxiety disorders can provide important information regarding the nature and extent of the burden associated with these disorders and may be useful in the development of strategies to deal with it (Mendlowicz & Stein, 2000). It also appears that patients who respond to placebo in PD treatment studies may show relief of symptoms but may not experience improvement in quality of life. Determinations of quality of life should be included as components of both standard clinical assessment and clinical treatment studies of patients with PD (Rapaport et al., 2000).

References

Abelson JL & Curtis GC. Hypothalamic-pituitary-adrenal axis activity in panic disorder. 24-hour secretion of corticotropin and cortisol. Arch Gen Psychiatry 53, 323, 1996

Agargün MY, Kara H, Algün E, Sekeroglu R & Tarakçioglu M. High cholesterol levels in patients with sleep panic. Biol Psychiatry 15, 1064–1065, 1996

Agargun MY & Kara H. Sleep panic attacks in patients with panic disorders: the association with major depression. Eur Psychiatry 12, 42–43, 1997

Albus M, Zahn TP & Breier A. Anxiogenic effects of yohimbine. I. Behavioral, physiological and biochemical measures. Eur Arch Psychiatry 241, 377–344, 1992

Altshuler LL. Fluoxetine-associated panic attacks. J Clin Psychopharmacol 14, 433–434, 1994

American Psychiatric Association. Diagnostic and statistical manual of mental disorders, 4th ed. Washington, DC: American Psychiatric Association, 1994

Andrade L, Eaton WW & Chilcoat HD. Lifetime co-morbidity of panic attacks and major depression in a population-based study: age of onset. Psychol Med 26, 991–996, 1996

Asmundson GJ, Norton GR, Wilson KG & Sandler LS. Subjective symptoms and cardiac reactivity to brief hyperventilation in individuals with high anxiety sensitivity. Behav Res Ther 32, 237–241, 1994

Ballenger JC. Medication discontinuation in panic disorder. J Clin Psychiatry 53S, 26–31, 1992

Ballenger JC. Comorbidity of panic and depression: implications for clinical management. Int. Clin Psychopharmacol 13 (Suppl 4), S13–S17, 1998

Ballenger JC, Davidson JRT, Lecrubier Y, Nutt DJ (International Consensus Group on Depression and Anxiety) and Baldwin DS, den Boer JA, Kasper S & Shear MK. Consensus Statement on Panic Disorder from the International Consensus Group on Depression and Anxiety. J Clin Psychiatry 59 (Suppl 8), 47–54, 1998

Bandelow B. Panic disorder – Diagnosis and differential diagnosis. Psycho 25 (12 Suppl 4), 178–184, 1999

Barlow DH, Craske MG, Cerney JA & Klosko JS. Behavioral treatment of panic disorder. Behav Ther 20, 261–282, 1989

Barlow DH. Cognitive-behavioral approaches to panic disorder and social phobia. Bull Menninger Clinic 56 (Suppl A), A14–A28, 1992

Barzega G, Maina G, Venturello S & Bogetto F. Gender-related distribution of personality disorders in a sample of patients with panic disorder. Eur Psychiatry 16, 173–179, 2001

Basoglu M, Marks IM, Kilic C, Swinson R,. Noshirvani H, Kuch K & O'Sullivan G. Relationship of panic, anticipatory anxiety, agoraphobia and global improvement in panic disorder with agoraphobia treated with alprazolam and exposure. Br J Psychiatry 164, 647–652, 1994

Battaglia M, Bernardeschi L, Politi E, Bertella S & Bellodi L. Comorbidity of panic and somatization disorder: A genetic-epidemiological approach. Compr Psychiatry 36 (6), 411–420, 1995
Battaglia M, Bertella S, Politi E, Bernardeschi L, Perna G, Gabriele A & Bellodi L. Age at onset of panic disorder: Influence of familial liability to the disease and of childhood separation anxiety disorder. Am J Psychiatry 152 (9), 1362–1364, 1995
Benkelfat C, Bradwejn J, Meyer E, Ellenbogen M, Milot S, Gjedde A & Evans A. Functional neuroanatomy of CCK4-induced anxiety in normal healthy volunteers. Am J Psychiatry 152 (8), 1180–1184, 1995
Berksun OE. Panic disorder and memory: does panic disorder result from memory dysfunction? Eur Psychiatry 14, 54–56, 1999
Birchall HM. Are gonadotrophic hormonal factors perceived to be important by women with panic attacks? Anxiety 1, 102, 1994
Black DW, Wesner RB, Gabel J, Bowers W & Monahan P. Predictors of short-term treatment response in 66 patients with panic disorder. J Affective Disord 30, 233–241, 1994
Booth R & Rachman S. The reduction of claustrophobia. I. Behav Res Ther 30, 207–221, 1992
Borden J, Clum GA, Broyles S & Watkins PL. Coping strategies and panic. J Anxiety Disord 2, 339–352, 1988
Boulenger J-P, Jerabek I, Jolicoeur FB, Lavallee YJ, Leduc R & Cadieux A. Elevated plasma levels of neuropeptide Y in patients with panic disorder. Am J Psychiatry 153, 114, 1996
Bradwejn J, Koszycki D & Meterissian G. Cholecystokinin tetrapeptide induces panic attacks in patients with panic disorder. Can J Psychiatry, 35, 83–85, 1990
Bradwejn J, Koszycki D & Shriqui C. Enhanced sensitivity to cholecystokinin tetrapeptide in panic disorder: clinical and behavioral findings. Arch Gen Psychiatry 48, 603–610, 1991
Bradwejn J, Koszycki J, Payeur D, Bourin M & Borthwick H. Replication of action of cholecystokinin tetrapeptide in panic disorder: clinical and behavioral findings. Am J Psychiatry 149, 962–964, 1992
Bradwejn J, Koszycki D, Couëtoux du Tertre A, van Megen HJGM, Westenberg HGM, Den Boer JA & Annable L. The panicogenic effects of CCK-tetrapeptide are antagonized by L-365, 260, a central CCK-tetrapeptide are antagonized by L-365, 260, a central CCK receptor antagonist in patients with panic disorder. Arch Gen Psychiatry 51, 486–493, 1994
Cassano GB, Perugi G & McNair DM. Panic disorder: review of the empirical and rational basis of pharmacological treatment. Pharmacopsychiatry 21, 157–165, 1988
Chambless DL, Caputo GC, Jasin SE, Gracely EJ & Williams C. The mobility inventory for agoraphobia. Behav Res Ther 23, 35–44, 1985
Chambless DL, Caputo GC, Bright P & Gallagher R. The assessment of fear in agoraphobics: the Body Sensations Questionnaire and the Agoraphobic Cognitions Questionnaire. J Consult Clin Psychol 52, 1090–1097, 1984
Charney DS, Grillon C & Bremner JD. The neurobiological basis of anxiety and fear: circuits, mechanisms, and neurochemical interactions, part I. Neuroscientist 4, 35–44, 1998
Charney DS, Heninger GR & Breier A. Noradrenergic function in panic anxiety: effects of yohimbine in healthy subjects and patients with agoraphobia and panic disorder. Arch Gen Psychiatry 41, 751–763, 1984

Charney DS, Heninger GR & Jatlow PI. Increased anxiogenic effects of caffeine in panic disorders. Arch Gen Psychiatry 42, 233, 1985

Chopin P & Briley M. Animal models of anxiety: The effect of compounds that modify 5-HT neurotransmission. Trends Pharmacol Sci 8, 383–388, 1987

Clark DM. Cognitive therapy for panic disorder. In: B Wolfe & JD Maser (eds): The treatment of panic disorder: A consensus development conference. Washington, DC: American Psychiatric Press, 1995

Clark DM. A cognitive approach to panic. Behav Res Ther 24, 461–470, 1986

Clum GA. Coping with panic. Pacific Grove, CA: Brooks/Cole Publishing, 1990

Clum GA, Broyles S, Borden J, Watkins PL & Hayes J. Validity and reliability of the Panic Attack Symptoms and Cognitions Questionnaires. J Psychopathol Behav Assesss 12, 233–245, 1990

Clum GA. CPP. Comprehensive Panic Profile. Unpublished manuscript, 1995

Crowe RR, Noyes R, Pauls DL & Slymen D. A family study of panic disorder. Arch Gen Psychiatry 40, 1065–1069, 1983

Coryell W, Noyes R & Clancy J. Excess mortality in panic disorder: a comparison with primary unipolar depression. Arch Gen Psychiatry 39, 701–703, 1982

Coryell W, Noyes R & Schlechte J. The significance of HPA-axis disturbance in panic disorder. Biol Psychiatry 25, 989–1002, 1989

Coryell W & Noyes R. Placebo response in panic disorder. Am J Psychiatry 145, 1138–1140, 1988

Coryell W, Noyes R Jr & Reich J. The prognostic significance of HPA-axis disturbance in panic disorder: A three-year follow-up. Biol Psychiatry 29, 96–102, 1991

Cross National Collaborative Panic Study, Second Phase Investigators. Drug treatment of panic disorder: comparative efficacy of alprazolam, imipramine and placebo. Br J Psychiatry 160, 191–202, 1993

David D, Giron A & Mellman TA. Panic-phobic patients and developmental trauma. J Clin Psychiatry 56, 113, 1995

Deci PA, Lydiard RB, Santos AB & Arana GW. Oral contraceptives and panic disorder. J Clin Psychiatry 53, 163, 1992

Deltito AN, Maier AP, Nutzinger AM, Ayuso RS & Bech P. The Panic-associated symptoms scale: measuring the severity of panic disorder. Acta Psychiatr Scand 83, 20–26, 1991

Di Nardo PA, O'Brien GT, Barlow DH, Waddell MT & Blanchard EB. Reliability of DSM-III anxiety disorder categories using a new structured interview. Arch Gen Psychiatry 40 (10), 1070–1074, 1983

Den Boer JA. Pharmacotherapy of panic disorder: Differential efficacy from a clinical viewpoint. J Clin Psychiatry 59 (Suppl 8), 30–36, 1998

Derogatis LR. SCL-90R Manual. Clinical Psychometric Research, Baltimore, MD. 1977

Dick CL, Bland RC & Newman SC. Epidemiology of psychiatric disorders in Edmonton: panic disorder. Acta Psychiatr Scand Suppl, 376, 45–53, 1994a

Dick CL, Sowa B, Bland RC & Newman SC. Epidemiology of psychiatric disorders in Edmonton. Phobic disorders. Acta Psychiatr Scand Suppl 376, 36–44, 1994b

Dorrow R, Horowski R, Paschelke M, Amin M & Braestrup C. Severe anxiety induced by FG714a b carboline ligand for benzodiazepine receptors. Lancet ii, 98–99, 1983

Dunner DL. The issue of comorbidity in the treatment of panic. Int Clin Psychopharmacol 13 (Suppl 4), S19–S24, 1998

Ehlers A & Breuer P. Increased cardiac awareness in panic disorder. J Abnorm Psychol 101, 371–382, 1992

Ester M. The autonomic nervous system and cardiac arrhythmias. Clin Auton Res 2, 133–135, 1992

Febbraro GAR, Clum GA, Roodman AA & Wright JH. The limits of bibliotherapy: A study of self-administered interventions in individuals with panic attacks. Behav Ther 30, 209–222, 1999

Flint AJ. Epidemiology and comorbidity of anxiety disorders in the elderly. Am J Psychiatry 151, 640–649, 1994

Fyer A, Mannuzza S, Chapman T, Lipsitz J, Martin L & Klein D. Panic disorder and social phobia: effects of comorbidity on familial transmission. Anxiety 2, 173–178, 1996

Goodman WK, Price LH, Rasmussen SA, Mazure C, Fleischmann RL, Hill CL, Heninger GR & Charney DS. The Yale-Brown Obsessive Compulsive Scale. I. Development, use, and reliability. Arch Gen Psychiatry 46 (11), 1006–1011, 1989

Goisman RM, Rogers MP, Steketee GS, Warshaw MG, Cuneo P & Keller MB. Utilization of behavioral methods in a multicenter anxiety disorders study. J Clin Psychiatry 54 (6), 213–218, 1993

Goldstein RB, Weissman MM, Adams PB et al. Psychiatric disorders in relatives of probands with panic disorder and / or major depression. Arch Gen Psychiatry 51, 383, 1994

Gorman JM, Cohen BS, Liebowitz MR, Fyer AJ, Ross D, Davies SO & Klein DF. Blood gas changes and hypophosphatemia in lactate-induced panic. Arch Gen Psychiatry 43 (11), 1067–1071, 1986

Gorman JM, Kent JM, Sullivan GM & Coplan JD. Neuroanatomical hypothesis of panic disorder, Revised. Am J Psychiatry 157 (4), 493–505, 2000

Gorman JM, Fyer MR, Goetz R, Askanazi J, Liebowitz MR, Fyer AJ, Kinney J & Klein DF. Ventilatory physiology of patients with panic disorder. [erratum appears in Arch Gen Psychiatry 48 (2), 181, 1991]. Arch Gen Psychiatry 45 (1), 31–39, 1988

Gorman JM, Papp LA, Coplan JD, Martinez JM, Lennon S, Goetz RR, Ross D & Klein DF. Anxiogenic effects of CO_2 and hyperventilation in patients with panic disorder. Am J Psychiatry 151 (4), 547–553, 1994

Gorman J & Wolkow R. Sertraline as a treatment for panic disorder (abstract). Neuropsychopharmacol 10 (Suppl 3), 197S, 1994

Gould RA, Clum GA & Shapiro D. The use of bibliotherapy in the treatment of panic: A preliminary investigation. Behav Ther 24, 241–252, 1993

Greenberg RL. Panic disorder and agoraphobia. In: J Scott, JMG Williams & AT Beck (eds): Cognitive therapy in clinical practice: An illustrative casebook. London, England: Routledge and Kegan Paul, 25–49, 1989

Hallfors DD & Saxe L. The dependence potential of short half-life benzodiazepines: a meta-analysis. Am J Public Health 83, 1300–1304, 1993

Hauri PJ, Friedman M & Ravaris CL. Sleep in patients with spontaneous panic attacks. Sleep 12, 323–337, 1989

Hollifield M, Katon W, Skipper B, Chapman T, Ballenger JC, Mannuzza S & Fyer AJ. Panic

disorder and quality of life: variables predictive of functional impairment. Am J Psychiatry 154 (6), 766–772, 1997
Iny LJ, Pecknold J, Suranyi-Cadotte BE, Bernier B, Luthe L, Nair NPV & Meaney MJ. Studies of a neurochemical link between depression, anxiety, and stress from (^{3}H) imipramine and (^{3}H) paroxetine binding on human platelets. Biol Psychiatry 36, 281–291, 1994
Jerabek I, Boulenger J-P, Bradwejn J, Lavallée Y-J & Jolicoeur FB. CCK_4-induced panic in healthy subjects I: psychological and cardiovascular effects. Eur Neuropsychopharmacol 9, 149–155, 1999
Johnston DG, Troyer IE & Whitsett SF. Clomipramine treatment of agoraphobic women. Arch Gen Psychiatry 45, 453–459, 1988
Kahn RS, Westenberg HGM, Verhoenen WMA, Gispen-de Wied CC & Kamerbeek WOJ. Effect of a serotonin precursor and uptake inhibitor in anxiety disorders: a double blind comparison of 5-hydroxytryptophan, clomipramine and placebo. Int Clin Psychopharmacol 2, 33–45, 1987
Kahn RS & Wetzler S. M-Chlorophenylpiperazine as a probe of serotonin function. Biol Psychiatry 30, 1139–1166, 1991
Kalus O, Asnis GM, Rubinson E, Kahn R, Harkavy JM, Iqbal N, Grosz D, Van Praag H & Cahn W. Desipramine treatment in panic disorder. J Affect Disord 21, 239–244, 1991
Katerndahl DA & Talamantes M. A comparison of persons with early-*versus* late-onset panic attacks. J Clin Psychiatry 61, 6, 422–427, 2000
Katerndahl DA & Realini JP. Where do panic attack sufferers seek care? J Fam Pract 40, 237–243, 1995
Katerndahl DA & Realini JP. Lifetime prevalence of panic states. Am J Psychiatry 150, 246–249, 1993
Katon W. Panic disorder and somatization. Review of 55 cases. Am J Med 77, 101, 1984
Katon W. Panic disorder: relationship to high medical utilization, unexplained physical symptoms, and medical costs. J Clin Psychiatry 57 (Suppl 10), 11–18, 1996
Katon W, Vitaliano PP, Russo J, Jones M & Anderson K. Panic disorder. Spectrum of severity and somatization. J Nerv Ment Dis 175, 12, 1987
Kawachi I, Sparrow D, Vokonas PS & Weiss ST. Symptoms of anxiety and coronary heart disease: the normative aging study. Circulation 90, 2225–2229, 1994
Keck PE, Taylor VE, Tugrul KC, McElroy SL & Bennett JA. Valproate treatment of panic disorder and lactate-induced panic attacks. Biol Psychiatry 33, 542–546, 1993
Kelsey JE. Venlafaxine in social phobia. Psychopharmacol Bull 31 (4), 767–771, 1995
Kendler KS, Walters EE, Truett KR, Heath AC, Neale MC, Martin NG & Eaves LJ. A twin-family study of self-report symptoms of panic-phobia and somatization. Behav Genet 25 (6), 499–515, 1995
Kent JM, Coplan JD & Gorman JM. Clinical utility of the selective serotonin reuptake inhibitors in the spectrum of anxiety. Biol Psychiatry 44, 812–824, 1998
King NJ, Ollendick TH & Mattis SG. Panic in children and adolescents: Normative and clinical studies. Aust Psychol 29, 89, 1994
King R, Margraf J, Ehlers A & Maddock R. Panic disorder-Overlap with symptoms of somatization disorder. In: I Hand & HV Wittchen (eds): Panic and phobias. Berlin: Springer-Verlag, 72, 1986

Klein DF. The pathophysiology of panic anxiety. J Clin Psychiatry 52, 2 (Suppl), 10–11, 1991
Klein DF. False suffocation alarms, spontaneous panics, and related conditions: an integrative hypothesis. Arch Gen Psychiatry 50, 306–317, 1993
Klein DF, Ross DC & Cohen P. Panic and avoidance in agoraphobia. Arch Gen Psychiatry, 44, 377–385, 1983
Klein DF. Anxiety reconceptualized. In: DF Klein & JG Rabkin (eds): Anxiety. New research and changing concepts. New York: Raven Press, 1981
Kramer MS, Cutler NR, Ballenger JC, Patterson WM, Mendels ,. Chenault A, Shrivastava R, Matzura-Wolfe D, Lines C & Reines S. A placebo-controlled trial of L-365,260, a CCKB antagonist, in panic disorder. Biol Psychiatry 37 (7), 462–466, 1995
Lecrubier Y & Judge R. Long-term evaluation of paroxetine, clomipramine and placebo in panic disorder. Collaborative Paroxetine Panic Study Investigators. Acta Psychiatr Scand 95 (2), 153–160, 1997
Lecrubier Y & Üstün TB. Panic and depression: a world-wide primary care perspective. Int. Clin Psychopharmacol 13 (Suppl 4), S7–S11, 1998
Lecrubier Y, Bakker A, Dunbar G, Judge R & the Collaborative Paroxetine Panic Study Investigators. A comparison of paroxetine, clomipramine and placebo in the treatment of panic disorder. Acta Psychiatr Scand 95, 145–152, 1997
LeDoux JE. The emotional brain: The mysterious underpinnings of emotional life. New York: Simon & Schuster, 1996
Lenox RH, Shipley JE, Peyser JM. Double-blind comparison of alprazolam *versus* imipramine in panic disorder. Psychopharmacol Bull 20, 79–82, 1984
Leon AC, Olfson M & Portera I. Service utilization and expenditures for the treatment of panic disorder. Gen Hosp Psychiatry 19, 82–88, 1997
Lepine JP, Chignon JM & Teherani M. Suicide attempts in patients with panic disorder. Arch Gen Psychiatry 50, 144–149, 1993
Lepola UM, Koponen H & Leinonen E. A naturalistic 6-year follow-up study of patients with panic disorder. Acta Psychiatr Scand 93, 181–183, 196, 1996
Lepola UM, Wade AG, Leinonen EV, Koponen HJ, Frazer J, Sjödin I, Penttinen JT, Pedersen T & Lehto HJ. A controlled, prospective, 1-year trial of citalopram in the treatment of panic disorder. J Clin Psychiatry 59, 528–534, 1998
Liebowitz MR, Fyer AJ, Gorman JM, Dillon D, Appleby IL, Levy G, Anderson S, Levitt M, Palij M & Davies SO. Lactate provocation of panic attacks. I. Clinical and behavioral findings. Arch Gen Psychiatry 41 (8), 764–770, 1984
Liebowitz MR, Gorman JM, Fyer A, Dillon D, Levitt M & Klein DF. Possible mechanisms for lactate's induction of panic. Am J Psychiatry 143 (4), 495–502, 1986
Lines C, Challenor J & Traub M. Cholecystokinin and anxiety in normal volunteers: an investigation of the anxiogenic properties of pentagastrin and reversal by the cholecystokinin receptor subtype B antagonist L-365-260. Br J Pharmacol 39, 235–242, 1995
Liskow B, Penick EC, Powell BJ, Haefele WF & Campbell JL. Inpatients with Briquet's syndrome: Presence of additional psychiatric syndromes and MMPI results. Compr Psychiatry 27, 461, 1986
Loerch B, Graf-Morgenstern M, Hautzinger M, Schlegel S, Hain C, Sandmann J & Benkert O. Randomised placebo-controlled trial of moclobemide, cognitive-bahavioural therapy

and their combination in panic disorder with agoraphobia. Br J Psychiatry 174, 205–212, 1999

Londborg PD, Wolkow R, Smith WT, DuBoff E, England D, Ferguson J, Rosenthal M & Weise C. Sertraline in the treatment of panic disorder. A multi-site, double-blind, placebo-controlled, fixed dose investigation. Br J Psychiatry 173, 54–60, 1998

Lydiard RB. Panic disorder and social phobia: possible implications of comorbid depression for drug therapy. Anxiety 2, 61–70, 1996

Maier W & Buller R. One-year follow-up of panic disorder: outcome and prognostic factors. Eur Arch Psychiatry Clin Neurosci 238, 105–109, 1988

Maier W, Lichtermann D, Minges J, Oehrlein A & Franke P. A controlled family study in panic disorder. J Psychiatric Res 27 (Suppl 1), 79–87, 1993

Malizia AL, Cunningham VJ, Bell CJ, Liddle PF, Jones T & Nutt DJ. Decreased brain GABA (A)-benzodiazepine receptor binding in panic disorder: preliminary results from a quantitative PET study. Arch Gen Psychiatry 55, 715–720, 1998

Marchesi C, Ampollini P, Signifredi R & Maggini C. The treatment of panic disorder in a clinical setting: A 12-month naturalistic study. Neuropsychobiol 36, 25–31, 1997

Marshall JR. Comorbidity and its effects on panic disorder. Bull Menninger Clin 60 (2, Suppl.), A39–A53, 1996

McNally RJ. Panic disorder. A critical analysis. New York: Guildford Press, 1994

Mendlowicz MV & Stein MB. Quality of life in individuals with anxiety disorders. Am J Psychiatry 157 (5), 669–682, 2000

Mendlewicz J, Papdimitriou G & Wilmotte J. Family study of panic disorder: comparison with generalized anxiety disorder, major depression and normal subjects. Psychiatr Gene 3, 73–78, 1993

Michelson D, Pollack M, Lydiard B, Tamura R, Tepner R, Tollefson G & the Fluoxetine Panic Disorders Study Group. Continuing treatment of panic disorder after acute response: randomised, placebo-controlled trial with fluoxetine. Br J Psychiatry 174, 213–218, 1999

Mrazek DA. Psychiatric complications of pediatric asthma. Ann Allergy 69, 285–290, 1992

Moisan D & Engels ML. Childhood trauma and personality disorder in 43 women with panic disorder. Psychol Rep 76, 1133, 1995

Noyes R, Crowe RR, Harris EL et al. Relationship between panic disorder and major depression. Arch Gen Psychiatry 43, 227–232, 1986

Nutt DJ, Glue P, Lawson C & Wilson S. Flumazenil provocation of panic attacks: evidence for altered benzodiazepine receptor sensitivity in panic disorder. Arch Gen Psychiatry 47, 917–925, 1990

Oehrberg S, Christiansen PE, Behnke K et al. Paroxetine in the treatment of panic disorder: a randomized, double-blind, placebo-controlled study. Br J Psychiatry 167, 374–379, 1995

Orenstein H. Briquet's syndrome in association with depression and panic: A reconceptualization of Briquet's syndrome. Am J Psychiatry 146, 334, 1989

Paniccia GS & Rapaport MH. Serotonin receptors, social phobia and panic disorder. Int. Rev Psychiatry 7, 131, 1995

Papp LA, Sinha SS, Martinez JM, Coplan JD, Amchin J & Gorman JM. Low-dose venlafaxine treatment in panic disorder. Psychopharmacol Bull 34 (2), 207–209, 1997

Papp LA, Klein DF & Gorman JM. Carbon dioxide hypersensitivity, hyperventilation, and panic disorder. Am J Psychiatry 150, 1149–1157, 1993

Papp LA, Martinez JM, Klein DF, Coplan JD, Norman RG, Cole R, de Jesus MJ, Ross D, Goetz R & Gorman JM. Respiratory psychophysiology of panic disorder: three respiratory challenges in 98 subjects. Am J Psychiatry 154, 1557–1565, 1997

Pauli P, Harti L, Marquardt C, Stalmann H & Strian F. Heartbeat and arrhythmia perception in diabetic autonomic neuropathy. Psychol Med 21, 413–421, 1991

Pecknold JC, Luthe L & Scott-Fleury M-H. Gepirone and the treatment of panic disorder: An open study. J Psychopharmacol 13 (2), 145–149, 1993

Perna G, Gabriele A, Caldirola D & Bellodi L. Hypersensitivity to inhalation of carbon dioxide and panic attacks. Psychiatry Res 57 (3), 267–273, 1995

Perna G, Bertani A, Caldirola D, Smeraldi E & Bellodi L. A comparison of citalopram and paroxetine in the treatment of panic disorder: A randomized, single-blind study. Pharmacopsychiatry 34, 85–90, 2001

Perna G, Battaglia M, Garberi A, Arancio C, Bertani A & Bellodi L. Carbon dioxide/oxygen challenge test in panic disorder. Psychiatry Res 52, 159–171, 1994

Perna G, Brambilla F, Arancio C & Bellodi L. Menstrual cycle-related sensitivity to 39% CO_2 in panic patients. Biol Psychiatry 37 (8), 528–532, 1995

Perna G, Bertani A, Caldirola D & Bellodi L. Family history of panic disorder and hypersensitivity to CO_2 in patients with panic disorder. Am J Psychiatry 153, 1060–1064, 1996

Peterson RA & Reiss S. Manual for the Anxiety Sensitivity Index, 2nd ed. Worthington, Ohio: International Diagnostic Services, Inc, 1992

Pilowsky DJ, Wu L-T & Anthony JC. Panic attacks and suicide attempts in mid-adolescence. Am J Psychiatry 156, 1545–1549, 1999

Pine DS, Weese-Mayer DE, Silvestri JM, Davies M, Whitaker AH & Klein DF. Anxiety and congenital central hypoventilation syndrome. Am J Psychiatry 151, 864–870, 1994

Pine DS, Coplan JD, Papp LA, Klein RG, Martinez JM, Kovalenko P, Tancer N, Moreau D, Dummit ES 3rd, Shaffer D, Klein DF & Gorman JM. Ventilatory physiology of children and adolescents with anxiety disorders. Arch Gen Psychiatry 55 (2), 123–129, 1998

Pine DS, Cohen P, Gurley D, Brook JS & Ma Y. The risk for early-adulthood anxiety and adolescents with anxiety disorders. Arch Gen Psychiatry 55, 123–129, 1998a

Pitts FN & McClure JN. Lactate metabolism in anxiety neurosis. N Engl J Med 227, 1329–1339, 1967

Pohl R, Yeragani VK, Balon R & Lycaki H. The jitteriness syndrome in panic disorder patients treated with antidepressants. J Clin Psychiatry 49, 100–104, 1988

Pollack M, Worthington JJ, Otto MW, Maki KM, Smoller JW, Manfro GG, Rudolph R & Rosenbaum JF. Venlafaxine for panic disorder: Results from a double-blind, placebo-controlled study. Psychopharmacol Bull 32 (4), 667–670, 1996

Pollack MH & Marzol PC. Panic: Course, complications and treatment of panic disorder. J Psychopharmacol 14 (2 Suppl 1), S25–S30, 2000

Pollack MH, Otto MW, Worthington JJ, Manfro GG & Wolkow R. Sertraline in the treatment of panic disorder. A flexible-dose multicenter trial. Arch Gen Psychiatry 55, 1010–1016, 1998

Pyke RE & Greenberg HS. Norepinephrine challenges in panic patients. J Clin Psychopharmacol 6, 279–285, 1986

Rachman S. Panics and their consequences: a review and prospect. In: S Rachman & JD Maser (eds): Panic: Psychological perspectives. Hillsdale, NJ: Lawrence A Erlbaum Associates, 259–303, 1988

Rago L, Kiivet RA, Harro J & Pold M. Behavioral differences in an elevated plus maze: correlation between anxiety and decreased number of GABA and benzodiazepine receptors in mouse cerebral cortex. Naunyn Schmiedebergs Arch Pharmacol 337, 675–678, 1988

Rainey JM JR, Pohl RB, Williams M et al. A comparison of lactate and isoproterenol anxiety states. Psychopathol 17 (Suppl. 1), 74–82, 1984

Raj BA, Corvea MH & Dagon EM. The clinical characteristics of panic disorder in the elderly: A rectrospective study. J Clin Psychiatry 54, 150–155, 1993

Rapaport MH, Pollack M, Wolkow R, Mardekian J, Clary C. Is placebo response the same as drug response in panic disorder? Am J Psychiatry 157 (6), 1014–1016, 2000

Rapee R, Brown T, Antony M & Barlow D. Response to hyperventilation and inhalation of 5.5% carbon dioxide-enriched air across the DSM-III-R anxiety disorders. J Abnorm Psychol 101, 538–552, 1992

Rapaport MH, Risch C, Gillin J, Golshan S & Janowsky D. Blunted growth hormone response to peripheral infusion of human growth hormone-releasing factor in patients with panic disorder. Am J Psychiatry 146, 92–95, 1989

Regier DA, Boyd JH, Burke JD Jr, Rae DS, Myers JK, Kramer M, Robins LN, George LK, Karno M & Locke BZ. One-month prevalence of mental disorders in the United States: based on five epidemiologic catchment area sites. Arch Gen Psychiatry 45, 977–986, 1988

Reiman EM, Raichle ME, Butler FK, Herscovitch &, Robins E. A focal brain abnormality in panic disorder, a severe form of anxiety. Nature 310 (5979), 683–685, 1984

Reiman EM, Raichle ME, Robins E, Butler FK, Herscovitch P, Fox P & Perlmutter J. The application of positron emission tomography to the study of panic disorder. Am J Psychiatry 143 (4), 469–477, 1986

Reiss S, Peterson RA, Gursky DM & McNally RJ. Anxiety sensitivity, anxiety frequency and the prediction of fearfulness. Behav Res Ther 24, 1–8, 1986

Robertson HA, Martin IL & Candy JM. Differences in benzodiazepine receptor binding in Maudsley reactive and Maudsley nonreactive rats. Eur J Pharmacol 50, 455–457, 1978

Roy-Byrne PP, Cowley DS, Greenblatt DJ, Shader RI & Hommer D. Reduced benzodiazepine sensitivity in panic disorder. Arch Gen Psychiatry 47, 259–272, 1990

Roy-Byrne PP, Stein MB, Russo J, Mercier E, Thomas R, McQuaid J, Katon WJ, Craske MG, Bystritsky A & Sherbourne CD. Panic disorder in the primary care setting: Comorbidity, disability, service utilization and treatment. J Clin Psychiatry 60, 492–499, 1990

Scheibe G & Albus M. Predictors of outcome in panic disorder: a 5-year prospective follow-up study. J Affective Disord 41, 111–116, 1996

Schmidt NB, Woolaway-Bickel K & Bates M. Evaluating panic-specific factors in the relationship between suicide and panic disorder. Behav Res Ther 39, 635–649, 2001

Schneier FR, Liebowitz MR, Davies SO, Fairbanks J, Hollander E, Campeas R & Klein DF. Fluoxetine in panic disorder. J Clin Psychopharmacol 10 (2), 119–121, 1990

Schneier FR, Garfinkel R, Kennedy B, Campeas R, Fallon B, Marshall R et al. Ondansetron in the treatment of panic disorder. Anxiety 2, 199–202, 1996
Shear MK, Brown TA, Barlow DH, Money R, Sholomskas DE, Woods SW, Gorman JM & Papp LA. Multicenter collaborative panic disorder severity scale. Am J Psychiatry 154 (11), 1571–1575, 1997
Shear MK & Maser JD. Standardized assessment for panic disorder research. Arch Gen Psychiatry 1951, 346–354, 1994
Sheehan DV, Raj BA, Trehan RR & Knapp EL. Serotonin in panic disorder and social phobia. Int Clin Psychopharmacol 8, 63, 1993
Sheehan DV & Sheehan KH. The classification of anxiety and hysterical states. Part I. Historical review and empirical delineation. J Clin Psychopharmacol 2, 235, 1982
Sheehan DV & Harnett-Sheehan K. The role of SSRIs in panic disorder. J Clin Psychiatry 57 (Suppl 10), 51–58, 1996
Shear MK & Masur JD. Standardized assessment for panic disorder research: a conference report. Arch Gen Psychiatry 51, 346–354, 1994
Shear MK. Factors in the etiology and pathogenesis of panic disorder: Revisiting the attachment-separation paradigm. Am J Psychiatry 153, 125, 1996
Shipherd JC, Beck JG & Ohtake PJ. Relationship between the anxiety sensitivity index, the suffocation fear scale, and responses to CO_2 inhalation. J Anxiety Disord 15, 247–258, 2001
Silove D, Harris M, Morgan A, Boyce P, Manicavasagar V, Hadzi-Pavlovic D & Wilhelm K. Is early separation anxiety a specific precursor of panic disorder-agoraphobia? A community study. Psychol Med 25 (2), 405–411, 1995
Simon GE & Vonkorff M. Somatization and psychiatric disorder in the NIMH Epidemiologic Catchment Area study. Am J Psychiatry 148, 1494–1500, 1991
Spitzer RL, Williams JBW, Kroenke K, Linzer M, deGruy III FV, Hahn SR, Brody D & Johnson JG. Utility of a new procedure for diagnosing mental disorders in primary care: The PRIME-MD 1000 study. JAMA 272 (22), 1749–1756, 1994
Stein MB, Walker JR, Anderson G, Hazen AL, Ross CA, Eldridge G & Forde DR. Childhood physical and sexual abuse in patients with anxiety disorders and in a community sample. Am J Psychiatry 153 (2), 275–277, 1996
Sutton SK & Davidson RJ. Prefrontal brain asymmetry: a biological substrate of the behavioral approach and inhibition systems. Psychol Sci 8, 204–210, 1997
Swales P, Solfrin J & Sheikh J. Cognitive-behaviour therapy in older panic disorder patients. Am J Geriatr Psychiatry 4, 46–60, 1996
Swartz M, Blazer D, George L & Landerman R. Somatization disorder in a community population. Am J Psychiatry 1143, 1403, 1986
Swinson RP, Cox BJ & Woszczyna CB. Use of medical services and treatment for panic disorder with agoraphobia and for social phobia. Can Med Assoc J 147, 878–883, 1992
Taylor S & Rachman S. Klein's suffocation theory of panic. Arch Gen Psychiatry 51, 505–506, 1994
Taylor CB, King R, Margraf J, Ehlers A, Telch M, Roth WT & Agras WS. Use of medication and *in vivo* exposure in volunteers for panic disorder research. Am J Psychiatry 146, 1423–1426, 1989

Telch MJ, Agras WS, Taylor CB, Roth WT & Gallen CC. Combined pharmacological and behavioral treatment for agoraphobia. Behav Res Ther 3, 325–335, 1985

Timmerman L. Panic disorder, a specific entity? An exploration into psychological and biochemical aspects (thesis). Rotterdam, the Netherlands: Erasmus University Rotterdam, 1995

Torgersen S. Genetic factors in anxiety disorders. Arch Gen Psychiatry 40, 1085–1089, 1983

Uhde T, Tancer M, Rubinow D, Roscow D, Boulenger J, Vittone B, Gurguis G, Geraci M, Black B & Post R. Evidence for hypothalamo-growth hormone dysfunction in panic disorder: Profile of growth hormone (GH) responses to clonidine, yohimbine, caffeine, glucose, GRF and TRH in panic disorder patients *versus* healthy volunteers. Neuropsychopharmacol 6, 101–118, 1992

Uhde TW, Boulenger JP, Vittone B et al. Human anxiety and noradrenergic function: preliminary studies with caffeine, clonidine and yohimbine. In: Proceedings of the 7th World Congress of Psychiatry. New York: Plenum, 1986

Uhde TW, Boulenger JP, Roy-Byrne PP, Geraci MF, Vittone BJ & Post RM. Longitudinal course of panic disorder: clinical and biological considerations. Progr Neuro-Psychopharmacol Biol Psychiatry 9 (1), 39–51, 1985

Van Megen HJGM, Den Boer JA, Westenberg HGM. Pentagastrin induced panic attacks: enhanced sensitivity in panic disorder patients. Psychopharmacol 114, 449–455, 1994

Van Megen HJGM, Westenberg HGM, den Boer JA, Slaap B & Scheepmakers A. Effect of the selective serotonin reuptake inhibitor fluvoxamine on CCK-4 induced panic attacks. Psychopharmacol 129, 357–364, 1997

Van Megen HJGM, Den Boer JA & Westenberg HGM. Single blind dose response study with cholecystokinin (CCK-4) in panic disorder patients. Eur Neuropsychopharmacol 6, 187–194,1996

Van Vliet IM, Slaap BR, Westenberg HG & Den Boer JA. Behavioral, neuroendocrine and biochemical effects of different doses of 5-HTP in panic disorder. Eur Neuropsychopharmacol 6, 103–110, 1996

Vieland V, Goodman D, Chapman T & Fyer A. New segregation analysis of panic disorder. Am J Med Genet 67, 147–153, 1996

Wade G, Lepola U, Koponen HJ, Perdersen V & Pedersen T. The effects of citalopram in panic disorder. Br J Psychiatry 170, 549–553, 1997

Wagner KD & Berenson AB. Norplant-associated major depression and panic disorder. J Clin Psychiatry 55, 478, 1994

Weissman MM. The epidemiology and genetics of panic disorder. Clin Neuropharmacol 15 (Suppl 1, pt A), 18A–19A, 1992

Weissman MM. Panic disorder: impact on quality of life. J Clin Psychiatry 52, 2 (Suppl), 6–11, 1991

Weissman MM, Markowitz JS, Ouellette R, Greenwald S & Kahn JP. Panic disorder and cardiovascular problems: results from a community survey. Am J Psychiatry 147, 1504–1508, 1990

Weissman MM. Family genetic studies of panic disorder. J Psychiatric Res 27, 69, 1993

Westenberg HGM. Developments in the drug treatment of panic disorder: what is the place of the selective serotonin reuptake inhibitors? J Affect Disord 40, 85–93, 1996

Weissman MM, Klerman GL, Markowitz JS & Ouellette R. Suicidal ideation and suicide attempts in panic disorder and attacks. N Engl J Med 321, 1209–1214, 1989
Weissman MM, Bland RC, Canino GJ, Faravelli C, Greenwald S, Hwu H-G, Joyce PR, Karam EG, Lee C-K, Lellouch J et al. The cross-national epidemiology of panic disorder. Arch Gen Psychiatry 54, 305–309, 1997
Welkowitz LA, Papp LA, Cloitre M, Liebowitz MR, Martin LY & Gorman JM. Cognitive-behavior therapy for panic disorder delivered by psychopharmacologically oriented clinicians. J Nerv Ment Dis 179, 473–477, 1991
Wiedemann G, Pauli P, Dengler W, Lutzenberger W, Birbaumer N & Buchkremer G. Frontal brain asymmetry as a biological substrate of emotions in patients with panic disorders. Arch Gen Psychiatry 56, 78–84, 1999
Wilkinson DJC Thompson JM, Lambert GW, Jennings GL, Schwarz RG, Jefferys D, Turner AG & Esler MD. Sympathetic activity in patients with panic disorder at rest, under laboratory mental stress, and during panic attacks. Arch Gen Psychiatry 55, 511–520, 1998
Wisner KL, Peindl KS & Hanusa BH. Effects of childbearing on the natural history of panic disorder with comorbid mood disorder. J Affect Disord 41, 173–180, 1996
Yonkers KA, Zlotnick C, Allsworth J, Warshaw M, Shea T, Keller MB. Is the course of panic disorder the same in women and men? Am J Psychiatry 155 (5), 596–602, 1998
Yonkers KA, Ellison JM, Shera DM, Pratt LA, Cole JO, Fierman E, Keller MB & Lavori PW. Description of antipanic therapy in a prospective longitudinal study. J Clin Psychopharmacol 16 (3), 223–232, 1996
Zajecka JM. The effect of nefazodone on comorbid anxiety symptoms associated with depression: experience in family practice and psychiatric out patient settings. J Clin Psychiatry 57 (Suppl 2), 10–14, 1996
Zitrin CM, Klein DF & Woerner MG. Behavior therapy, supportive psychotherapy, imipramine and phobias. Arch Gen Psychiatry 35, 307–316, 1978
Zitrin CM, Klein DF & Woerner MG. Treatment of agoraphobia with group exposure *in vivo* and imipramine. Arch Gen Psychiatry 37, 63–72, 1980
Zoccolillo M & Cloninger CR. Somatization disorder: Psychologic symptoms, social disability, and diagnosis. Compr Psychiatry 27, 65, 1986

Chapter 6
Obsessive-compulsive disorder

1 Introduction

OCD is characterised by recurrent, unpleasant thoughts which enter consciousness against the will of the individual, termed obsessions, and repetitive, unwanted behaviours, which may be ritualistic, termed compulsions, that lead to severe impairment in daily functioning. One of the most common compulsions is cleaning. Some individuals concerned about contamination will spend hours showering or bathing, others will wash their hands almost constantly, and some will spend hours and hours of each day cleaning their home. In addition to cleaning there are a number of other compulsions including checking (e.g., individuals may check hundreds of times if all doors at home are locked), repeating (e.g., some people may wish to ease anxiety by repeating a name or phrase over and over), slowness (being overly meticulous and tidy and spending hours organising and arranging objects and possessions) and fear of contamination (e.g., a person may devote hours of the day to washing their hands and avoids any social contact with others due to the fear of contamination).

At one time, it was speculated that OCD resulted from family attitudes or childhood experiences including a harsh discipline by demanding parents. Recent evidence indicates that biological factors may contribute to the development of OCD. Various lines of evidence suggest that fronto-striatal systems of the brain are involved in this disorder (Savage, 1998; Tallis, 1997). Although symptoms of anxiety and depression commonly occur, there is growing recognition that OCD should be separated from the other anxiety disorders and from depression. OCD shows a distinctive response to drug treatments and does not share the same biological markers as many of the other anxiety disorders (Fineberg & Montgomery, 1992). There is a close association with other neuropsychiatric disorders, such as Gilles de la Tourette's syndrome, which suggests organic factors may play a role in some patients (Holzer et al., 1994).

2 Diagnostic

OCD is a clinical diagnosis, the diagnostic criteria for which are shown in Table 6.1 (APA, 1994; WHO, 1993). Obsessions are ideas, thoughts, or impulses that are experienced as senseless and intrusive and persist despite attempts to suppress them.

Table 6.1: A comparison of DSM-IV and ICD-10 diagnostic criteria for OCD

DSM-IV	
A.	Either obsessions or compulsions Obsessions as defined by (1), (2), (3) and (4) (1) Recurrent and persistent thoughts, impulses or images that are experienced, at some time during the disturbance, as intrusive and inappropriate and that cause marked anxiety distress. (2) The thoughts, impulses or images are not simply excessive worries about real-life problems. (3) The person attempts to ignore or suppress such thoughts, impulses or images, or to neutralize them with some other thoughts or action. (4) The person recognises that the obsessional thoughts, impulses or images are a product of his or her own mind (not imposed from without as in thought insertion). Compulsions as defined by (1) or (2) (1) Repetitive behaviours (e.g. hand washing, ordering, checking) or mental acts (e.g., praying, counting, repeating words silently) that the person feels driven to perform in response to an obsession, or according to rules that must be applied rigidly. (2) The behaviours or mental acts are aimed at preventing or reducing distress or preventing some dreaded event or situation; however, these behaviours or mental acts either are not connected in a realistic way with what they are designed to neutralise or prevent or are clearly excessive.
B.	At some point during the course of the disorder, the person has recognised that the obsessions or compulsions are excessive or unreasonable. Note: This does not apply to children.
C.	The obsessions or compulsions cause marked distress, are time consuming (take more than 1 h a day), or significantly interfere with the person's normal routine, occupational (or academic) functioning, or usual social activities or relationships.
D.	If another Axis I disorder is present, the content of the obsessions or compulsions is not restricted to it (e.g., preoccupation with food in the presence of an eating disorder; hair pulling in the presence of dysmorphic disorder; preoccupation with drugs in the presence of a substance use disorder; preoccupation with having a serious illness in the presence of hypochondriasis; preoccupation with sexual urges or fantasies in the presence of a paraphilia; or guilty ruminations in the presence of major depressive disorder).
E.	The disturbance is not due to the direct physiological effects of a substance (e.g., a drug of abuse, a medication) or a general medical condition.

Some of the more common obsessions include fear of contamination, need for order or symmetry, pathologic doubt, and recurrent aggressive or horrific images. Compulsions are repetitive, purposeful behaviours performed in response to obsessions or in a stereotypical fashion, with the goal of reducing distress or preventing some dreaded event or situation. The activity is either not connected in a realistic way with what it is designed to prevent or is clearly excessive (e.g., ritualised hand-washing, repeated checking). The most common compulsive behaviour includes washing, checking, counting, ordering, and repeating words or actions. For example, a patient with OCD who has contamination obsessions may spend hours washing until the skin becomes raw in order to neutralise certain obsessive thoughts. Not surprisingly, obsessions and compulsions are time consuming and can significantly interfere with normal daily routine and occupational functioning. OCD is classified

Table 6.1 (continued)

ICD-10	
A.	Either obsessions or compulsions (or both) are present on most days for a period of at least 2 weeks.
B.	Obsessions (thoughts, ideas, or images) and compulsions (acts) share the following features, all of which must be present:
(1)	They are acknowledged as originating in the mind of the patient, and are not imposed by outside persons or influences.
(2)	They are repetitive and unpleasant, and at least one obsession or compulsion that is acknowledged as excessive or unreasonable must be present.
(3)	The patient tries to resist them (but resistance to very long-standing obsessions or compulsions may be minimal). At least one obsession or compulsion that is unsuccessfully resisted must be present.
(4)	Experiencing the obsessive thought or carrying out the compulsive act is not in itself pleasurable. (This should be distinguished from the temporary relief of tension or anxiety).
C.	The obsessions or compulsions cause distress or interfere with the patient's social or individual functioning, usually by wasting time.
D.	Most commonly used exclusion clause. The obsessions or compulsions are not the result of other mental disorders, such as schizophrenia and related disorders (F20-F29) or mood (affective) disorders (F30-F39).

as a neurosis because patients generally retain insight. It is, though, frequently a distressing and disabling condition precluding normal social and occupational functions.

Recent studies suggest that OCD has overlapping features with major depression in terms of natural history, family history and some neurotransmitter functions (Sciuto et al., 1995; Insel et al., 1984). One study has made a direct comparison of personality features between OCD and major depressive (MD) patients, showing that there was no difference between the two groups in the frequency of personality disorders or personality disorder scores (Joffe et al., 1988). Nevertheless, there is a possibility that personality disorder scores are not very sensitive to the personality differences between the two disorders. Another study used the Temperament and Character Inventory (TCI) personality dimensions to compare personality features among patients with OCD and MD (Kusunoki et al., 2000). The TCI, a 240-item self-rating questionnaire, is designed to measure four temperament dimensions (novelty seeking, harm avoidance, reward dependence, persistence) as well as three character dimensions (self-directedness, co-operativeness, self-transcendence). It was shown that compared to controls, the OCD and MD patients scored significantly higher on harm avoidance and significantly lower on self-directedness and co-operativeness. However, the OCD patients scored significantly lower on novelty seeking than the MD patients and controls. The finding that OCD was distinguishable from MD on novelty seeking suggests that the two disorders may be, at least in part, different in the biopsychological backgrounds underlying the aetiology. Although a conclusion regarding a truly specific relationship cannot yet be drawn, low novelty seeking may have a profound relationship to the specific aetiology of OCD.

2.1 Comorbidity

OCD is often comorbid with other anxiety disorders, depression, anorexia nervosa, tic disorders and trichotillomania, and probably also with autistic spectrum disorders (Hollander & Wong, 1995; Kopp & Gillberg, 1992). Patients with OCD and concomitant anorexia nervosa may exhibit autistic traits or obsessive-compulsive personality disorder (Gillberg et al., 1995). OCD and anorexic patients tend to have personality traits such as high harm avoidance, perfectionism and obsessionality (Kaye et al., 1992).

The connection between OCD and dissociative identity disorder (DID or multiple personality disorder) was reported when a subgroup of OCD patients with prominent dissociative features was noted (Ross & Anderson, 1988). It was recommended that all OCD patients should be screened for dissociative phenomenology. Further research suggests that the patients with the highest dissociation scores also had the most severe OCD symptoms (Goff et al., 1992). Depersonalisation was the most commonly reported dissociative symptom among the OCD patients. Amnestic experiences were also reported as fairly common experiences.

There are several patterns of comorbidity that have been associated in children with OCD. In a study of 70 children diagnosed as having OCD, only 26% had OCD as their only diagnosis (Swedo et al., 1989). Tic disorders (30%), major depression (26%), and specific developmental disorders (24%) were the most common comorbidities found. Other diagnoses included simple phobias, overanxious disorder, adjustment disorder with depressed mood, oppositional disorder, all with rates between 10% and 17% (Swedo et al., 1989).

2.2 Epidemiology

The lifetime prevalence of OCD is estimated to be 1–3%, based on population-based surveys conducted in many communities nationally and internationally (Karno & Golding, 1991; Weissman et al., 1994). Although the disorder affects individuals of all ages, the period of greatest risk is from childhood to middle adulthood (Nestadt et al., 1994; 1998). Patients experience a chronic or episodic course with exacerbations that can substantially impair social, occupational, and academic functioning. According to the WHO, OCD is among the ten most disabling medical conditions world-wide (Murray & Lopez, 1996).

Epidemiologic studies interested in gender-related clinical differences in OCD have shown that the lifetime prevalence of this disorder ranges between 0.9 and 3.4% in women and between 0.5 and 2.5% in men with a female/male ratio ranging between 0.8 to 3.8 (Weissman et al., 1994). In addition, all studies have reported an earlier age at onset in males together with insidious onset and chronic course (Castle et al., 1995; Lensi et al., 1996; Ravizza et al., 1997). Gender-related differences have also been observed in obsessive-compulsive symptomatology. In general, women have been noted to exhibit more aggressive and contamination obsessions and cleaning rituals, while men tend to report more frequently primary obsessive slowness, sexual, exactness and symmetry obsessions and odd rituals (Fischer et al., 1997; Lensi et al., 1996; Marks, 1987; Ronchi et al., 1992). A recent study in Italy showed that males had an earlier age at onset with a lower impact of precipitant events in triggering the disorder (Bogetto et al., 1999). OCD seemed to occur in a relative high proportion of males who already have phobias and/or tic disorders. A surfeit of chronic course of the illness in males in comparison with females was also observed. The relatively high frequency of tic disorders that precede the onset of OCD and the male preponderance may support the hypothesis that organic factors play a significant role in the onset of the disorder among the male population. Preliminary research suggests that the symptoms of this illness do not change markedly as people grow older (Kohn et al., 1997).

Although most studies suggest that women are 1.5 times more likely than men to develop OCD during their lifetime, 3 times as many prepubertal boys as girls are diagnosed with OCD (Karno et al., 1988; Weissman et al., 1994). OCD has a later age at onset in women (mean age = 25 years) than in men (mean age = 20 years) (Neziroglu et al., 1994; Thomsen, 1995). Boys are more likely than girls to develop OCD classified as early onset (before 6 years of age) (Swedo et al., 1989). However, the incidence of OCD markedly increases in women and eventually surpasses that in men after puberty (Weissman et al., 1994). Past history of an eating disorder, depression, panic attacks, aggressive obsessions, or cleaning rituals also are more commonly associated with women with OCD (Castle et al., 1995; Lensi et al., 1996; Thomsen & Mikkelsen, 1995). In contrast to the finding reported in GAD and social anxiety disorder, women with OCD may have an episodic and less severe clinical course than men (Thomsen, 1995; Hantouche & Lancrenon, 1996).

Pre-menstrual changes in the severity of symptoms of anxiety disorders are often clinically apparent. The pre-menstrual period has been consistently reported to elicit exacerbations in OCD symptoms (Williams & Koran, 1997; Yaryura Tobias et al., 1995). In the largest study to date, the impact of the menstrual cycle was retrospectively examined in 57 women with OCD (Williams & Koran, 1997). Nearly half (42%) of the women reported pre-menstrual worsening of OCD symptoms, and a substantial number (21%) also noted pre-menstrual dysphoria. Menopause and oestrogen-depletion states as well as the use of oral contraceptives or hormone replacement therapy (HRT) have also been associated with the onset of, or substantial changes in OCD and PD (Shear, 1997; Arpels, 1996; Warnock & Bundren, 1997).

In retrospective reports, substantial portions (13–36%) of women with OCD have noted the onset of OCD during pregnancy or the postpartum period (Altshuler et al., 1998; Williams & Koran, 1997). Several reports also suggest that women with pre-existing OCD experience worsening symptoms during pregnancy (Altshuler et al., 1998; Chelmow & Halfin, 1997; Weiss et al., 1995). However, recent large-scale investigations have not demonstrated that most women with OCD experience a substantial change in OCD symptoms during pregnancy. These studies support the finding that the postpartum period is often associated with an exacerbation in pre-existing OCD. Results suggest that more than 30% of women with OCD experience postpartum worsening of symptoms (Sichel, 1993; 1996).

2.3 Natural history

Systematic studies of course of illness in OCD using standardised diagnostic criteria are relatively rare. In a study that assessed predictors of course of illness, 100 patients diagnosed with OCD were prospectively followed for up to 5 years (Steketee et al., 1999). The results showed that approximately 20% of patients had full remission and 50% had partial remission during follow-up. Significant predictors of partial remission included being married and having lower global severity scores at baseline. The presence of major depression was marginally predictive of poorer course.

A recent study which performed a 40-year follow-up of patients with OCD reported that improvement was observed in 83%, including recovery (completely recovered, 20%; recovery with subclinical symptoms, 28%) (Skoog & Skoog, 1999). Early age of onset, having both obsessive and compulsive symptoms, low social functioning at baseline, and a chronic course at initial examination were correlated with a worse outcome. Although all monosymptomatic patients showed improvement by the time of the second examination, magical obsessions and compulsive rituals were among the worst outcome. These symptoms are less understandable, more bizarre and stereotypical than other symptoms and perhaps more resistant to intellectual, emotional and therapeutic coping.

3 Physiopathology

OCD is currently thought to be a neuropsychiatric illness associated with dysfunction in a circuit involving the basal ganglia and prefrontal cortex. Evidence supporting this model derived predominantly from neuroimaging, genetic and clinical studies has accumulated (Aylward et al., 1996; Baxter, 1994; Cummings, 1993). There is particular interest in the effect of the serotonin system on the basal ganglia-prefrontal cortical circuit. This is consistent with the noted efficacy of serotonin reuptake blockers in the disorder.

3.1 Neurobiology

A study examined the cyclic adenosine monophosphate (cAMP) protein kinase A, a serine-threonine kinase, in platelets from unmedicated patients with OCD and healthy comparison subjects (Perez et al., 2000). The data show that patients have significantly higher levels of platelet regulatory subunits type I (108.6 ± 11.0 vs. 96.7 ± 7.3, $p < 0.0005$) and II (165.4 ± 52.9 vs. 100.3 ± 15.3, $p < 0.00002$) and lower levels of the catalytic subunit (67.9 ± 10.7 vs. 99.6 ± 11.3, $p < 0.00001$) than healthy subjects. The results suggest that protein kinase A is affected in patients with OCD. Whether the alterations of the proteins involved in cAMP signalling reflect a primary or secondary response to neurohormonal perturbations remains unclear. Although the main limitation of peripheral models is that blood cells are exposed to a different environment, this finding is in line with other studies showing abnormalities of cAMP signalling in patients with affective diseases such as bipolar disorder and major depression (Shelton et al., 1996; Perez et al., 1999). Further replication in other studies may help to clarify the relevance of these preliminary data in the pathophysiology of OCD.

A study designed to investigate whether there is HPA response to acute apomorphine (a dopamine agonist) stimulation in OCD patients and in healthy volunteers and whether the responses differ in the two groups measured the cortisol responses to stimulation (Brambilla et al., 2000). This study showed that there are no significant alterations of the central dopaminergic function connected with the regulation of the HPA axis in OCD. However, this study needs confirmation in larger groups of patients using other DA-dependent parameters.

There is strong evidence for serotonergic system involvement in OCD. Recent studies have shown that sumatriptan, a selective ligand of the 5-$HT_{1D\beta}$ autoreceptor, modifies OCD symptoms (Mundo et al., 2000). These data suggest that there may be important implications for the 5-$HT_{1D\beta}$ receptor gene in the pathogenesis and treatment of OCD. Recently, a 5-HT_{2A} $-1438 > G$ promoter polymorphism has been reported to be associated with OCD in women but not in men, strengthening the hypothesis that there may be fundamental gender differences in the genetic differences in the genetic susceptibility to OCD (Enoch et al., 2001). However, these findings need confirmation in larger samples of OCD patients.

Attention has been recently focused on CNS neuropeptides as potential mediators of the symptoms profile of OCD. A study which assessed circadian endocrine variables in OCD patients reported a decrease of melatonin plasma levels and an increase of cortisol plasma levels, compared to those of healthy subjects (Monteleone et al., 1994). However, these results have not been confirmed (Millet et al., 1998). A recent study in which CSF oxytocin and NPY in OCD patients and healthy normal volunteers were measured showed that the results do not support a prior finding of elevated CSF oxytocin in OCD patients (Altemus et al., 1999). The data do not provide any evidence for an abnormality of NPY regulation in OCD.

3.2 Brain imaging

Advances in neuroimaging were more clear-cut, with emerging conceptualisations of OCD as a disorder of corticostriatal dysfunction (Owens et al., 1982). Resting or neutral state studies of OCD have indicated hyperactivity within the orbitofrontal and anterior cingulate cortex as well as the caudate nucleus, which is accentuated during symptom provocation and attenuated following successful treatment (Saxena et al, 1998). Further, whereas healthy subjects reliably recruit the right striatum during an implicit sequence-learning task, patients with OCD fail to do so. They instead exhibit aberrant medial temporal activation that may serve a compensatory function (Rauch et al., 1997). It has been proposed that the striatum may be the principal site of primary pathology in OCD and related disorders. This hypothesis finds support from models of pathogenesis related to autoimmune processes known to cause striatal damage (Rauch et al., 1998; Swedo et al., 1998).

In general, functional and structural neuroimaging studies confirm the hypothesis that dysfunctions in the orbitofrontal-striatal circuit may be involved in the pathophysiology of OCD (Rauch & Savage, 1997). As the structures within a particular pathway are all interconnected, disturbances in different areas of the pathway could produce similar obsessive-compulsive symptoms. This is further supported by studies of patients who have acquired OCD as a result of focal brain lesions. In support of this observation, a study reported that single or multiple lesions in various areas along the orbitofrontal-striatal circuit, including lesions involving exclusively the cerebral cortex (e.g., frontal, temporal or cingulate regions), the basal ganglia or both were associated with the development of OCD (Berthier et al., 1996). Thus, striatal abnormalities may represent a primary area of disturbance in child-onset OCD, whereas disturbances in other, related areas of the orbitofrontal-striatal pathway may be involved in adult-onset cases of the disorder.

A recent study designed to measure neuroanatomical changes in the thalamus of paediatric patients with OCD near the onset of illness, before and after treatment conducted volumetric MRI studies in 21 psychometric drug-naïve children, aged 8 to 17 years with OCD and 21 case-matched healthy comparison subjects (Gilbert et al., 2000). The results showed that thalamic volumes were significantly greater in treatment-naïve patients with OCD than in controls but declined significantly with pharmacological treatment comparable with those of controls. Decrease in thalamic volume in patients with OCD was associated with reduction in OCD symptom severity.

Although activation of the anterior cingulate after provocation of symptoms is shared with other anxiety disorders (e.g., simple phobia), metabolic changes in the caudate nuclei and orbitofrontal cortex appear to be unique to OCD, and are normalised by treatment with SSRI or behaviour therapy (Rauch et al., 1995).

3.3 Genetics

The role of heredity in OCD has long been suspected by clinicians. Several twin studies have reported that the concordance for obsessive-compulsive symptoms is substantially greater in monozygotic twin pairs (80–87%) than dizygotic twin pairs (47–50%) (Inyoue, 1965; Carey & Gottesman, 1981). A recent study designed to determine whether OCD is familial and to investigate clinical characteristics that might influence the familial aggregation of the disorder reported that the lifetime prevalence of OCD was significantly higher in cases compared with control relatives (11.7% vs. 2.7%, $p < 0.001$) (Nestadt et al. 2000). The first-degree relatives of probands diagnosed with OCD had a nearly 5-fold higher lifetime prevalence of OCD. Case relatives had higher rates of both obsessions and compulsions. However, this finding is more robust for obsessions. Earlier age at onset of the symptoms of OCD indicates a more familial subgroup. The relationship between younger ages at onset and familiarity of medical conditions is a well-recognised phenomenon confirmed by this study (Pauls et al., 1995; Childs & Scriver, 1986). Indeed, no occurrence of OCD in the relatives of probands who had an age at onset of OCD older than 17 years was found.

The results of these various studies encourage a molecular genetic approach to identify a genetic aetiology for OCD. Clarification of the range of psychopathology that is transmitted in these families, as well as identification of etiologically homogeneous clinical subtypes, will increase the ability of association studies and genome-wide searches to detect genes involved in the pathogenesis of OCD.

Perhaps the most dramatic evidence implicating a basal ganglia-prefrontal circuit in childhood OCD derives from studies that demonstrate an association between poststreptococcal autoimmune reactions and a complex psychiatric syndrome that involves motoric, emotional, attentional and profound obsessive-compulsive features (Allen et al., 1995). Both the motoric and obsessive-compulsive aspects of this syndrome have been attributed to dysfunction of basal ganglia arising as a result of the production of anticaudate antibodies.

3.4 Cognitive dysfunctions

A number of studies have provided evidence for deficits in learning and memory, especially for non-verbal information (Savage et al., 1996; Dirson et al., 1995). A study suggests that OCD patients' impairments in free recall are also associated with deficits in the ability to organise information during encoding, especially when complex non-verbal information is involved (Savage et al., 1999). That is, despite their ability to copy a complex geometric figure (Rey-Osterrieth) accurately, individuals with OCD tended to assemble the figure by copying small unrelated details rather than core elements such as a basic rectangle. Poor organisational strategies strongly predicted subsequent deficits in immediate free recall (Savage et al., 1999).

A study designed to study the cognitive dysfunction in OCD patients and to identify its correlation with both the clinical picture and the severity of the disorder examined neuropsychological and electrophysiological event-related potentials in 30 OCD patients compared to 30 normal controls (Raffat et al., 2000). The results showed a defective visuospatial recognition, which worsens with chronicity. Deteriorated set-shifting abilities, overfocused attention to irrelevant stimuli and delayed selective attention to relevant tasks were also observed. Mild cases showed better selective attention than severe cases. This study demonstrates that OCD patients have a characteristic pattern of cognitive dysfunction that differs among patients of varied severity, chronicity and symptom type. It was suggested that such dysfunctions may be related to a striato-frontoparietal neural pathophysiology. A recent study which aimed to determine the pattern of memory deficits in OCD showed that these patients were impaired in immediate and delayed free recall, exhibited slowed rates of verbal learning and deficits in organisation over long delays, and had preserved verbal recognition memory (Deckersbach et al., 2000). The results show that OCD patients were significantly impaired in both verbal and non-verbal memory performance and suggest that deficits in organisation in OCD are not restricted to the non-verbal domain but extend to verbal information and memory as well.

Deficits in organisational strategies are consistent with fronto-striatal dysfunction models in OCD. Neuropsychological deficits were observed in patients with OCD that were not observed in matched patients with PD or unipolar depression (Purcell et al., 1998). As such, the cognitive dysfunction in OCD appears to be related to the specific illness processes associated with the disorder.

Individuals with OCD tend to hide their problem rather than to seek help. They are often extremely successful in hiding their behaviour and may delay therapy for many years. Unfortunately, this delay reduces the chance of successful treatment because the obsessive-compulsive habits have become more deeply ingrained with time.

4 Treatment

Many patients with OCD benefit from a form of behaviour therapy in which they are gradually exposed to circumstances that trigger their compulsive behaviour. Such therapy works best when the feared situation can be easily simulated. It is more difficult if the anxiety-provoking situation is hard to recreate. Medication also plays a prominent role in the treatment of OCD and is particularly helpful for patients who are bothered by obsessions.

4.1 Psychological treatment

Prolonged exposure *in vivo* coupled with response or ritual prevention are the critical elements of modern effective behaviour therapy of OCD. Exposure involves prolonged confrontations with stimuli that normally provoke obsessional thoughts or compulsive behaviours. Patients agree not to engage in their usual ritualistic behaviour or cognitions and to remain in the situation for 60-90 minutes until their discomfort wanes. Homework extensions are generally used outside the therapist contact. Success rates vary (50–80%) (Hand, 1995). Generally, an average of 70% maintain their acute gains at one-year follow-up (Foa et al., 1985).

Various behavioural techniques (e.g. exposure *in vivo* with response prevention for treating compulsions and thought stopping for treating obsessions) have been suggested in the treatment of OCD, from aversion therapy to systematic desensitisation. OCD patients seem to respond best to a combination of clomipramine and either cognitive therapy or behaviour therapy (DeRubeis & Crits-Christoph, 1998). A recent study designed to examine the effectiveness of cognitive-behaviour therapy for OCD in a private setting concluded that it can be effectively delivered in routine clinical practice (Warren & Thomas, 2001). In this study, 26 consecutive patients who were referred to a private anxiety disorders speciality clinic began treatment for OCD. Of the 19 (73%) patients who completed treatment, 84% were treatment responders. Such results are interesting as they demonstrate that findings from controlled studies of the effects of cognitive-behaviour therapy in OCD patients can be generalised to everyday clinical practice.

The only reports on treating OCD in older adults are case studies. One article describes 3 years of psychodynamic therapy to treat OCD in an 84-year-old man (Weiner & White, 1985). Other reports document cognitive-behavioral approaches with imaginal and *in vivo* exposure paired with response prevention to break the cycle of engaging in ritualised or inappropriate behaviour to reduce anxiety. Additional treatment elements include education, social reinforcement, spouse involvement and assertiveness training as needed.

4.2 Pharmacological treatment

4.2.1 *Clomipramine*

Clomipramine and SSRIs reduce the whole spectrum of obsessional symptoms, including obsessional thoughts, compulsive behaviours, anxiety and depression. The treatment effect emerges slowly and gradually, increasing over several weeks (Fineberg et al., 1994). However, some reports have suggested that clomipramine administered i.v. is effective for OCD and that it may act more rapidly and be more effective even among patients who have not responded to oral clomipramine (Warneke, 1989; Fallon et al.,1998).

Although clomipramine is as effective as the SSRIs, anticholinergic and antiadrenergic adverse effects may limit its utility in clinical practice (Leonard, 1997).

4.2.2 *SSRI and the 5-HT receptors*

All the various SSRIs have been studied in the treatment of OCD, and each has proven effective in many cases (Laird, 1996; Stein et al., 1995; Zohar et al., 1996). Paroxetine, fluoxetine, fluvoxamine and sertraline have shown efficacy in the treatment of OCD, and all four drugs have been approved by the U.S. Food and Drug Administration for use in patients with OCD (Goodman et al., 1997; Greist et al., 1995a, 1995b; Tollefson et al., 1994). Although there are no data to suggest that one medication is more effective than another, some patients may respond specifically to one product (Rasmussen & Eisen, 1997: Leonard, 1997; Mundo et al., 1997).

Both pre-and postsynaptic $5\text{-HT}1_{B/D}$ receptors could be supersensitive in OCD. The therapeutic actions of SSRIs would be to down-regulate these presynaptic autoreceptors allowing increased synaptic levels of serotonin, possibly resulting in a subsequent down-regulation of postsynaptic 5-HT receptors. These postsynaptic receptors may be of the $5\text{-HT}_{1B/D}$, 5-HT_{2c} or another subtype. Antagonists at the $5\text{-HT}_{1B/D}$ receptor are thus likely to be potent and reliably acting anti-obsessive medications.

Although the SSRI and clomipramine were similarly efficacious in the management of OCD, clomipramine typically was associated with higher rates of adverse effects, particularly anticholinergic effects (Freeman et al., 1994; Jenike et al., 1990; Pigott et al., 1990).

On the basis of beneficial effects in depressed patients, several researchers have begun to evaluate the use of adjunctive pindolol (a β-blocker that inhibits 5-HT_{1A})

to initiate a more rapid onset of SSRI effects in patients with OCD (Maes et al., 1996; Moreno et al., 1997). However, preliminary data suggest that adjunctive pindolol is ineffective in treatment-resistant OCD.

4.2.3 Addition of atypical neuroleptics

One of the most recent polypharmacotherapy approaches to evolve is the addition of the atypical antipsychotic medication risperidone (Risperdal) to a regimen already including one of the SSRIs or clomipramine (Saxena et al., 1996; Jacobsen, 1995). Risperidone blocks both dopamine and serotonin receptors, but it can have the paradoxical effect of exacerbating OCD symptomatology when used alone. Although it is contraindicated as a monotherapy, it has been surprisingly effective in treating those patients whose OCD has been refractory to both clomipramine and fluvoxamine or any of their related agents when it has been added. Risperidone in combination with SSRIs seems to work best with that subset of OCD patients troubled by horrific mental imagery and those with symptoms falling within the schizo-obsessive spectrum (Saxena et al., 1996; McDougle et al., 2000). This regimen has been found to work less well with OCD patients than with comorbid tic disorders.

Although haloperidol and pimozide are commonly used in treatment augmentation strategies for severe OCD, the role of atypical neuroleptics is unclear (Baker et al., 1997). A case report of two patients with severe OCD who dramatically improved after olanzapine was added to treatment with SSRI was discussed (Marazziti & Pallanti, 1999). It was suggested that olanzapine may help otherwise untreated patients with OCD and that having a family history of bipolar disorder might predict a good response to olanzapine. Therefore, these data suggest that further assessment of the potential benefits of olanzapine treatment in a defined subgroup of treatment-resistant patients with OCD is warranted.

4.2.4 Course of therapy

When initiating pharmacologic treatment, medications should be titrated gradually. The standard pharmacologic regimen is a 10- to 12-week trial with an SSRI in adequate doses before initiating alternative therapy (Rasmussen & Eisen, 1997).

Initial response to medications in OCD can take 4 to 8 weeks, and maximal response may take as long as 20 weeks. Therapy should be continued for at least 6 months to 1 year once a therapeutic response is achieved (Rasmussen & Eisen, 1997). Medications should be tapered slowly during discontinuation and should be restarted if symptoms reappear (Leonard, 1997). In one study, the risk of relapse was 2.7 times greater in patients who discontinued therapy compared with patients who remained on therapy (Steiner et al., 1995).

4.2.5 Children

With respect to its clinical presentation, OCD in children and adolescents is quite similar to that observed in adults (Swedo et al., 1989). Studies of OCD in childhood and adolescence have revealed a high frequency of obsessions involving fears of contamination, fears of potential harm to oneself or loved ones, aggressive or sexual obsessions, or obsessions involving a concern with symmetry, order or exactness. Common compulsions noted in this age group have included excessive or ritualised washing or cleaning behaviours, counting, ordering and arranging rituals (Flament et al., 1988, Wever & Rey, 1997). These same obsessions and compulsions are among those most frequently observed in adult cases.

Despite similarities in clinical presentation, notable differences have been found between childhood OCD and that observed in adulthood. One such difference is the predominance of boys represented among child cases of OCD. The majority of studies investigating childhood OCD in clinically referred samples have found that boys outnumber girls (Toro et al., 1992; Wever & Rey, 1997; Thomsen & Mikkelsen, 1991). This contrasts with studies of OCD in adults, which have generally found either an equal distribution of men and women or a predominance of women with this disorder (Kolada et al., 1994; Ristvedt et al., 1993). The overrepresentation of boys among referred children and adolescents with OCD seems to reflect a tendency for males to have an earlier onset of the disorder than women. An onset of OCD between 5 and 15 years of age was more common in boys, whereas a later onset between the ages of 26 and 35 was twice as common in women (Noshirvani et al., 1991). The bimodal onset of OCD in childhood and in later adulthood suggests that different etiological factors, differentially affecting boys and women may underlie child- and adult-onset cases. In particular, early-onset cases are likely to have a stronger genetic and biological component that late-onset cases with boys potentially being more vulnerable to these influences than women (Goldstein et al., 1997). A hypothesis receiving growing empirical support is that at least some forms of early-onset OCD may be related to Tourette's syndrome and other tic disorders that are more prevalent in boys (Leckman et al., 1997).

The first drug trials for OCD in children in the 1980s demonstrated clomipramine hydrochloride to be efficacious (Flament et al., 1985). Subsequent research has shown that medications with potent effects on serotonin reuptake have been shown to be clearly efficacious in childhood OCD, as they are in adult OCD (Greist et al., 1995). This conclusion is based on clinical trials of fluoxetine, clomipramine and fluvoxamine (Leonard et al., 1989, 1991; Riddle et al., 1992; 1996). Data are also emerging on the efficacy of psychotherapeutic treatments for childhood anxiety disorders. Open studies suggest that similar treatment for OCD in children is well tolerated, but there are no data available from randomised clinical trials (March 1995).

4.2.6 *Some cultural differences in treatment practice*

Some differences in the approach to treat OCD may be discussed. In the US, there tends to be agreement that the most effective treatment is a combination of drug and behaviour therapies. Typically, a US psychiatrist first prescribes drug therapy, looks for a medication response and then recommends behaviour therapy. The majority of OCD patients receive drug therapy for their symptoms, but a much smaller group undergo behaviour therapy because it is time-consuming for both clinician and patient. The pharmacological therapies of choice include the tricyclic antidepressants, clomipramine and four SSRIs: fluoxetine, fluvoxamine, sertraline and paroxetine. Frequently, clomipramine is the first-line therapy because it is less expensive than the SSRIs. In settings less restricted by cost, however, doctors are more likely to prescribe one of the SSRIs as the first-line drug therapy. All these drugs are used at higher doses for treating OCD than they are for treating depression. Generally, the physician prescribes a relatively low dose initially and increases it over a period of weeks. If the patient tolerates the drug, the doctor aims for a daily maintenance dose in the following ranges: clomipramine, 200–250 mg; fluoxetine, 80 mg; fluvoxamine, 300 mg; sertraline, 200–300 mg and paroxetine, 60 mg. If the patient cannot take the prescribed medication without unacceptable side effects, the prescriber may change medications, reduce the dose or split the dose so that the patient takes a half-dose twice a day.

In France, once the diagnosis is confirmed, the majority of OCD patients receive pharmacological treatment. French doctors tend to favour fluoxetine together with behaviour therapy as first-line treatment. Treatment typically starts with a low dose to test patient tolerance and is gradually increased over a period of weeks. The targeted maintenance doses for fluoxetine are similar to those prescribed in the US, but in France there is a tendency to prescribe higher doses of clomipramine – up to 350 mg per day for as long as 2 months. If the patient requires a third-line treatment, the doctor may use any one of the variety of pharmacological treatments. He may prescribe paroxetine or fluvoxamine, or tricyclics with an SSRI.

In Germany, psychiatrists diagnose OCD patients often in specialised OCD clinics. When the diagnostic procedures are completed and the OCD diagnosis is confirmed, a case conference is usually held for each patient. Psychiatrists and psychologists jointly design behavioural therapy programs aimed at distracting patients from their compulsions by gradually increasing their involvement in other activities. Social workers help patients who have difficulties coping at work. In addition to psychotherapy, most patients also receive drug therapy, although some psychiatrists prefer to rely solely on psychodynamic treatment approaches. Clomipramine is the most common first-line drug therapy for OCD treatment in Germany. However, it is anticipated that in the next five years, SSRI will replace clomipramine as first-line drug therapy because their side effects are more easily tolerated.

In Spain, once the OCD diagnosis is confirmed, the majority of OCD patients undergo drug therapy. Behaviour therapy is not widely used in Spain. Clomipramine (75 mg/day) remains the most commonly prescribed first-line drug therapy for OCD. However, the SSRIs, particularly fluoxetine (40 mg/day) are currently gaining favour as first-line OCD treatment. Spanish physicians also commonly prescribe anxiolytics with BDZs at the start of the patient's OCD drug therapy.

In the UK, GPs, psychiatrists and behavioural psychotherapists treat OCD patients. Frequently, GPs attempt to control comorbid conditions, such as depression, before referring the patient to a specialist for OCD treatment. Because patients in the UK often fail to report obsessions and compulsions, GPs frequently misdiagnose OCD as an anxiety or depressive disorder. A GP who does discern OCD symptoms makes a referral to a specialist. Frequently, psychiatrists in the UK work jointly with behavioural psychotherapists. Clomipramine, fluoxetine and sertraline are commonly prescribed first-line drug therapies for OCD in the UK.

In Japan, Japanese doctors suspect that OCD is significantly underdiagnosed because the culture tends to accept some methodical behaviours that would be regarded as obsessive-compulsive elsewhere. For example, repeated checking is not considered abnormal. When a patient is diagnosed with OCD, physicians initiate both pharmacological and behavioural therapies. Bromazepam (6-14 mg/day) and clomipramine (20 mg/day) are common first-line drug treatments for OCD patients. As a second-line regimen, some physicians prescribe a combination of imipramine (20 mg/day) and bromazepam (10 mg/day). Some physicians may prescribe levomepromazine or fluphenazine as third line drug therapy.

5 Methodology for clinical investigation

In the selection of patients for clinical studies, it is a sine qua non that volunteers should meet some set of recognised diagnostic criteria; either the DSM-IV or ICD-10 would be appropriate. When specifying inclusion and exclusion criteria for future OCD studies, attention should be paid to the following: presence and severity of comorbid depression, age at disease onset, baseline disease severity, presence of comorbid tic disorders, presence and nature of comorbid personality disorder. Age of onset of the disease appears to be a very strong predictor of response (Ackerman et al., 1994). The younger the patient at disease onset, the less likely a response, independent of the duration of illness. A baseline score below 16 on the 10-item Y-BOCS is a very good prognostic indicator, irrespective of drug or placebo treatment.

The duration of therapy, experimental design (cross over *versus* parallel group) and issues surrounding comparative efficacy should be carefully considered. In conditions such as major depression and GAD, it is conventional and clinically reasonable to test for efficacy in studies of 4 to 6 weeks duration. However, studies in OCD have rarely been successful with such a short duration. The results of a study suggest that a "short term" efficacy and safety evaluation in OCD should include three months of active treatment (Tollefson et al., 1994). Since carry-over effects in cross over studies become unmanageable, most successful studies have used a parallel group design. If 3 months may present "acute" treatment, questions concerning long-term efficacy studies have been raised. A good approach could be to offer patients who had responded in a short-term study the possibility of a consolidation phase treatment (perhaps another 3 months of treatment) and then randomly continue on active drug or be switched double blind, with appropriate down titration, to continue on placebo. Relapse rates over the subsequent 6 months could then be compared between those continuing on active medication and those on placebo.

It would seem reasonable to perform a three-way parallel group active reference and placebo controlled study of a new drug. When both active treatments separate from placebo, their relative degrees of separation can be a useful measure by which to evaluate the clinical value of a new treatment.

5.1 Psychometric scales

A number of rating scales for measuring disease severity in OCD have been developed. The two gold standard instruments are the 10-item Y-BOCS and the National Institute of Mental Health Global Obsessive Compulsive Scale (NIMH-OC) (Goodman et al., 1989; Kim et al., 1990; Murphy et al., 1982). They have proven to be reliable and sensitive to drug effects. The 10-item Y-BOCS is a useful tool for identifying OCD and monitoring severity of illness (Goodman et al., 1989; Kim et al., 1990). Using inclusion criteria such that patients had a minimum disease severity of 16 points on the Y-BOCS would more or less guarantee that patients had clinically relevant obsessions and compulsions and does not allow investigation of mildly ill patients or patients with only obsessions or compulsions. There remains some debate as to whether 25 or 35% reductions on the Y-BOCS should be used to define responders.

The Padua Inventory-Revised (PI-R) is used to measure obsessive compulsive symptoms (Van Oppen et al., 1995). The dimensional structure of the PI-R was investigated by means of large clinical groups (i.e. OCD patients, PD patients and social phobics). A five-factor solution emerged which could be interpreted as (1) impulses, (2) washing, (3) checking, (4) rumination and (5) precision. Looking at the phenomenology, the subscales of the PI-R adequately reflect the different symptoms of OCD. The reliability of these subscales proved to be satisfactory to excellent. With regard to discriminant validity, apart from the subscale impulses, the scales were able to differentiate between obsessive compulsives from patients with PD, social phobics and normals. This instrument was tested in various large clinical samples and turned out to be both reliable and valid in terms of construct and discriminant validity (Van Oppen et al., 1995). Moreover, of the existing self-report measures of OCD that have been clinically validated, the PI-R appears to assess more heterogeneous symptoms of OCD.

The Dissociative Experience Scale (DES) is an instrument which is particularly useful in uncovering therapeutically relevant subjective experience and should be considered whenever a patient speaks of subjective memory loss or lost portions of time, especially when co-existent with a history of childhood trauma, to screen for possible dissociative disturbances (Bernstein & Putnam, 1986).

In summary, relevant scales to measure efficacy in OCD trials exist although the definition of clinically relevant responses remains difficult.

6 Discussion

OCD is a disabling illness characterised by time-consuming, intrusive, recurrent obsessions and compulsions that cause marked distress and significant life impairment. Symptoms are similar across cultures (Weissman et al., 1994). Of all the anxiety disorders, OCD may well be the most disabling as well as the least understood (Karno & Golding, 1991). It is far more idiosyncratic, in that in addition to problems of increased anxiety associated with all anxiety disorders, it also consists of unusual patterns of behaviour (repetitive behaviours) and highly intrusive and often bizarre ideation (obsessive thoughts). Little is known about its association with other anxiety problems or the degree to which its various components relate to interference with daily living or readiness to seek treatment. A recent study showed that when "full screen" OCD (patients with both obsessions and compulsions) is viewed as a single entity in which there is no comorbid anxiety problem, incidence of OCD appears very low (Welkowitz et al., 2000). However, when comorbidity is taken into account, the incidence rates rise dramatically. Thus for patients who meet full-screen criteria for OCD and any other anxiety disorders (GAD, PTSD, SP or PD), the prevalence rate of OCD rises from 0.7 to 3.3%. The presence of GAD appears to give the OCD the largest comorbid numbers, suggesting that most patients are also experiencing significant problems in general worrying and nervousness.

One observation receiving growing empirical support is that some forms of early-onset OCD may be related to Tourette's syndrome and other tic disorders. Tic disorders are more prevalent in boys (Leckman et al., 1997). Therefore, a relationship between some forms of early-onset OCD and tic disorders could account for the preponderance of boys among child cases of OCD. Evidence supporting the relationship between Tourette's syndrome and early-onset OCD comes also from studies reporting a high degree of comorbidity between OCD and tics among child-onset cases. Although unusual obsessions and compulsions appear to be more frequent in those children with OCD and comorbid tic disorders, some children with OCD who do not have comorbid tics also display these tic-like rituals. In the absence of comorbid tics, there appears to be a higher frequency of both comorbid tic disorders and tic-like rituals in childhood cases of OCD (Rettew et al., 1992). However, such unusual obsessions and compulsions have not been reported in studies of OCD in adults (Rasmussen & Eisen, 1992; Rasmussen & Tsuang, 1986). Thus, it appears that onset of OCD does typically occur in childhood or adolescence in patients with tic disorders.

Dosages of pharmacological treatments have often been described as being significantly higher than antidepressant dosages (e.g., 60–80 mg once a day (qd) of fluoxetine). However, in controlled trials, there has been no observed significant difference between response to higher and lower dosages for the SSRIs (e.g., 50 and 200 mg qd of sertraline). This clinical impression may well relate to the slow onset of efficacy with many patients taking 10 to 12 weeks to improve, during which time the prescriber continues to increase the patient's doses, mistakenly thinking it was the increased dose, not time, that was responsible for improvement. Many patients will not respond to the first SSRI but will respond to another antiobsessional drug. Therefore, sequential trials are frequently necessary, which easily can take up to a year to accomplish. Patients who have not responded to large dosages of each of these medications occasionally improve on extremely low dosages (e.g., 5–10 mg/

day of fluoxetine or 25 mg/day of clomipramine) (Jenike, 2001). These patients have not been carefully studied. If patients fail to improve with high dosages, it may be worth trying a very low dose.

Relapse prevention programs have proved beneficial in maintaining the gains of acute treatment (Hiss et al., 1994). In routine practice, some combination of pharmacotherapy and behavioural therapy is often employed. Available research is not yet clear on potential benefits of combined medication and behavioural therapy, either on response or on relapse prevention. Nonetheless, most OCD patients on pharmacological treatment should probably be encouraged to practice exposure prevention.

Clomipramine is as effective as SSRIs in the treatment of OCD. In very elderly patients, it is best to avoid clomipramine as the initial drug, since it has adverse effects that can interfere with thinking and cause confusion or worsen confusion. Other drugs like SSRIs can be used in elderly patients, but reduced dosages are often necessary (Salzman, 1982). Although relatively pure noradrenergic re-uptake inhibitors such as desipramine are inactive in OCD, compounds inhibiting the re-uptake of both serotonin and noradrenaline, such as venlafaxine and milnacipran may be superior to the SSRIs in OCD (Schatzberg, 2000, Ninan, 1999). A study of a small series of patients suggested that venlafaxine may also be effective (Rauch et al., 1996). Clearly placebo-controlled studies are warranted to demonstrate the potential of SSRIs and SNRIs in OCD.

Current hypotheses regarding the pathophysiological features of OCD emphasise the involvement of the prefrontal cortex, subcortical structures and the distributed neural circuits that connect these regions (Insel, 1992; Cummings, 1993; Rauch et al., 1996). Future neuroimaging studies of OCD will benefit from the use of cognitive activation paradigms to examine activation while controlling the mental state of patients.

References

Ackerman DL, Greenland S, Bystritsky A, Morgernstern H & Katz RJ. Predictors of treatment response in obsessive-compulsive disorder: Multivariate analyses from a multicenter trial of clomipramine. J Clin Psychopharmacol 14, 247–254, 1994

Allen AJ, Leonard HL & Swedo SE. A new infection-triggered autoimmune subtype of pediatric OCD and Tourette's syndrome. J Am Acad Child Adolesc Psychiatry 34, 307–311, 1995

Altemus M, Jacobson KR, Debellis M, Kling M, Pigott T, Murphy DL & Gold PW. Normal CSF oxytocin and NPY levels in OCD. Biol Psychiatry 45 (7), 931–933, 1999

Altshuler LL, Hendrick V & Cohen LS. Course of mood and anxiety disorders during pregnancy and the postpartum period. J Clin Psychiatry 59 (Suppl 2), 29–33, 1998

American Psychiatric Association. Diagnostic and Statistical manual of mental disorders, 4th ed. Washington, DC: American Psychiatric Association, 1994

Arpels JC. The female brain hypoestrogenic continuum from the premenstrual syndrome to menopause: a hypothesis and review of supporting data. J Reprod Med 41, 633–639, 1996

Aylward EH, Harris GJ, Hoehn-Saric R, Barta PE, Machlin SR & Pearlson GD. Normal caudate nucleus in obsessive-compulsive disorder. Arch Gen Psychiatry 53, 577–584, 1996

Baker RW, Bermazonn PC, Wirshing DA & Chengappa KN. Obsessions, compulsions, clozapine and risperidone. Central Nervous System Spectrums 2, 6–36, 1997

Baxter LR Jr. Positron emission tomography studies of cerebral glucose metabolism in obsessive compulsive disorder. J Clin Psychiatry 55 (Suppl), 54–59, 1994

Bernstein E & Putnam F. Development, reliability and validity of a dissociation scale. J Nerv Ment Dis 174, 727–735, 1986

Berthier ML, Kulisevsky J, Gironell A & Heras JA. Obsessive-compulsive disorder associated with brain lesions: Clinical phenomenology, cognitive function, and anatomic correlates. Neurology 47, 353–361, 1996

Bogetto F, Venturello S, Albert U, Maina G & Ravizza L. Gender-related clinical differences in obsessive-compulsive disorder. Eur Psychiatry 14, 434–441, 1999

Carey G & Gottesman II. Twin and family studies of anxiety, phobic, and obsessive disorders. In: DF Klein, JG Rabkin (eds): Anxiety: New research and changing concepts. New York, NY: Raven Press, 117–136, 1981

Castle DJ, Deale A & Marks IM. Gender differences in obsessive compulsive disorder. Aus N Z J Psychiatry 29, 114–117, 1995

Chelmow D & Halfin VP. Pregnancy complicated by obsessive-compulsive disorder. J Matern Fetal Med 6, 361–34, 1997

Childs B & Scriver CR. Age at onset and causes of disease. Perspect Biol Med 29 (3, pt 1), 437–460, 1986

Cummings JL. Frontal-subcortical circuits and human behavior. Arch Neurol 500, 873–880, 1993

Deckersbach T, Otto MW, Savage CR, Baer L & Jenike MA. The relationship between semantic organization and memory in obsessive-compulsive disorder. Psychother Psychosom 69, 101–107, 2000

DeRubeis R & Crits-Christoph P. Empirically supported individual and group psychological treatments for adult mental disorders. J Consult Clin Psychol 66, 37–52, 1998

Dirson S, Bouvard M, Cottraux J & Martin R. Visual memory impairment in patients with obsessive-compulsive disorder. J Neuropsychiatry 6, 22–31, 1996

Enoch M-A, Greenberg BD, Murphy DL & Goldman D. Sexually dimorphic relationship of a 5-HT_{2A} promoter polymorphism with Obsessive-Compulsive Disorder. Biol Psychiatry 49, 385–388, 2001

Fallon BA, Liebowitz MR, Campeas R, Schneier FR, Marshall R, Davies S, Goetz D & Klein DF. Intravenous clomipramine for obsessive-compulsive disorder refractory to oral clomipramine. Arch Gen Psychiatry 55, 918–924, 1998

Fineberg NA & Montgomery SA. Are serotonin receptors involved in obsessive compulsive disorder? Eur Neuropsychopharmacol 2 (3), 179–181, 1992

Fineberg NA, Roberts A & Montgomery SA. Are higher doses more effective in OCD? Eur Neuropsychopharmacol 3, 264–265, 1994

Fischer DJ, Himle JA & Hanna GL. Age and gender effects on obsessive compulsive symptoms in children and adults. Depress Anxiety 4, 237–239, 1997

Flament MF, Whitaker A, Rapoport JL, Davies M, Berg CZ, Kalikow K, Sceery W & Shaffer D. Obsessive compulsive disorder in adolescence: An epidemiological study. J Am Acad Child Adolesc Psychiatry 27, 764–771, 1988

Flament MF, Rapoport JL, Berg CJ, Sceery W, Kilts C, Mellstrom B & Linnoila M. Clomipramine treatment of childhood obsessive-compulsive disorder. A double-blind controlled study. Arch Gen Psychiatry 42 (10), 977–983, 1985

Foa EB, Steketee GS & Ozarow BJ. Behavior therapy with obsessive-compulsive: from theory to treatment. In: M Mavissakalian, SM Turner SM & L Michelson (eds): Obsessive-compulsive disorder: psychological and pharmacological treatment. New York: Plenum Press, 49–129, 1985

Freeman CPL, Trimble MR, Deakin JFW et al. Fluvoxamine *versus* clomipramine in the treatment of obsessive compulsive disorder: a multicenter, randomized, double-blind, parallel group comparison. J Clin Psychiatry 55, 301–305, 1994

Gilbert AR, Moore GJ, Keshavan MS, Paulson LAD, Narula V, Mac Master FP, Stewart CM & Rosenberg DR. Decrease in thalamic volumes of pediatric patients with obsessive-compulsive disorder who are taking paroxetine. Arch Gen Psychiatry 57, 449–456, 2000

Gillberg I, Rastam M & Gillberg C. Anorexia nervosa 6 years after onset. Part 1. Personality disorders. Compr Psychiatry 36, 61–69, 1995

Goff D, Olin J, Jenike M, Baer L & Buttolph M. Dissociative symptoms in patients with obsessive-compulsive disorder. J Nerv Ment Dis 180, 332–337, 1992

Goldstein RB, Wickramaratne PJ, Horwath E & Weissman MM. Familial aggregation and phenomenology of "early"-onset (at or before age 20 years) panic disorder. Arch Gen Psychiatry 54, 271–278, 1997

Goodman WK, Ward H, Kablinger A & Murphy T. Fluvoxamine in the treatment of obsessive-compulsive disorder and related conditions. J Clin Psychiatry 58 (Suppl 5), 32–49, 1997

Goodman WK, Price LH, Rasmussen SA, Mazure C, Delgado P, Heninger CR & Charney DS. The Yale-Brown Obsessive Compulsive Scale. Arch Gen Psychiatry 46, 1006–1016, 1989

Greist JH, Chouinard G, DuBoff E, Halaris A, Kim SW, Koran L, Liebowitz M, Lydiard RB, Rasmussen S & White K. Double-blind parallel comparison of three dosages of sertraline and placebo in outpatients with obsessive-compulsive disorder. Arch Gen Psychiatry 52, 289–295, 1995a

Greist JH, Jefferson JW, Kobak KA, Katzelnick DJ & Serlin RC. Efficacy and tolerability of serotonin transport inhibitors in obsessive-compulsive disorder. Arch Gen Psychiatry 52, 53–60, 1995

Hand I. Ambulante Verhaltenstherapie bei Zwansstorungen. Fortschr Neurol Psychia 63 (1), 12–18, 1995

Hantouche EG & Lancrenon S. Modern typology of symptoms and obsessive-compulsive syndromes: results of a large French study of 615 patients. Encephale 1, 9–21, 1996

Hiss H, Foa EB & Kozak MJ. Relapse prevention program for treatment of obsessive-compulsive disorder. J Consult Clin Psychol 62, 801–808, 1994

Hollander E & Wong C. Body dysmorphic disorder, pathological gambling and sexual compulsions (review). J Psychiatry 4, 7–12, 1995

Holzer JC, Goodman WK, McDougle CJ, Baer L, Boyarsky BK, Leckman JF & Price LH. Obsessive compulsive disorder with and without a chronic tic disorder. Br J Psychiatry 164, 469–473, 1994

Insel TR, Mueller EA, Gillin JC & Siever LJ. Biological markers in obsessive-compulsive and affective disorders. Biol Psychiatry Res 18, 407–420, 1984

Insel TR. Toward a neuroanatomy of obsessive-compulsive disorder. Arch Gen Psychiatry 49, 739–744, 1992

Inyoue E. Similar and dissimilar manifestations of obsessive-compulsive neurosis in monozygotic twins. Am J Psychiatry 121, 1171–1175, 1965

Jacobsen F. Risperidone in the treatment of affective illness and obsessive-compulsive disorder. J Clin Psychiatry 56, 423–439, 1995

Jenike MA. A 45-year-old woman with obsessive-compulsive disorder. JAMA 285, 2121–2128, 2001

Jenike MA, Baer L & Greist JH. Clomipramine *versus* fluoxetine in obsessive-compulsive disorder: a retrospective comparison of side effects and efficacy. J Clin Psychopharmacol 10, 122–124, 1990

Joffe RT, Swinson RP & Regan JJ. Personality features of obsessive-compulsive disorder. Am J Psychiatry 145, 1127–1129, 1988

Karno M, Golding J, Sorenson S & Burnam MA. The epidemiology of obsessive-compulsive disorder in five US communities. Arch Gen Psychiatry 45, 1094–1099, 1988

Karno M & Golding JM. Obsessive compulsive disorder. In: LN Robins, DA Regier (eds): Psychiatric disorders in America. New York, NY: Free Press, 204–219, 1991

Kaye WH, Weltzin TE, Hsu LKG, Bulik CM, McConaha C & Sobkiewicz T. Patients with anorexia nervosa have elevated scores on the Yale-Brown Obsessive-Compulsive Scale. Int J Eat Disord 12, 57–62, 1992

Kim SW, Dysken MW & Kuskowski M. The Yale-Brown Obsessive-Compulsive Scale: a reliability and validity study. Psychiatry Res 34, 99–104, 1990

Kohn R, Westlake RJ, Rasmussen SA, Marsland RT & Norman WH. Clinical features of obsessive-compulsive disorder in the elderly patients. Am J Geriatr Psychiatry 5, 211–215, 1997

Kolada JL, Bland RC & Newman SC. Obsessive-compulsive disorder. Acta Psychiatr Scand 376, 24–35, 1994

Kopp S & Gillberg C. Girls with social deficits and learning problems: autism, atypical Asperger syndrome or a variant of these conditions. Eur Child Adolesc Psychiatry 1, 89–99, 1992

Kusunoki K, Sato T, Taga C, Yoshida T, Komori K, Narita T, Hirano S, Iwata N & Ozaki N. Low novelty-seeking differentiates obsessive-compulsive disorder from major depression. Acta Psychiatr Scand 101, 403–405, 2000

Laird L. Issues in the monopharmacotherapy and polypharmacotherapy of obsessive-compulsive disorder. Psychopharmacother Bull 32, 569–578, 1996

Leckman JF, Peterson BS, Pauls DL & Cohen DJ. Tic disorders. Psychiatr Clin North Am 20, 839–861, 1997

Lensi P, Cassano GB, Correddu G, Ravagli S, Kunovac JL & Akiskal HS. Obsessive-compulsive Disorder: familial-developmental history, symptomatology, comorbidity and course with special reference to gender-related differences. Br J Psychiatry 169, 101–107, 1996

Leonard HL, Swedo SE, Rapoport JL et al. Treatment of obsessive-compulsive disorder with clomipramine and desipramine in children and adolescents. A double-blind cross-over comparison. Arch Gen Psychiatry 46, 1088–1092, 1989

Leonard HL, Swedo SE, Lenane MC et al. A double-blind desipramine substitution during long-term clomipramine treatment in children and adolescents with obsessive-compulsive disorder. Arch Gen Psychiatry 48, 922–927, 1991

Leonard HL. New developments in the treatment of obsessive-compulsive disorder. J Clin Psychiatry 58 (Suppl 14), 39–45, 1997

March JS. Cognitive-behavioral psychotherapy for children and adolescents with OCD: a review and recommendation for treatment. J Am Acad Child Adolesc Psychiatry 34, 7–18, 1995

Maes M, Vandoolaeghe E & Desnyder R. Efficacy of treatment with trazodone in combination with pindolol or fluoxetine in major depression. J Affect Disord 41, 201–210, 1996

Marazziti D & Pallanti S. Effectiveness of olanzapine treatment for severe obsessive-compulsive disorder. Am J Psychiatry 156, 11, 1834–1835, 1999

Marks IM. Fears, phobias and rituals. New York: Oxford University Press, 1987

McDougle CJ, Epperson CN, Pelton GH, Wasylink S & Price LH. A double-blind, placebo-controlled study of Risperidone addition in serotonin reuptake inhibitor-refractory obsessive-compulsive disorder. Arch Gen Psychiatry 57, 794–801, 2000

Millet B, Touitou Y, Poirier MF et al. Plasma melatonin and cortisol in patients with obsessive-compulsive disorder: relationship with axillary temperature, physical activity, and clinical symptoms. Biol Psychiatry 44, 874–881, 1998

Monteleone P, Catapano F, Del Buono G & Maj M. Circadian rhythms of melatonin, cortisol and prolactin in patients with obsessive-compulsive disorder. Acta Psychiatr Scand 89, 411–415, 1994

Moreno FA, Gelenberg AJ, Bachar K & Delgado PL. Pindolol augmentation of treatment-resistant depressed patients. J Clin Psychiatry 58, 437–439, 1997

Mundo E, Richter MA, Sam F, Macciardi F & Kennedy JL. Is the 5-HT (1Dbeta) receptor gene implicated in the pathogenesis of obsessive-compulsive disorder? Am J Psychiatry 157 (7), 1160–1161, 2000

Mundo E, Bianchi L & Bellodi L. Efficacy of fluvoxamine, paroxetine, and citalopram in the treatment of obsessive-compulsive disorder: a single-blind study. J Clin Psychopharmacol 17 (4), 267–271, 1997

Murray CL & Lopez AD. The global burden of disease: A comprehensive assessment of mortality and disability from diseases, injuries and risk factors in 1990. Cambridge, Mass: Harvard University Press, 1996

Murphy DL, Pickar D & Alterman IS. Methods for the quantitative assessment of depressive and manic behaviour. In: ET Burdock, A Sudilousky & S Gersho (eds): The behavior of psychiatric patients. New York: Marcel Dekker Inc, 355–391, 1982

Neziroglu FA, Yaryura Tobias JA, Lemli JM & Yaryura RA. [Demographic study of obsessive compulsive disorder]. Acta Psiquiatr Psicol Am Lat 40 (3), 217–223, 1994

Nestadt G, Samuels JF, Romanoski AJ, Folstein MF & McHugh PR. Obsessions and compulsions in the community. Acta Psychiatr Scand 55 (Suppl), S5–S10, 1994

Nestadt G, Bienvenu OJ, Cai G, Samuels J & Eaton WW. Incidence of obsessive-compulsive disorder in adults. J Nerv Ment Dis 186, 401–406, 1998

Nestadt G. Samuls J, Riddle M, Bienvenu IIIJ, Liang K-Y, LaBuda M, Walkup J, Grados M & Hoehn-Saric R. A family study of obsessive-compulsive disorder. Arch Gen Psychiatry 57, 358–363, 2000

Ninan PT. The functional anatomy, neurochemistry, and pharmacology of anxiety. J Clin Psychiatry 60 (Suppl 22), 12–17, 1999

Noshirvani HF, Kasvikis Y, Marks IM, Tsakiris F & Monteiro WO. Gender-divergent aetiological factors in obsessive-compulsive disorder. Br J Psychiatry 158, 260–263, 1991

Owens DG, Johnstone EC & Frith CD. Spontaneous involuntary disorders of movement: their prevalence, severity, and distribution in chronic schizophrenics with and without treatment with neuroleptics. Arch Gen Psychiatry 39, 452–461, 1982

Pauls DL, Cohen DJ, Kidd KK & Leckman JF. Tourette syndrome and neuropsychiatric disorder: Is there a genetic relationship? Am J Hum Genet 43, 206–217, 1988

Pauls DL, Alsobrook JP, Goodman W, Rasmussen S & Leckman JF. A family study of obsessive-compulsive disorder. Am J Psychiatry 152, 76–94, 1995

Perez J, Tardito D, Ravizza L, Racagni G, Mori S & Maina G. Altered cAMP-dependent protein kinase A in platelets of patients with obsessive-compulsive disorder. Am J Psychiatry 157, 284–286, 2000

Perez J, Tardito D, Mori S, Racagni G, Smeraldi E & Zanardi R. Abnormalities of cyclic adenosine monophosphate signaling in platelets from untreated patients with bipolar disorder. Arch Gen Psychiatry 56, 248–253, 1999

Pigott TA, Pato MT, Bernstein SE et al. Controlled comparison of clomipramine and fluoxetine in the treatment of obsessive-compulsive disorder. Arch Gen Psychiatry 47, 926–932, 1990

Purcell R, Maruff P, Kyrios M & Pantelis C. Neuropsychological deficits in Obsessive-Compulsive Disorder. A comparison with unipolar depression, panic disorder, and normal controls. Arch Gen Psychiatry 55, 415–423, 1998

Rafaat OA, Mahallawy N, El Nahas G, Seld El Dawla A, Sayed M & El Kholi S. Cognitive dysfunction in obsessive-compulsive disorder. Acta Psychiatr Scand 101, 281–285, 2000

Rasmussen SA & Eisen JL. The epidemiology and clinical features of obsessive compulsive disorder. Psychiatr Clin North Am 15, 743–758, 1992

Rasmussen SA & Tsuang MT. Clinical characteristics and family history in DSM-III obsessive-compulsive disorder. Am J Psychiatry 143, 317–322, 1986

Rasmussen SA & Eisen JL. Treatment strategies for chronic and refractory obsessive-compulsive disorder. J Clin Psychiatry 58 (Suppl 13), 9–13, 1997

Rauch SL, Savage CR, Alpert NM, Miguel EC, Breiter HC, Fishman AJ, Manzo P, Moretti C & Jenike MA. A positron emission tomographic study of simple phobic symptoms provocation. Arch Gen Psychiatry 52, 20–28, 1995

Rauch SL, O'Sullivan RL, Jenike MA. Open treatment of obsessive-compulsive disorder with venlafaxine: a series of ten cases. J Clin Psychopharm 16, 81–84, 1996

Rauch SL & Savage CR. Neuroimaging and neuropsychology of the striatum: Bridging basic science and clinical practice. Psychiatr Clin North Am 20, 741–768, 1997

Rauch SL, Savage CR, Alpert NM, Dougherty D, Kendrick A, Curran T, Brown HD, Manzo P, Fischman AS & Jenike MA. Probing striatal function in obsessive-compulsive disorder using PET and a sequence learning task. Neuroimage 3 (Suppl), S507, 1996

Rauch SL, Whalen PJ, Dougherty DD & Jenike MA. Neurobiological models of obsessive

compulsive disorders. In: MA Jenike, L Baer & WE Minichiello (eds): Obsessive compulsive disorders: practical management. Boston: Mosby, 222–253, 1998
Rauch SL, Savage CR, Alpert NM, Dougherty D, Kendrick A, Curran T et al. Probing striatal function in obsessive compulsive disorder. A PET Study of implicit sequence learning. J Neuropsychiatry 9, 568–573, 1997
Ravizza L, Maina G & Bogetto F. Episodic and chronic obsessive-compulsive disorder. Depress Anxiety 6, 154–158, 1997
Rettew DC, Swedo SE, Leonard HL, Lenane MC & Rapoport JL. Obsessions and compulsions across time in 79 children and adolescents with obsessive-compulsive disorder. J Am Acad Child Adolesc Psychiatry 31, 1050–1056, 1992
Riddle MA, Scahill L, King RA, Hardin MT, Anderson GM, Ort SI, Smith JC, Leckman JF & Cohen DS. Double-blind, crossover trial of fluoxetine and placebo in children and adolescents with obsessive-compulsive disorder. J Am Acad Child Adolesc Psychiatry 31, 1062–1069, 1992
Riddle MA, Claghorn J, Gaffney G et al. Fluvoxamine for children and adolescents with obsessive-compulsive disorder: a controlled multicenter trial. Proc Am Acad Child Adolesc Psychiatry, 80–87, 1996
Ristvedt SL, Mackenzie TB & Christenson GA. Cues to obsessive-compulsive symptoms: Relationships with other patient characteristics. Behav Res Ther 31, 721–729, 1993
Ronchi P, Abruzzese M, Erzegovesi S, Diaferia G, Sciuto G & Bellodi L. The epidemiology of obsessive-compulsive disorder in an Italian population. Eur Psychiatry 7, 53–59, 1992
Ross C & Anderson G. Phenomenological overlap of multiple personality disorder and obsessive-compulsive disorder. J Nerv Ment Dis 176, 295–299, 1988
Shelton RC, Manier DH & Sulser F. cAMP-dependent protein kinase activity in major depression. Am J Psychiatry 153, 1037–1042, 1996
Salzman C. A primer on geriatric psychopharmacology. Am J Psychiatry 139, 67–76, 1982
Saxena S, Wang D, Bystritsky A & Baxter L. Risperidone augmentation of SRI treatment for refractory obsessive-compulsive disorder. J Clin Psychiatry 57, 303–306, 1996
Saxena S, Brody AL, Schwartz JM & Baxter LR Jr. Neuroimaging and frontal-subcortical circuitry in obsessive-compulsive disorder. Br J Psychiatry 173 (Suppl 35), 26–38, 1998
Savage CR. Neuropsychology of OCD: Research findings and treatment implications. In: MA Jenike, L Baer & WE Minichiello (eds): Obsessive compulsive disorders: practical management. Boston: Mosby, 254–275, 1998
Savage CR, Baer L, Keuthen NJ, Brown HD, Rauch SL & Jenike MA. Organizational strategies mediate nonverbal memory impairment in obsessive-compulsive disorder. Biol Psychiatry 45 (7), 905–916, 1999
Savage CR, Keuthen NJ, Jenike MA, Brown H, Baer L, Kendrick AD, Miguel EC, Rauch SL & Albert MS. Recall and recognition in obsessive-compulsive disorder. J Neuropsychiatry 8, 99–103, 1996
Schatzberg AF. New indications for antidepressants. J Clin Psychiatry 61 (Suppl 11), 9–17, 2000
Sciuto G, Pasquale L & Bellodi L. Obsessive compulsive disorder and mood disorders: a family study. Am J Med Genet 60, 475–479, 1995
Shear MK. Anxiety disorders in women: gender-related modulation of neurobiology and behavior. Semin Reprod Endocrin 15, 69–76, 1997

Sichel DA, Cohen LS, Dimmock JA et al. Postpartum obsessive compulsive disorder: a case series. J Clin Psychiatry 54, 156–159,1993

Sichel D, Cohen L, Rosenbaum J et al. Postpartum onset of obsessive-compulsive disorder. Psychosomatics 34, 277–279, 1996

Skoog G & Skoog I. A 40-year follow-up of patients with obsessive-compulsive disorder. Arch Gen Psychiatry 56, 121–127, 1999

Stein D, Spadaccini E & Hollander E. Meta-analysis of pharmacotherapy trials for obsessive-compulsive disorder. Int Clin Psychopharmacol 10, 11–18, 1995

Steiner M, Bushnell WD & Gergel I. Long-term treatment and prevention of relapse of obsessive-compulsive disorder with paroxetine. Presented at the 1995 annual meeting of the American Psychiatric Association; May 20–25, 1995, Miami, Fla.

Steketee G, Eisen J, Dyck I, Warshaw M & Rasmussen S. Predictors of course in obsessive-compulsive disorder. Psychiatry Res 89, 229–238, 1999

Swedo SE, Leonard HL, Garvey M, Mittleman B, Allen AJ, Perlmutter S et al. Pediatric autoimmune neuropsychiatric disorders associated with streptococcal infections: Clinical description of the first 50 cases. Am J Psychiatry 155, 164–271, 1998

Swedo S, Rapaport J, Leonard H et al. Obsessive-compulsive symptoms in children and adolescents: Clinical phenomenology of 70 consecutive cases. Arch Gen Psychiatry 46, 335–341, 1989

Thomsen PH & Mikkelsen HU. Course of obsessive-compulsive disorder in children and adolescents: a prospective follow-up study of 23 Danish cases. J Am Acad Child Adolesc Psychiatry 34, 1432–1440, 1995

Thomsen PH & Mikkelsen HU. Children and adolescents with obsessive-compulsive disorder: The demographic and diagnostic characteristics of 61 Danish patients. Acta Psychiatr Scand 83, 262–266, 1991

Thomsen PH. Obsessive-compulsive disorder in children and adolescents: predictors in childhood for long-term phenomenological course. Acta Pschiatr Scand 92, 255–259, 1995

Tollefson GD, Rampey AH, Potvin JH et al. A multicenter investigation of fixed-dose fluoxetine in the treatment of obsessive-compulsive disorder. Arch Gen Psychiatry 51, 559–567, 1994

Toro J, Cervera M, Osejo E & Salamero M. Obsessive-compulsive disorder in childhood and adolescence: A clinical study. J Child Psychol Psychiatry 33, 1025–1037, 1992

Van Oppen P, Hoekstra RJ & Emmelkamp PMG. The structure of obsessive compulsive symptoms. Behav Res Ther 33, 15–23, 1995

Warneke LB. Intravenous chlorimipramine therapy in obsessive-compulsive disorder. Can J Psychiatry 34, 853–859, 1989

Warnock J & Bundren J. Anxiety and mood disorders associated with gonadotropin-releasing hormone agonist therapy. Psychopharmacol Bull 33, 311–316, 1997

Warren R & Thomas JC. Cognitive-behavior therapy of obsessive-compulsive disorder in private practice: An effectiveness study. J Anxiety Disord 15, 277–285, 2001

Weiner MB & White MT. The use of a self-psychology approach in treating a compulsive 84-year-old man. Clin Gerontol 3, 64–67, 1985

Weiss M, Baerg E, Wisebord S et al. The influence of gonadal hormones on periodicity of obsessive-compulsive disorder. Can J Psychiatry 40, 205–207, 1995

Weissman MM, Bland RC, Canino GJ, Greenwald S, Hwu HG, Kyoon C, Newman SC, Oakley-Browne MA, Rubio-Stipec M, Wickramaratne PJ et al. for the Cross National Collaborative Group. The Cross national epidemiology of obsessive-compulsive disorder. J Clin Psychiatry 55 (Suppl), S5–S10, 1994

Welkowitz LA, Struening AL, Pittman J, Guardino M & Welkowitz J. Obsessive-compulsive disorder and comorbid anxiety problems in a National Anxiety Screening sample. J Anxiety Disord 14 (5), 471–482, 2000

Wever C & Rey JM. Juvenile obsessive-compulsive disorder. Aust NZ J Psychiatry 31, 105–113, 1997

Williams KE & Koran LM. Obsessive-compulsive disorder in pregnancy, the puerperium, and the premenstrum (CME). J Clin Psychiatry 58, 330–334, 1997

World Health Organization. The ICD-10 Classification of Mental and behavioural Disorders. Diagnostic Criteria for Research. Geneva: WHO Office of Publications, 1993

Yaryura Tobias JA, Neziroglu FA & Kaplan S. Self-mutilation, anorexia, and dysmenorrhea in obsessive compulsive disorder. Int J Eat Disord 17, 33–38, 1995

Zohar J, Judge R & the OCD Paroxetine Study Investigators. Paroxetine vs. Clomipramine in the treatment of obsessive-compulsive disorder. Br J Psychiatry 169, 468–474, 1996

Chapter 7
Posttraumatic stress disorder

1 Introduction

In 1980, the APA added PTSD to the third edition of its DSM-III nosologic classification scheme. The DSM-III chose to define PTSD as a final common pathway occurring in response to many different types of catastrophic stressors, including burn injury, concentration camps, combat, and natural disasters. In fact, this approach was in opposition to the idea of the uniqueness of individual traumas such as "Vietnam syndrome" or "post-rape syndrome". Although a controversial diagnosis when first introduced, the concept of PTSD is today regarded as having filled an important gap in neuropsychiatric theory and practice. The DSM-III diagnostic criteria for PTSD were revised in DSM-IIIR (1987) and DSM-IV (APA, 1994). Diagnostic criteria for PTSD include a history of exposure to a "traumatic event" and symptoms from each of three symptom clusters: intrusive recollections, avoidant/numbing symptoms and hyperarousal symptoms. Another criterion concerns duration of symptoms (see Tab. 7.1). There are three subtypes of PTSD. The first is the acute subtype which corresponds to duration of symptoms of less than 3 months. The second is the chronic subtype which corresponds to a duration of symptoms of more than 3 months. The third subtype has a delayed onset, which corresponds to onset of symptoms at least 6 months following the stressor, but may be much later. Indeed, there have been cases in which PTSD re-emerged after 20, or even 40 years. PTSD is unique among other psychiatric diagnoses because of the great importance placed upon the etiologic agent, the traumatic stressor. In fact, one cannot make a diagnosis unless the patient has actually met the stressor criterion that means that he or she has been exposed to a historical event that is considered traumatic. Another hallmark is the alternation between re-experiencing and avoiding trauma-related memories. The memories that are particularly associated with PTSD appear rapidly and spontaneously, often intruding into consciousness with high frequency. The intrusive memories may consist of images accompanied by high levels of physiological arousal and are experienced as re-enactments of the original trauma (flashbacks). Flashbacks are qualitatively different from memories of the trauma which are retrievable through a normal search of long-term memory. They may be distinguished from normal memories by the original intensity of the emotions that accompany the flashbacks (Terr, 1991; Van der Kolk & Fisler, 1995).

Traumatic events are commonly associated with a cascade of secondary stresses (Pynoos et al., 1998). They constitute additional sources of distress and increase the risk of comorbidity of PTSD reactions with other adverse reactions. They complicate efforts at adjustment and may interfere with normal opportunities for develop-

Table 7.1: DSM-IV criteria for PTSD

A.	The person has been exposed to a traumatic event in which both of the following have been present:
(1)	The person has experienced, witnessed, or been confronted with an event or events that involve actual or threatened death or serious injury, or a threat to the physical integrity of oneself or others
(2)	The person's response involved intense fear, helplessness, or horror. Note: in children, it may be expressed instead by disorganised or agitated behaviour.
B.	The traumatic event is persistently reexperienced in at least one of the following:
(1)	Recurrent and intrusive distressing recollections of the event, including images, thoughts, or perceptions. Note: in young children, repetitive play may occur in which themes or aspects of the trauma are expressed.
(2)	Recurrent distressing dreams of the event. Note: in children, there may be frightening dreams without recognisable content
(3)	Acting or feeling as if the traumatic event were recurring (includes a sense of reliving the experience, illusions, hallucinations, and dissociative flashback episodes, including those that occur upon awakening or when intoxicated). Note: in young children, trauma-specific re-enactment may occur
(4)	intense psychological distress at exposure to internal or external cues that symbolise or resemble an aspect of the traumatic event
(5)	physiologic reactivity upon exposure to internal or external cues that symbolise or resemble an aspect of the traumatic event
C.	Persistent avoidance of stimuli associated with the trauma and numbing of general responsiveness (not present before the trauma), as indicated by at least three of the following:
(1)	efforts to avoid thoughts, feelings, or conversations associated with the trauma
(2)	efforts to avoid activities, places, or people that arouse recollections of the trauma
(3)	inability to recall an important aspect of the trauma
(4)	markedly diminished interest or participation in significant activities
(5)	feeling of detachment or estrangement from others
(6)	restricted range of affect (e.g., unable to have loving feelings)
(7)	sense of a foreshortened future (e.g., does not expect to have a career, marriage, children, or a normal life span)
D.	Persistent symptoms of increased arousal (not present before the trauma), as indicated by at least two of the following:
(1)	difficulty falling or staying asleep
(2)	irritability or outbursts of anger
(3)	difficulty concentrating
(4)	hypervigilance
(5)	exaggerated startle response
E.	Duration of the disturbance (symptoms in B, C, and D) is more than one month.
F.	The disturbance causes clinically significant distress or impairment in social, occupational, or other important areas of functioning.

Specify if:
ACUTE: if duration of symptoms is less than three months.
Specify if:
With delayed onset: onset of symptoms at least six months after the stressor.

mental maturation or initiate maladaptive coping responses that, over time, may be associated with chronic psychopathology other than PTSD.

Several approaches have been used to explain PTSD, including biological theories, psychological paradigms, learning theory, cognitive models and models that integrate both psychological and biological perspectives (Horowitz, 1986; Kolb, 1987; Fairbank & Brown, 1987; Jones & Barlow, 1990). Although all of these approaches encompass theories that offer valid insights into the nature of the dysfunction underlying PTSD, it is the cognitive model that is perhaps the most fully developed and offers the greatest explanation and predictive power. There is a clear clinical need to understand PTSD, both to devise effective treatments and to gain some insight into its prevention. Claims for efficacy have been made for various drugs including tricyclics, MAOIs, fluoxetine, lithium, carbamazepine, BDZs, β-blockers, α_2-agonists and neuroleptics. In December 1999, sertraline (Zoloft) was approved by the FDA for the treatment of PTSD. As pharmacotherapy occupies an important place in PTSD, there is a need to devise rigorous clinical trials to assess short- and long-term efficacy treatment in PTSD patients. In this chapter, the aetiology of PTSD will be discussed. Emphasis will be laid on the cognitive dysfunctions associated with PTSD as well as current potential pharmacological treatments as revealed by psychopharmacology research. A discussion on the physiological and neurological abnormalities associated with PTSD will also be included.

2 Epidemiology

Epidemiological studies suggest that a lifetime prevalence of PTSD in the general population is currently estimated to range from 7.8 to 9.2% (Breslau et al., 1991; Davidson et al., 1991; Kessler et al., 1995). Approximately 60% of these cases seem to become chronic. A recent study in New York found that 39% of patients who sought medical attention after a road traffic accident met criteria for PTSD (Blanchard et al., 1995). The initial onset of PTSD may occasionally be delayed by many years and a large percentage of patients (70%) recalled traumatic events at 2 years that they had not reported at 1 month after the trauma (Hales & Zatzick, 1997; Blank, 1993). However, the development of PTSD at 1 year can be predicted as early as 1 week after the accident on the basis of the existence and severity of early PTSD-related symptoms (Koren et al. 1999). The first 3 months following the accident appear to be the critical period for the development of PTSD. Its longitudinal course has multiple variations, namely acute, delayed, chronic, intermittent, residual and reactivated patterns (Zeiss & Dickman, 1989). A Vietnam readjustment study reported that 19 years after combat exposure, 15% of veterans still suffered from PTSD (Kulka et al., 1990).

Lifetime prevalence of exposure to traumatic events and number of traumatic events did not vary by sex but the risk for PTSD after exposure to traumatic events was more than two-fold higher in women than in men (Breslau et al., 1997). Gender differences have been identified in the acute, as well as delayed, response to severe trauma and abuse. A large study of a treated study group with PTSD showed a rate of 11% in women and 7% in men (Yonkers & Ellison, 1996). The investigators extrapolated from their data to estimate that 31% of women and 19% of men who are exposed to major trauma develop PTSD symptoms. In other words, when exposed to a traumatic event, more women than men develop PTSD. In addition, women make up 85% of the group whose symptoms last for over a year. Women victimised by domestic violence are more likely to develop anxiety symptoms, whereas men may be at greater risk of developing substance use disorders in the context of ongoing abuse or violence (Magdol et al., 1997). Although physical symptoms and emotional distress are common sequelae of domestic violence, the presence of severe or life-threatening physical injuries does not reliably predict that psychiatric symptoms or PTSD will subsequently emerge (Sutherland et al., 1998). Instead, "perceived threat", the victim's perception of danger during an assault, may be more important than objective or realistic assessments in the formation of PTSD. Most studies suggest that women are not at greater risk for traumatic exposure, but are more likely to develop PTSD when exposed to trauma (Breslau et al., 1995; 1997; Kesler & McLeod, 1984). This difference is also noted when all other socio-demographic factors were controlled, with the rate in women being more than two-fold higher than in men (Breslau et al. 1996). The reason that women seem more vulnerable to PTSD and other anxiety disorders remains largely undetermined.

Considering the types of trauma involved in PTSD, the most frequent traumata reported by people who had PTSD were (1) threat or close call, (2) seeing someone hurt or killed, (3) physical attack, (4) accident, and (5) combat (Helzer et al., 1987). In women, a study reported assault and rape as the most frequent trauma leading ot PTSD (Resnick et al., 1993). There are no data on the period prevalence of PTSD in the general elderly population.

3 Comorbidity

PTSD is highly comorbid with other psychiatric disorders including drug dependence. Studies of Vietnam veterans provided some evidence of the comorbidity between PTSD and drug abuse disorders (Breslau et al., 1998; McFall et al., 1991; Davidson et al., 1990; Escobar et al., 1983). Little is known about the causal pathways that might explain the observed comorbidity. However, a recent study which investigated PTSD and drug disorders indicated that PTSD is correlated with an increased risk of drug abuse or dependence whereas exposure to traumatic events in the absence of PTSD did not increase the risk of drug abuse or dependence (Chilcoat & Breslau, 1998). The risk for abuse or dependence was the highest for prescribed psychoactive drugs. There was no evidence that pre-existing drug abuse or dependence increased the risk of subsequent exposure to traumatic events or the risk of PTSD after traumatic exposure. The relationship between PTSD and drug abuse disorders is complex but it is likely that in many cases, the drug abuse disorder may develop as an attempt to self-medicate painful symptoms of PTSD. In any individual case, the relationship between these disorders, both in order of onset and symptom exacerbation and presentation, should be explored to provide individually tailored treatment.

Across a number of studies, major depressive disorder and dysthymia are the psychiatric disorders most likely to co-occur with PTSD. A study reported that 48% of men and 49% of women with PTSD had lifetime major depressive disorder, making it the most common co-occurring disorder (Kessler et al., 1995). High rates of comorbid PTSD and depression have been found among preadolescents and adolescents after catastrophic natural, transportation disasters and violence (Goenjian et al., 1995). Most studies suggest that individuals with both PTSD and depression were more distressed, had more major role impairment and were less likely to experience symptom remission during the 6-month follow-up (Blanchard et al., 1998; Shalev et al., 1998). PTSD with major depression appears to be an important risk factor for suicidality (Wonderlich et al., 1997). In general, PTSD and depressive disorders are closely related, but the nature of this relationship is complex and variable and must be examined on a case-by-case basis.

Considering PTSD and comorbid anxiety disorders, a study reported that 69% of treatment-seeking patients with trauma histories reported experiencing panic attacks (Falsetti & Resnick, 1997). There was no indication that PD was related to the type of traumatic experience. The panic symptoms most frequently reported were rapid heart rate or palpitations and fear of going crazy or losing control. In differential diagnosis, it is helpful to keep in mind that in PD, fear and avoidance have more to do with physical symptoms associated with panic attacks (e.g., palpitations, sweating, chest pains, fear of having a heart attack), whereas in PTSD, fear and avoidance are specifically related to trauma-related memories and cues.

The association between SP and PTSD has only recently been appreciated. A study reported that 72% of Vietnam veterans who met criteria for PTSD also met criteria for SP (Orsillo et al., 1996). Significantly more veterans with PTSD met criteria for SP compared with a group of veterans without PTSD. It was postulated that fear of disapproval and lack of a supportive posttrauma environment contributed to social anxiety.

The comorbidity of PTSD and psychotic disorders is a relatively unexplored area. However, several investigators have studied the presence of psychotic symptoms in individuals with PTSD. A study showed that 40% of veterans consecutively admitted to a PTSD inpatient rehabilitation unit reported psychotic symptoms (David et al., 1999). These psychotic symptoms included auditory hallucinations, visual hallucinations, and delusions. The hallucinations were nonbizarre and consisted of trauma-related themes. These patients had no formal thought disorders. In fact, 81% of the chronic PTSD veterans met criteria for current major depression, suggesting the psychotic symptoms were associated with major depression.

4 Physiological and neurological abnormalities associated with PTSD

Neurobiological research indicates that PTSD may be associated with significant alterations in both the autonomic nervous and central nervous system. Psychophysiological alterations with PTSD include hyperarousal of the sympathetic nervous system, increased sensitivity and augmentation of the acoustic-startle eyeblink reflex, a reducer pattern of auditory evoked cortical potentials, and sleep abnormalities.

4.1 Physiological abnormalities

Neurophysiological abnormalities have been detected in the noradrenergic, HPA and endogenous opioid systems of PTSD patients (see Tab. 7.2). Much clinical evidence also suggests that in many of these victims such chronic alterations persist even 25 years after exposure to the trauma (Southwick et al., 1992; Friedman et al., 1995). Trauma survivors with PTSD show evidence of a highly sensitised HPA axis characterised by decreased basal cortisol levels and increased negative feedback regulation. Cortisol levels are equally low in men and women with PTSD (Yehuda et al., 1995). The physiological effects of cortisol depend on the ability of cortisol to bind to glucocorticoid receptors. Current research suggests that PTSD patients have more type II glucocorticoid receptors on circulating lymphocytes compared to normals whereas depressed patients have fewer receptors (Yehuda et al., 1995; Whalley et al., 1986). Consistent with both low cortisol and increased glucocorticoid receptor number, PTSD patients have shown a significant augmented cortisol suppression in response to dexamethasone (8:00 am postdexamethasone cortisol levels at or above 5.0 µg/dl) compared to normals. This finding is opposite to the classic cortisol non-suppression typically observed in depressed patients (Carroll et al., 1981; Bauer et al., 1994). The finding of enhanced cortisol suppression in response to dexamethasone has been confirmed in several other PTSD populations including adult survivors of childhood sexual abuse, adult sexual abuse and children exposed to natural disasters (Goenjian et al., 1996; Heim et al., 1997; Stein et al., 1997).

Another neuroendocrine method, the metyrapone test, has been used to provide information about basal adrenocorticotropic hormone (ACTH) release in PTSD (Yehuda et al., 1996). Metyrapone temporarily prevents adrenal steroidogenesis by blocking the conversion of 11-deoxycortisol to cortisol. In this way, it unmasks the pituitary gland from the influences of negative feedback inhibition. Therefore, metyrapone administration permits a direct evaluation of pituitary release of ACTH while excluding the potentially confounding effects of differing ambient cortisol levels or glucocorticoid receptor responsiveness. When metyrapone (2500 mg) is administered in the morning when HPA axis activity is quite high, maximal pituitary activity can be achieved. It is possible to assess group differences in pituitary activity. The results of this study are consistent with an enhanced feedback sensitivity in PTSD in that PTSD patients showed a greater ACTH and 11-deoxycortisol increase following metyrapone administration compared to normal controls. The metyrapone test clearly differentiates between PTSD and normal controls. The unusual HPA axis profile noted in PTSD validates the suggestion that PTSD is a distinct disorder that can be differentiated from other neuropsychiatric illnesses. It

Table 7.2: Some abnormal physiological parameters observed in PTSD. REM: rapid eye movement

Some abnormal decrease
Blood and urinary cortisol
Platelet α_2-adrenergic receptor binding
Platelet monoamine oxidase activity
Platelet serotonin uptake
Sleep time
P300 event-related potential response to target stimuli
Hippocampal volume
Some abnormal increase
Physiological (e.g. catecholaminergic and electromyographic) responses to trauma-related stimuli
Physiologic responses to trauma-unrelated stimuli (e.g. loud tones)
Baseline heart rate and blood pressure
HPA axis negative feedback
Lymphocyte glucocorticoid receptors
Blood triiodothyronine (T3)
Sleep movements & awakenings
REM density

requires the development of specific treatment strategies for effective therapy of PTSD patients.

Investigations of neuroendocrine and peripheral catecholamine receptor systems also provide evidence for a dysregulation of sympathetic nervous system activity in PTSD. Twenty-four hour urine noradrenaline excretion has been reported as significantly increased, while platelet α_2-adrenergic receptor number and lymphocyte adenylate cyclase activity have been reported as significantly decreased compared with that in controls (Perry et al., 1987; Yehuda et al., 1992). This decrease in receptor number and adenylate cyclase activity may represent an adaptive down-regulation in response to persistently elevated levels of circulating catecholamines. Furthermore, lower basal cyclic AMP and lower basal adenylate cyclase levels among combat veterans as compared to controls were also reported (Lerer et al., 1987; 1990). Neuroendocrine challenge strategies have also been used to probe catecholamine systems in PTSD patients.

Sodium lactate infusion (10 ml/kg of 0.5 M administered over a period of 20 min) has been observed to induce flashbacks in individuals with PTSD without comorbid PD as compared to patients with PD or normal subjects (Jensen et al., 1997). Induced flashbacks were rated as very similar to spontaneous flashbacks. Cortisol levels were significantly lower in the PTSD group than in the comparison group at the end of the infusion.

The administration of intravenous (i.v.) yohimbine (0.4 mg/kg), an α_2-adrenergic blocker, produced panic attacks (70%) and flashbacks (40%) in a subgroup of PTSD patients (Southwick et al., 1993). In addition, in the patients with PTSD, yohimbine induced significant increases in core PTSD symptoms, such as intrusive traumatic thoughts, emotional numbing, and grief. A recent study investigating the effect of yohimbine and *m*-CPP (1.0 mg/kg i.v.; a probe of serotonergic activity) confirmed the effects of yohimbine in PTSD patients (Southwick et al., 1997). On the other hand, *m*-CPP induced panic attacks in PTSD patients who also showed significantly greater increases in anxiety, panic and PTSD symptoms compared to controls. Yohimbine-induced panic attacks tended to occur in patients different from those with *m*-CPP-induced panic attacks. The results of this study suggest that there are at least two different neurobiological subgroups of PTSD patients. Whereas the first group tends to have a sensitised noradrenergic system, the other group has a sensitised serotonergic system. Such a finding is important for the discovery and research of effective psychopharmacological treatment. Matching biological subtypes with appropriate pharmacological products may considerably increase the efficacy of the pharmacological treatment of PTSD.

Such clinical investigations may further clarify our understanding of PTSD and the pathophysiological mechanisms involved. For example, such approach has led to the suggestion that the hypersecretion of endogenous opioids results in the psychopathological condition of emotional numbing (Glover, 1992). All these hypotheses may hopefully lead to the discovery of innovative effective new pharmacological entities.

4.2 Neurobiology and brain abnormalities

Neurological changes in the neuronal pathways and synaptic clefts are hypothesised to occur as a consequence of excessive traumatic stimulation. An interesting finding was recently made when MRI scans of brains of combat veterans with PTSD were compared with those of civilians who did not have the disorder (Gurvits et al., 1996). Scans of the veterans' brains showed that the right hippocampus, a structure that plays a key role in memory, was slightly smaller than normal. This may indicate the possibility of neuronal death in this brain region. Hippocampal neuronal death in cells with high glucocorticoid receptors was also observed (Sapolsky et al. 1984). Such an observation was interpreted as being the result of a response to stress over time. This may also suggest that war, rape or torture induces psychiatric impairment as well as neurological dysfunctions.

Subtle neurologic impairment or neurologic soft signs (NSSs) has been reported in PTSD (Gurvits et al., 1999). NSSs reflect subtle abnormalities of language, motor coordination, perception and other CNS functions. This study showed that patients with PTSD had more neurodevelopmental problems and more childhood attention deficit/hyperactivity disorder symptoms. They had lower intelligence quotients, all of which were significantly correlated with NSSs. It is possible that the presence of antecedent neurologic abnormalities makes it less likely that patients with PTSD will recover. They are thus predisposed to a chronic course. Neurologic vulnerabilities may play a lesser role in acute PTSD. However, these hypotheses will need to be validated by further investigation.

Studies of PET scans also revealed clear neurological disturbances in PTSD patients (Shin et al., 1994; Rauch et al., 1996). The right amygdala was observed to be abnormally active while PTSD patients were reliving traumatic memories. As the amygdala is the key to the conditioned-fear response in animal studies, these studies indicate that traumatic memories are activating this learning centre. They also suggest that stress hormones stimulate these memories in the brain, inducing flashbacks. In a randomised, double-blind study of Vietnam combat veterans with PTSD and age-matched controls which used PET to measure brain metabolism after yohimbine (0.4 mg/kg) or placebo, it was reported that yohimbine resulted in a significant increase in anxiety in the patients with PTSD, but not in healthy volunteers (Bremner et al., 1997). There was a significant difference in brain metabolic response to yohimbine in patients with PTSD compared with healthy subjects in prefrontal, temporal, parietal, and orbitofrontal cortexes. Metabolism tended to decrease in patients with PTSD and increase in healthy subjects following administration of yohimbine. Another study that used PET investigation in combat veterans with PTSD reported that patients with PTSD had increased rCBF in ventral anterior cingulate gyrus and right amygdala when generating mental images of combat-related pictures. When viewing combat pictures, patients with PTSD showed decreased rCBF in Broca's area (Shin et al., 1997).

Recently, the event-related potentials (ERP) which provide a physiological index of central processing in PTSD patients were also studied (Paige et al., 1991). P300 and contingent negative variation (CNV) are ERP which are obtained in recording EEG from patients submitted to cognitive tasks. While P300 is related to "context updating" and working memory, CNV is more influenced by attention, motivation and motor preparation (Tecce & Cattanach, 1993). CNV and P300 amplitude were noted to be significantly lower in PTSD victims as compared to non-PTSD patients (McFarlane et al., 1993; Charles et al., 1995; Boudarene & Timsit-Berthier, 1997). This reduced ERP amplitude obtained in PTSD patients may be considered as physiological indicator of attentional deficits and the dynamics of the cerebral defence system after stressful events.

Considering the plasticity of the CNS and the results from animal model studies of brain trauma, the relationship between trauma and neurological deficit appears reciprocal. Trauma may cause alterations in neurological functioning while brain damage may precipitate behaviours that provoke PTSD symptoms. Obviously, further research is needed to provide a better understanding of the relationship between psychologic trauma and the development of neurological deficits.

Among adults, one model of PTSD focuses on abnormalities in the HPA axis. PTSD is associated with enhanced feedback control of this axis. Signs of such enhanced feedback include increased density of lymphocyte glucocorticoid receptors, low levels of resting cortisol and enhanced cortisol sensitivity to dexamethasone (Yehuda et al., 1995). Some evidence indicates that such abnormalities are tied to circadian rhythm disturbances, as reflected in the 24-h cortisol secretory pattern.

Preliminary neuroimaging studies among adults suggest a role for the hippocampus in PTSD (Bremner et al., 1995). Consistent with the close interplay between HPA and noradrenergic axes, there is also interest in the direct contribution of the noradrenergic axis to PTSD (Charney et al., 1993; Southwick et al., 1993).

Studies are beginning to extend these findings to children with PTSD. Children with PTSD exhibit both a blunted ACTH response to CRH challenge and abnormalities in peripheral catecholamine metabolism, suggesting HPA-and noradrenergic-axis abnormalities (DeBellis & Putnam, 1994). Childhood PTSD is also associated with signs of circadian rhythm disturbances (Glod & Teicher, 1996).

5 Cognitive dysfunction associated with PTSD

Current research suggests that certain cognitive alterations occur in PTSD. These changes are generally characterised by a preferential bias or increased attention associated with the presentation of threat-related stimuli (see Fig. 7.1). A stepwise discriminant analysis including all neuropsychological variables in neuropsychological tests identified attention and memory factors as the major cognitive dysfunctions associated with PTSD (Gilbertson et al., 1997). Studies on memory in PTSD patients also indicate that PTSD victims tend to overgeneralise on tasks involving personal recall, suggesting limitations in their ability to distinguish effectively among various salient cues. Various neuropsychological approaches have been attempted to assess PTSD.

5.1 Assessment of PTSD

Since 1980 there has been a great deal of attention devoted to the development of instruments/questionnaires to assess PTSD. Both psychometric and psychophysiologic assessment techniques that have proven to be reliable and valid have been devised (Keane et al., 1987).

The Impact of Event Scale (IES) which measures intrusion and avoidance symptomatology characteristics of PTSD is widely used in PTSD research and clinical practice (Horowitz et al., 1979). Although it does not strictly follow DSM diagnostic criteria, the IES does evaluate the three main symptom domains: intrusion, avoidance and hyperarousal (Weiss & Marmar, 1997). The IES quantifies 22 current (past week) symptoms, each on a severity rating of 0 to 5, and is fairly extensive to changes in symptoms between two time points. The IES yields a total score but can also be divided into three subscales, corresponding to the above-mentioned symptom domains. The IES can adequately discriminate between PTSD and non-PTSD groups for both re-experiencing and avoidance factors with a reported sensitivity of 74% and specificity of 78% (Woodfolk & Grady, 1988; Schwarzwald et al., 1987). Thus, its factor structure is indeed robust and has been shown to be consistent across studies (Shalev, 1997). The IES has been translated into many languages and

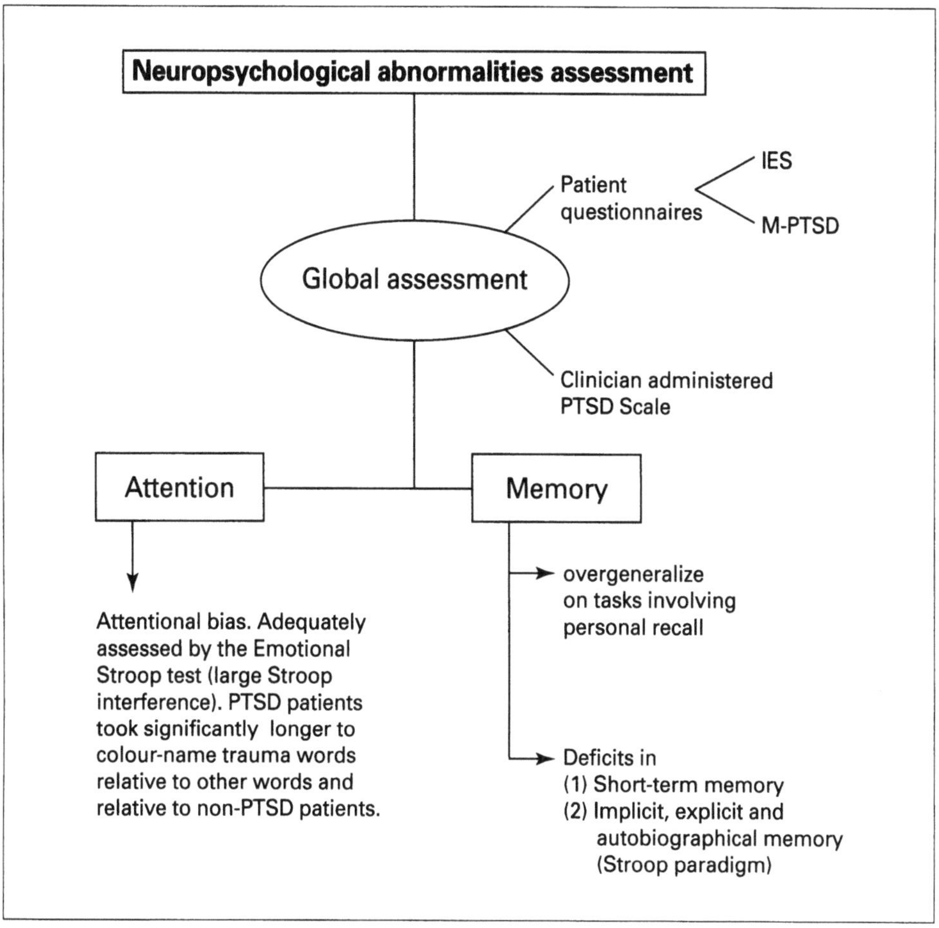

Figure 7.1
Some main neuropsychological dysfunctions in PTSD and their assessment methods. IES: Impact Event Scales; M-PTSD: Mississippi Scale for Combat-related PTSD

validated in several studies (Schwarzwald et al., 1987). It has been used extensively in treatment studies.

Considerable work has been conducted on the applicability of the Minnesota Multiphasic Personality Inventory (MMPI) to PTSD patients. The MMPI test has distinguished veterans with heavy combat experience from those with light combat experience (Penk et al., 1981). The MMPI test has also clearly differentiated PTSD from non-PTSD veterans seeking help for psychological problems (Foy et al., 1984).

The Mississipi Scale for Posttraumatic Stress Disorder (MISS) is a 35-item self-report questionnaire that focuses on the symptomatology found specifically after trauma (Keane et al., 1988). The MISS has both a civilian and a combat-related version (Vreven et al., 1995). The MISS does not follow DSM-IV symptoms but has been used in numerous epidemiologic studies of PTSD from which a cutoff score has been derived to indicate the presence or absence of PTSD. Respondents indicate that frequency with which they experience each symptom on a Likert scale ranging from 1 ("Never") to 5 ("Very Frequently"). Items include, for example: "It seems as if I have no feelings" (emotional numbing) and "I wonder why I am alive when others died in the military" (survival guilt). Scores can range from 35 to 175, and scores of 107 or higher generally indicate the presence of PTSD. The MISS test has a high test-retest reliability and excellent sensitivity (test sensitivity = 0.93, specificity = 0.93, overall hit rate = 0.90) when used to differentiate between a PTSD and a non-PTSD group (Keane et al., 1988).

Specifically designed for PTSD, the Duke Global Rating of PTSD (DGRP) offers a global evaluation of PTSD by an observing clinician. As does the CGI measurement, the DGRP refers to the clinician's total clinical experience with this particular population as a basis for a global evaluation of four items: intrusive phenomena, avoidant behaviour, hyperarousal and overall severity. Each item is rated on a severity scale of 1 to 7.

The Clinician Administered PTSD Scale (CAPS) is a structured clinical interview dedicated to PTSD (Blake et al., 1990; 1995). The CAPS has been widely used in clinical studies of PTSD, including treatment studies. The CAPS examines all three symptom clusters of PTSD, quantifying symptom frequency and intensity for each PTSD symptom during the past month or past 2 weeks, depending on the version used. The CAPS yields both a continuous measure of symptom severity and a dichotomous diagnosis of PTSD. However, it requires clinical skills, judgement and experience. The interview takes between 25 and 45 min. The CAPS has been used effectively to assess change in symptom intensity over time. The Davidson Trauma Scale is a self-rating questionnaire that requires the subject to rate the frequency and the intensity of his or her PTSD symptoms during the last week on a scale of 0 (not at all) to 5 (every day; extreme) (Davidson et al., 1997). The instrument assesses 17 DSM-IV PTSD symptoms and yields a continuous measure of global severity, as well as partial measures of each cluster of symptoms (intrusions, avoidance and hyperarousal).

Davidson's TOP-8 is a brief structured interview, based on eight PTSD symptoms that have been shown to better respond to treatment interventions (Davidson & Colket, 1997). The items evaluate the following symptoms: (1) intrusive images, thoughts of memories of traumatic events, (2) physiological responsivity to reminders of the traumatic event, (3) avoidance of places, people, activities or conversations that remind the patient of the traumatic events, (5) loss of interest in other people and estrangement, (6) numbing and loss of feelings towards others, (7) being on guard, watchful and on edge, and (8) exaggerated startle response. These items belong to all three symptom clusters for PTSD, and showed an improved ability to detect drug *versus* placebo differences. Each symptom is evaluated on a 1–4 intensity scale. The instrument yields a continuous measure of symptom severity.

However, due to limitations in the definition of the criterion diagnosis of PTSD as well as the uncertainty with which respective cutoff points were chosen for some of the existing scales, further research is necessary to analyse the validity of screening measures to assess PTSD. There is a crucial need to develop instruments to assess PTSD diagnosis among highly traumatised populations other than American Vietnam veterans. It also appears that the CAPS has a better prediction of clinical observation of PTSD, which possibly captures additional components of the patient's behaviour (Gelpin et al., 1996). However, whether the difference is due to specific properties of the CAPS or whether it represents some generic advantage of clinical observation over self-report psychometrics deserves further study.

5.2 Attentional bias: the emotional Stroop test

It is acknowledged that anxious individuals show bias in selective attention. Such individuals are prone to attend to material whose content is threatening in preference to neutral or positive material. The Stroop colour-word task has been a valuable tool to study attentional bias and in the classic Stroop test, the subject is required to name the colour of ink in which an incompatible colour word is printed (e.g. the word "green" is printed in red ink) (Stroop, 1935). Subjects take longer to name the ink colour in this case than in a control condition in which the word "red" is printed in red. This phenomenon is referred to as Stroop interference. The emotional Stroop test that is the principal method to demonstrate attentional bias is a modified version of this classical paradigm.

Research on cognitive dysfunction in PTSD has focused on two types of information-processing studies. Valence-independent studies require patients to process information that varies in complexity, but not in emotional valence (e.g. experiments on intelligence and short-term memory) (McNally & Shin, 1995). Valence-dependent studies require patients to process affectedly charged information related to trauma (e.g. experiments on attentional and memory biases favouring processing of trauma-relevant information). In the studies using valence-dependent processing biases in PTSD, the technique of emotional Stroop colour-naming paradigm seems promising. In this attentional paradigm, patients are shown words of varying emotional significance that are printed in different colours. They are asked to name the colours in which the words appear while ignoring the meanings of the words. Delayed colour naming (Stroop interference) occurs when the meaning of a word captures the patient's attention despite his effort to focus on its colour. Because colour-naming delays reflect involuntary activation of meaning, interference produced by trauma-related material may provide a quantitative index of intrusive cognition: PTSD patients ought to take longer to name the colours of trauma-related words relative to other words, whereas patients without PTSD should not. Current research suggests the confirmation of this hypothesis in studies in which it was observed that PTSD patients took significantly longer to name the colours of all the words on a single card (McNally et al., 1990). In addition, PTSD patients took significantly longer to colour-name trauma words relative to other words and relative to non-PTSD patients who did not respond differentially as a function of word type. Interference for trauma words was also significantly related to the severity of the PTSD symptoms.

Stroop studies confirmed that words closely related to trauma produce more interference than words that are less related to trauma (Cassiday et al., 1992;

Thrasher et al., 1994; Kaspi et al., 1995). Trauma-related words are a sensitive measure of clinical state, thus indicating the potential utility of the emotional Stroop paradigm as a convenient measure for evaluating response to treatment. However, it may be suggested from the fact that the size of the Stroop interference effect is much stronger in PTSD (115–400 ms) as compared to interference effects in other psychopathology (e.g. panic attack: 24–57 ms; OCD: 24–108 ms; SP: 24–113 ms; depression: 18–116 ms) that different or additional cognitive mechanisms might underlie colour-naming disruption in PTSD conditions (Williams et al., 1996). Although it may be argued that such large Stroop interference effect in PTSD patients may be due to their particular clinical pathology in which highly frequent and severe intrusive thoughts and flashbacks are a major diagnostic feature, further future studies to better understand such observation are necessary.

The interpretation of the findings with the emotional Stroop paradigm in anxiety states in terms of selective attention to threatening information seems relatively straightforward. However, interests in the explanation of the mechanisms underlying Stroop interference have led to the propositions of some models. The most common explanatory models have been Beck's schema theory or Bower's network theory (Beck et al., 1985; Bower, 1981). Recent studies have suggested different explanations for the attentional bias hypothesis (Dawkins & Furnham, 1989; Carter et al., 1992). It was observed, for example that PD patients displayed interference on threat words but also on other emotional words including positively valenced words and that "repressors" showed even greater interference than high trait anxious subjects. The findings that colour-naming interference may be shown on emotionally valent stimuli whether positive or negative is very important. This observation calls into questions those explanations of the emotional Stroop test that assume that emotionally disturbed individuals have increased accessibility only to threat information. Such observations have led to the proposition of an alternative hypothesis in which both attentional bias and cognitive avoidance are assumed to function in the emotional Stroop test but in which the cognitive avoidance is suggested to be mainly responsible for the greater interference effects found in PTSD victims, anxious subjects and "repressors" (De Ruiter & Brosschot, 1994). It was also suggested that future research should use, in addition to the Stroop task, other paradigms such as dichotic listening and attention deployment task to further unravel the cognitive biases associated with anxiety states of the patients concerned.

5.3 Memory

Significant deficits in short-term memory have been reported in PTSD patients (Bremner et al., 1993). In a study comparing Vietnam veterans with combat-related PTSD to physically healthy subjects and using a battery of neuropsychological tests (e.g. Wechsler adult intelligence scale, Wechsler memory scale, selective reminding test), severe memory deficits were observed in PTSD patients. The PTSD patients scored significantly lower on the logical memory component of the Wechsler memory scale (44% lower on immediate recall and 55% lower on delayed recall). Interestingly, a significant negative correlation was also observed between the percentage of retention for the Wechsler memory scale figural memory component and the current level of PTSD symptoms as measured by the Mississippi scale for combat-related PTSD ($r = -0.62$).

The Stroop paradigm has been used to study memory impairment (implicit, explicit and autobiographical memory) in PTSD patients. The Stroop methodology employed was based on the hypothesis that explicit memory is revealed when task performance requires conscious recollection of previous experiences. Explicit memory may be usually accessed by direct tests such as recognition, free recall, and cued recall. Implicit memory is revealed when previous experiences enhance performance on a task that does not require effortful, conscious recollection of these experiences. It is usually measured by indirect tests such as word-stem completion, lexical decision, and tachistoscopic word identification. The results suggest that patients with PTSD seem characterised by explicit and implicit memory biases favouring trauma-relevant information, yet also exhibited poor recall for all but trauma words.

Studies dealing with autobiographical memory suggest that this type of memory is also impaired in the PTSD patients who exhibited difficulties retrieving specific personal memories in response to cue words having either positive (e.g. kindness), neutral (e.g. appearance), or negative (e.g. panic) valence (McNally et al. 1993; Kaspi et al., 1995). When asked to retrieve an autobiographical memory triggered by a cue, PTSD patients tended to retrieve general memories that did not reference any specific event, suggesting that trauma-related thoughts may hamper access to other memories. A relative inability to retrieve specific personal memories having positive emotional valence may be related to emotional numbing, and to the extent that inability to retrieve episodes from the past handicap an individual's ability to envision the future. Overgenerality may be implicated in the problem-solving deficits that occur in PTSD patients (Nezu & Carnevale, 1987).

At present, no generally acceptable method is available to diagnose PTSD when the causal event has resulted in neurogenic amnesia. PTSD and neurogenic amnesia may not be diagnosed concurrently since memory for the trauma is assumed to be a necessary condition for the manifestation of PTSD (the unitary memory theory, Sbordone, 1992). However, the multiple memory systems which divide memory into declarative memory (refers to stored experience that actually or potentially is accessible to conscious recollection-memory system disrupted in amnesia) and nondeclarative memory (mediates a variety of phenomena, none of which are accessible to consciousness) suggest that declarative memory for a traumatic event is not a necessary condition for development of PTSD (Layton & Wardi-Zonna, 1995). It is suggested that the operation of a nondeclarative memory system is a sufficient condition for the development of PTSD. Two case reports with posttraumatic amnesia that developed PTSD illustrate this hypothesis. One of the cases reported was a subject (GR) who denied memory of the accident but developed nightmares with images of motorcycles crashing. Such observation also questions the belief that neurogenic amnesia may be protective with respect to posttraumatic emotional reactions.

For problems of amnesia not directly related to physical neurological concussion or brain damage, several terms that include "repression", "dissociative amnesia" and "psychogenic amnesia" have been used to describe such memory deficits (Freud, 1914; American Psychiatric Committee on Nomenclature and Statistics, 1994; Spiegel, 1995). In DSM-IV, dissociative amnesia is defined as "inability to recall important personal information, usually of a traumatic or stressful nature, that is too important to be explained by ordinary forgetfulness". In a review of evidence from prospective studies to test whether individuals can develop amnesia for traumatic experiences, it was argued that the data failed to demonstrate that individuals can develop dissociative amnesia for traumatic events (Pope et al., 1998). In studies in which patients were asked directly about a past traumatic experience, they consistently reported memories. Non-reporting occurred only in studies where patients were not asked directly about the experience. In a recent study that aimed to investigate the profile of PTSD after severe traumatic brain injury during which the patients had no cohesive recall of events occurring in the first months after the trauma, it was observed that 27.1% of the patients met the criteria for PTSD (Bryant et al., 2000). This study indicates that emotional (96.2%) and physiological reactivity (50%) mediate trauma re-experiencing. The low incidence of intrusive memories (19.2%) in this group of patients contrasts with the rate of intrusive memories in PTSD after assault (93%) and terrorist activity (85%) (Foa et al., 1995; Loughrey et al., 1993). However, this observation provides strong evidence against the claim that PTSD cannot occur after a severe traumatic brain injury (Sbordone & Liter, 1995).

6 Treatment of PTSD

Many therapeutic approaches have been proposed for the treatment of PTSD, including psychodynamic therapy (Marmar et al., 1995), cognitive-behavioral therapy (Foa et al., 1995), pharmacotherapy (Friedman & Southwick, 1995) and treatment for patients dually diagnosed with PTSD and alcoholism (Kofoed et al., 1993). Psychotherapy is considered to be a major part of the treatment. However, there are times when the distress and discomfort from the hyperarousal of the sympathetic nervous system may inhibit or impede a psychotherapeutic treatment. Treatment of PTSD is generally multimodal, with pharmacotherapy medication that may be helpful in controlling the trauma-related symptoms playing an important role (Shalev et al., 1996). There can also be a beneficial effect of both psychotherapy and pharmacologic therapy (Friedman, 1988; Van der Kolk, 1988).

6.1 Psychotherapeutic approach

According to a survey of 52 experts on psychotherapy treatment, three psychotherapy techniques (exposure therapy, cognitive therapy and anxiety management) are considered to be the most useful in the treatment of PTSD (The Expert Consensus Guidelines Series, 1999) (see Tab. 7.3). The most successful interventions are those implemented immediately after an incident such as civilian disaster or war zone

Table 7.3: Preferred psychotherapy techniques for different target symptoms. Treatment of choice for target symptoms of either intrusive thoughts or flashbacks or trauma-related fears or panic and avoidance is exposure therapy. For guilt/shame, it is cognitive therapy (The Expert Consensus Guidelines Series, 1999).

Most prominent symptom	Recommended techniques	Also consider
Intrusive thoughts	Exposure therapy	Cognitive therapy Anxiety management Psychoeducation Play therapy for children
Flashbacks	Exposure therapy	Anxiety management Cognitive therapy Psychoeducation
Trauma-related fears, panic and avoidance	Exposure therapy Cognitive therapy Anxiety management	Psychoeducation Play therapy for children
Numbing/detachment from others/loss of interest	Cognitive therapy	Psychoeducation Exposure therapy
Irritability/angry outbursts	Cognitive therapy Anxiety management	Psychoeducation Exposure therapy
Guilt/shame	Cognitive therapy	Psychoeducation Play therapy for children
General anxiety (hyperarousal, hypervigilance, startle)	Anxiety management Exposure therapy	Cognitive therapy Psychoeducation Play therapy for children
Sleep disturbance	Anxiety management	Exposure therapy Cognitive therapy Psychoeducation
Difficulty concentrating	Anxiety management	Cognitive therapy Psychoeducation

trauma. This is often referred to as critical incident stress debriefing (CISD). The best outcomes are obtained when the trauma survivors receive CISD within hours or days of exposure. Such interventions not only attenuate the acute response to the trauma but also often forestall the latter development of PTSD.

6.1.1 *Exposure therapy*

Traditional learning theory and bio-informational theory suggest that exposure to conditioned stimuli, while preventing escape or avoidance, results in habituation of anxiety. Behaviour therapy proceeds either by gradual (desensitisation) or by massive (flooding) re-exposure to the conditioned stimuli. The bio-informational theory emphasises the necessity of activating the fear memory and of providing information which is incompatible with that existing in the fear memory so that a new memory can be formed (Foa et al., 1989). Thus programs of exposure therapy vary in duration of exposure (short *versus* prolonged), the number of low-level anxiety situations that precede the introduction of the most feared situation, and the arousal level experienced (low *versus* high). Exposure therapy is a relatively easy treatment to master and instructions to patients are relatively straightforward.

An exposure treatment called "image habituation training" for patients suffering from PTSD has been proposed (Vaughan & Tarrier, 1994), the objective of which is to expose the patient to self-evoked images in order to produce habituation of anxiety. This was achieved by the use of audiotaped descriptions of the trauma which were to be used during self-directed homework sessions. The use of audiotapes in habituation training has been suggested as a method of maximising exposure to cognitive events (Salkovskis & Kirk, 1989). The benefit of this method is its economy in clinician's time and its use of an audiotape to facilitate self-directed exposure to trauma-related images and thoughts. This approach also permits frequent exposure sessions to be carried out by the patient at home and decreases problems of anticipatory anxiety. Several studies have investigated the effects of exposure therapy in veterans from the Vietnam War with PTSD (Foa & Meadows, 1997). These studies indicate that exposure therapy is effective in reducing PTSD symptoms in this population, but the therapeutic effects were modest (Keane et al., 1989). However, a recent study designed to predict response to exposure treatment in PTSD patients (rape victims) emphasised the impact of mental defeat and alienation on treatment outcome (Ehlers et al., 1998). It was suggested that patients who experienced mental defeat, alienation or permanent change may require cognitive restructuring in addition to exposure.

6.1.2 Anxiety management programs

Anxiety management programs emerged from the view that pathologic anxiety stems from a deficit in skills required to cope with anxiety. These programs provide patients with management skills to help them reduce anxiety when it occurs. Anxiety management programs include relaxation training, controlled breathing, positive imagery, cognitive restructuring and distraction techniques. One of the most commonly used anxiety management programs for PTSD is stress inoculation training (Meichenbaum, 1974; Veronen & Kilpatrick, 1982). Some uncontrolled studies have examined the efficacy of stress inoculation training in women who had been raped (Kilpatrick et al., 1982; Veronen & Kilpatrick, 1983). Although these studies provided encouraging results, the absence of a control group prevented definitive conclusions.

Desensitisation therapy is another method of treatment using relaxation responses to counter stimuli that previously elicited anxiety (Rawlins et al., 1993). This is accomplished through relaxation training, which involves the construction of a hierarchy of situations that elicit anxiety in varying degrees, and working to remain relaxed through each situation in the hierarchy until the most anxiety-producing situation is reached.

6.1.3 *Cognitive therapy*

Cognitive therapy postulates that certain dysfunctional thinking patterns produce pathologic emotions that culminate in the manifestations of psychiatric disorders, including PTSD. Cognitive therapy teaches the patients to identify their dysfunctional cognitions, challenge them, and replace them with functional, realistic beliefs. One kind of cognitive therapy designed for rape victims with PTSD is cognitive processing therapy (Resick & Schnicke, 1992). The goal of cognitive processing therapy is to correct specific maladaptive cognitions with focus on five issues thought to be associated with rape victims: safety, trust, power, esteem and intimacy. The program also includes an exposure component, an instruction to write down a detailed account of the traumatic memory and read it back to the therapist. Preliminary results suggest that this treatment is highly effective in ameliorating PTSD (Resick et al., 1999). However, a drawback of the cognitive processing therapy is that it requires the therapist to undertake extensive training and place considerable intellectual demands on the patients.

6.1.4 *Eye movement and desensitisation reprocessing*

Much interest has recently been generated by case reports of rapid improvements measurements in PTSD patients using eye-movements as described in eye-movement desensitisation-reprocessing procedure (EMD-R) (Spector & Huthwaite, 1993; Wolpe & Abrams, 1991). With this approach, patients imagine the traumatic event together with associated thoughts and somatic reactions while they visually track the therapist's finger that moves rapidly from side to side across the visual field. It appears that this treatment reduced anxiety, changed the way patients thought about the traumatic event, and stopped their flashbacks, intrusive thoughts and sleep disturbances (Shapiro, 1989). Analysis of eye movement data in the laboratory with normal volunteers provides an explanation as to the mechanism involved. All data seem to suggest that if EMD-R works, this may be due to the reduction of the vividness and emotiveness of traumatic images *via* the visuospatial sketchpad system of working memory which processes visual and spatial information (Andrade et al., 1997). Although criticisms argue that EMD-R will not fulfil its promise of being a treatment approach superior to existing exposure treatments (Herbert & Mueser, 1992), current research suggests the development of the technique of EMD-R in PTSD has triggered a re-examination of exposure in anxiety and PTSD. It is likely that results from such research will provide methodology to improve the current version of the EMD-R into a very effective treatment approach in PTSD patients.

Controlled trials of cognitive-behavioral treatments of patients with PTSD have demonstrated the clinical benefit of exposure and cognitive therapy (Marks et al., 1998; Tarrier et al., 1999). A study which investigated whether treatment benefits and equivalence are maintained at 12-month follow-up in patients with chronic PTSD treated with either imaginal exposure or cognitive therapy showed that there was significant clinical improvement at 12 months compared with pre-treatment (Tarrier et al., 1999a). However, 39% of those followed up still met criteria for

PTSD. There were no significant differences between the two treatments. Victims of crime showed higher levels of symptoms at follow-up than accident victims.

6.2 Biofeedback

A study in 29 Vietnam veterans with a 12 to 15 year history of chronic combat-related PTSD was performed (Peniston & Kulkosky, 1991). Alpha (8–13 Hz)-theta (4–8 Hz)-enhancement training of 15 patients was compared with traditional medical treatment of 14 patients. The 15 alpha-theta feedback patients improved on all ten clinical MMPI scales: hypochondriasis, depression, conversion hysteria, psychopathic deviate, masculinity-femininity, paranoia, psychasthenia, schizophrenia, hypomania, and social introversion. The traditional treatment group improved in only one, the schizophrenia scale. The 14 alpha-theta feedback patients who were medicated all required less medication, compared with only 1 of 13 traditional treatment patients who were medicated. At 30 months three alpha-theta feedback patients had relapsed, compared with all 14 traditional treatment patients.

6.3 Pharmacological approach

It is important to distinguish between acute and chronic PTSD since this will affect both the selection and the duration of drug therapy. In managing acute PTSD, pharmacologic therapy may help to enable the repressed traumatic events to be brought to the surface, to be accepted and integrated by the patient so that he is no longer afraid. For acute PTSD, diazepam has been used (Sargant & Slater, 1972). Positive results with propranolol in children with acute PTSD were noted where a dose of 2.5 mg/kg was observed to reduce symptoms of hyperarousal and hypervigilance (Famularo et al., 1988).

Chronic PTSD has been the most intensely studied form of PTSD from the standpoint of pharmacotherapy. Drug treatment may be expected to accomplish a number of positive effects such as to reduce intrusive and avoidant symptoms, decrease hyperarousal, improve sleep, better regulate aggressive and uncontrollable impulses, control psychotic symptoms and treat comorbid psychopathology. Despite having a theoretical appeal based upon their antiarousal effects, BDZs have received very little attention in PTSD. This is probably due to the fact that this class of compounds may induce tolerance and a patient is likely to abuse this medication.

6.3.1 Tricyclics

Double-blind trials of tricyclic drugs indicated positive effects on PTSD symptoms (Frank et al., 1988; Davidson et al., 1990). Tricyclic antidepressants (TCAs) are often considered a first-line medication for symptoms involving re-experiencing and numbing, and other symptoms such as hyperalertness, sleep disturbance and memory difficulties. Amitriptyline was found to be helpful with nightmares and in treating symptoms such as insomnia, depressed mood and flashbacks (Falcon et al., 1985). Imipramine was observed to be beneficial in relieving the intrusion symptoms to a greater degree than the avoidance symptoms (Burstein, 1984). Neuroleptics were suggested to be generally inferior to antidepressants in PTSD, possibly due to greater neuroleptic-associated behavioural deficits which would indicate a need for some caution regarding their use (Casella & Davis, 1985). In general, although the use of these antidepressants suggests that they may improve PTSD symptoms of intrusion and avoidance as well as depression, insomnia and anxiety, the magnitude of the effect is far less than that obtained with these medications in major depression. No study has demonstrated a full remission of PTSD symptoms as is often the case in major depression.

6.3.2 *Selective serotonin reuptake inhibitors*

Fluoxetine, an SSRI, was reported to be an effective treatment for some patients with chronic PTSD (see Tab. 7.4). In an open, 10-week trial of fluoxetine in 19 PTSD patients and using a battery of assessment scales (the Clinician-Administered PTSD scale-diagnostic/weekly version, Keane combat exposure scale, IES, Hamilton depression scale and Hamilton anxiety scale), positive beneficial effects of fluoxetine were noted in reducing re-experiencing, avoidance and hyperarousal symptoms of PTSD (Nagy et al., 1993). In other studies, fluoxetine was also noted to have some efficacy in decreasing numbing in PTSD and dosages indicating some efficacy ranged from 20–80 mg/day (McDougle et al., 1990; Davidson et al., 1991). Moreover, responders after fluoxetine treatment showed most improvement in the avoidance symptom cluster, which has been the most resistant symptom cluster in the majority of PTSD patients treated with an antidepressant (Southwick et al., 1990). The use of fluoxetine was also reported to allow psychotherapeutic gains to occur more rapidly and to decrease explosive outbursts of rage and explosiveness in PTSD patients (Davidson et al., 1991; Shay, 1992). A double blind, placebo-controlled study of fluoxetine in a larger population of PTSD patients (22 women and 42 men) confirmed the efficacy of fluoxetine in PTSD treatment (van der Kolk et al., 1994). The average dose of fluoxetine was two capsules (40 mg/day). Positive changes were most apparent in the arousal and numbing symptoms. Significant adverse effects of fluoxetine in this study were diarrhoea, sweating and headaches.

Two other SSRIs, fluvoxamine and sertraline, were also reported to show some beneficial effects in PTSD. In a small open pilot study with a treatment period of 12 weeks in 24 Dutch world war II resistance veterans, fluvoxamine was reported to alleviate chronic PTSD symptoms, in particular insomnia, nightmares, anxiety, intrusive recollections, guilt feelings and tiredness (De Boer et al., 1992). Sertraline was also observed to be beneficial in an open-label trial in male Vietnam veterans (Kline et al., 1994). Positive responders (63%) after sertraline treatment (mean daily dose = 98.5 mg, range = 50–150 mg) after a minimum of 3 months suggest that there was a significant decrease in dysphoria, irritability and anger as measured by monthly scores on the Beck depression inventory, IES, STAI, clinical global evaluation and impression scales. However, in these clinical trials, although a good signif-

Table 7.4: Treatment of PTSD by SSRI and other drug. OT: Open trial; DB: double blind; PC: placebo controlled

Drugs (mg/day)	Design and time of study	Populations	Sample size	Conclusions	References
SSRI					
Fluoxetine (20–80)	Case report	4 women (26–35 years) and 1 man (42 years)	5	Marked improvement in both intrusive and avoidant symptoms. Allow psycho-therapeutic gains to occur more rapidly.	Davidson et al. 1991
Fluoxetine (20–80)	OT, up to 27 months	Male veterans	26	Reduced explosiveness, improved mood and insomnia in 16 (61%) patients	Shay, 1992
Fluoxetine (20-80)	OT, 10 weeks	Male veterans (45.1 ± 8.2 years)	19	Significant decrease in PTSD symptoms, mostly after 6 weeks. 50% decrease in frequency of panic attacks, 30% drop out due to adverse effects (e.g. anxiety)	Nagy et al., 1993
Fluoxetine (20–60) vs. placebo	DB, PC, 5 weeks	31 veterans and 33 civilian with PTSD/ 22 women and 42 men (22–55 years)	64	Decrease in arousal numbing and depression. No significant effect on intrusion, dissociation or hostility. Better results in recent civilian PTSD.	Van der Kolk et al., 1994
Fluvoxamine (up to 300 mg)	OT, 12 weeks	Male veterans	24	Modest improvement of PTSD symp-toms, particularly insomnia, nightmares, anxiety & intrusive recollections.	De Boer et al., 1992
Sertraline (50-150)	OT, > 3 months	Male veterans with co-occurring major depression	19	Significantly decreased dysphoria, irritability and anger in 12 (63% patients although 9 (47%) still complained of pre-existing insomnia.	Kline et al., 1994
5-HT_{2a} antagonist					
Nefazodone (up to 600 mg/day)	OT, 8 weeks	Veterans with chronic PTSD (49 ± 9 years).	36	Nefazodone treatment improved the symptoms of PTSD, including the core symptoms. It was well tolerated with only 4 patients discontinuing because of adverse effects.	Davis et al., 2000

icant improvement in PTSD symptoms was observed in the "responders", the patients did not achieve a full remission with complete absence of PTSD symptoms. The observed gradual and incomplete improvement did not lead to total functional recovery as in most of these studies considerable functional impairment persisted. Recently, sertraline was approved by the FDA for the treatment of PTSD.

6.3.3 *Anticonvulsants*

Lipper et al. (1986) have suggested clinical efficacy for carbamazepine, an anticonvulsant, in patients with PTSD, particularly upon symptoms of hyperarousal, intrusive recollections, sleep impairment and hostility. A second open trial showed alleviation of impulsivity, violent behaviour, and angry outbursts in Vietnam combat veterans with PTSD (Wolf et al., 1988).

6.3.4 *β-blocker and α_2-agonist*

It was reported that propranolol, a β-blocker, and clonidine, an α_2-agonist, are helpful in treating PTSD. Propranolol was studied at 120–160 mg/day in 12 Vietnam combat veterans (Kolb et al. 1984). The patients reported lessened explosiveness, fewer nightmares and dreams, improved sleep, fewer startle responses and less hyperalertness, less intrusive thoughts and improved psychosocial functioning. Adverse effects included depression, fatigue, forgetfulness, sexual impairment, bradycardia, hypotension and mental confusion. It was suggested that antiaggressive properties of β-blockers might also be beneficial in some patients.

With clonidine, doses of 0.1–0.4 mg were observed in an open trial among Vietnam veterans to produce encouraging results. Clonidine was also observed to attenuate PTSD-driven self-mutilatory behaviour when given on a p.r.n. basis (Van der Kolk, 1987). The addition of clonidine to an antidepressant regime to treat the hyperactivity, startle reactions and nightmares has been suggested (Kinzie, 1986; Kinzie & Leung, 1989). The utility of the use of clonidine (0.1 – 0.2 mg/day) in preschool children suffering from PTSD and in patients whose PTSD symptoms of hyperarousal, impulsivity and aggression remained severe and had not abated with other therapeutic approaches was noted in an open clinical trial (Harmon & Riggs, 1996). The use of a clonidine patch (Catapres-TTS®) which was replaced every 5 days was tolerated better than oral clonidine with less initial sedation. The results of this study indicated the efficacy of clonidine in reducing symptoms of aggression, hyperarousal and sleep difficulties in children with severe PTSD. However, it was pointed out for safety concerns that parental/guardian compliance is important in the use of clonidine in children because abrupt discontinuation of clonidine can be dangerous. It should be used only in children free from cardiac or other major medical illness, to follow closely target symptoms and to perform regular follow-up ECG and blood pressure.

Guanfacine, another α_2-agonist, was observed to be beneficial in PTSD symptoms as an addition to an antidepressant such as sertraline (Horrigan & Barnhill, 1996). Due to its prolonged half-life in adults (18–22 h) as compared to clonidine, beneficial effects of guanfacine in PTSD were particularly on the suppression of nightmares throughout the night.

6.3.5 *α_1-antagonists*

The preferential distribution of human α_1-adrenergic receptors in hippocampus, amygdala and other brain areas relevant to PTSD in the modulation of sleep and startle provide the neurobiological rationale for exploring the efficacy of α_1-adrenergic antagonist therapy in this disorder (Gross-Isseroff et al., 1990; Stevens et al., 1994). A small open-label study in chronic PTSD patients showed that treatment with prazosin, an α_1-antagonist, was effective in eliminating or reducing nightmares (Raskind et al., 2000). The two patients who achieved a daily prazosin dose of at least 5 mg were markedly improved, with complete elimination of trauma nightmares and resumption of normal dreaming. The other two patients who limited the dose to 2 mg due to side effects of decrease of blood pressure improved with at lest 50% reduction in nightmare severity. Placebo-controlled studies are needed to assess the efficacy of prazosin and other antiadrenergic medications in the symptomatic management of PTSD.

6.3.6 *Buspirone*

Buspirone may be effective in treating some PTSD symptoms when used alone (LaPorta & Ware, 1992; Wells et al., 1991) (see Tab. 7.5). The onset of efficacy was observed to range from 5-29 days after buspirone administration with dosage of 15-35 mg daily (Wells et al., 1991). Symptoms that responded to treatment included insomnia, nightmares, flashbacks, anxiety and depressed mood. Recently, buspirone was added to the regimen of patients judged to be unresponsive or only partially responsive to antidepressant treatment (Hamner et al., 1997). Response to buspirone was evaluated at baseline and after potentiation using a clinical global impression change. A positive response to buspirone addition was observed in 11 of 14 patients (73%). Buspirone was discontinued in four patients, two due to adverse effects and two due to lack of efficacy. No patients experienced a worsening of symptoms. The average buspirone daily dose was 40 mg in responders (30–60 mg/day). Given the positive preliminary results of the study, future research should devise a controlled trial in a larger sample of PTSD patients to establish the efficacy of buspirone combination therapy. The mechanism of action of buspirone in alleviating symptoms of PTSD also awaits clarification.

6.3.7 *Other drugs*

Recently, an open study showed that nefazodone, a presynaptic serotonin reuptake inhibitor and 5-HT_{2A} antagonist, improved the symptoms of PTSD, including the core symptoms in chronic PTSD patients (Davis et al., 2000). However, the total mean improvement in symptoms as measured by both the CAPS and the Hamilton rating scales during this 8-week trial was modest (25–30%). These promising results

Table 7.5: Treatment of PTSD by buspirone. OT: open trial

Drugs (mg/day)	Design and time of study	Populations	Sample size	Conclusions	References
Buspirone (35–60 mg/day)	Case report	Males, 45–68 years old with a DSM-IIIR diagnosis of PTSD	3	Symptoms that responded to treatment included insomnia, nightmares, flash-backs, anxiety and depressed mood. Onset of clinical efficacy: 5–29 days	Wells et al. 1991
Buspirone (30 mg/day)	Case report	Females, 37 and 21 years old with a DSM-IIIR criteria for PTSD	2	Reduction in insomnia, recollections, nightmares and anxiety; improved concentration daily functioning.	LaPorta & Ware, 1992
Buspirone (30–60 mg/day; prescribed to patients unresponsive to antidepressants)	Open trial	Male Vietnam combat veterans meeting DSM-IV criteria for PTSD	15	A positive response to buspirone augmentation occurred in 11 of 14 patients (73%). Buspirone was dis-continued in 4 patients, 2 due to adverse effects and 2 due to lack of efficacy (symptoms unchanged)	Hamner et al., 1997

suggest that blinded placebo-controlled trials are needed to further define the efficacy of nefazodone for the treatment of PTSD.

6.3.8 New research strategy in pharmacotherapy of PTSD

The tendency for yohimbine to elicit traumatic memory recall and flashbacks in PTSD patients may relate to β-adrenergic receptor stimulation in the amygdala and cortical structures (Cahil et al., 1994). If the possibility that PTSD patients' memories of disturbing images can be blunted by drugs that block a type of receptor (e.g. noradrenaline), then these drugs may produce a new generation of medications for treating PTSD. The idea to avoid PTSD by interrupting the memory-consolidation process before those traumatic memories become pathological looks attractive. The observation that nalmefene, an opiate antagonist, may significantly induce a favourable response with a marked decrease of emotional numbing and other symptoms of PTSD, including startle response, nightmares, flashbacks, intrusive thoughts, rage and vulnerability in PTSD patients is interesting and warrants further confirmation. This approach may also lead to new drug development strategies in pharmacotherapy of PTSD (Glover, 1993).

7 Discussion

Exposure to trauma in itself is not sufficient for subsequent development of PTSD. Only low to moderate proportions of individuals exposed to trauma develop PTSD (e.g. 15.2% of Vietnam veterans, 23.6% of urban adults and 39% of traffic accident victims) (Kulka et al., 1990; Breslau et al., 1991; Blanchard et al., 1996). The relative lack of knowledge about the nature of the relationship between PTSD and the traumatic stressor or about the course of PTSD development suggests that further research in these areas is urgently needed. Longitudinal studies, starting immediately after exposure to the trauma and using repeated assessments at multiple points in time are critically important for the clarification of the development course of PTSD. It is possible that low socio-economic and educational status, previous neuropsychiatric morbidity and personality traits such as neuroticism could be implicated as pre-traumatic risk factors but these assumptions need to be confirmed (McFarlane, 1989; Solomon, 1989; Green, 1994). Although recent research has focused on combat, rape, and other assaultive violence as causes of PTSD, sudden unexpected death of a loved one is also a significant cause of PTSD in the community, accounting for nearly one third of PTSD cases (Breslau et al., 1998). Such findings highlight the need for further research on this heterogeneous category of trauma and the vulnerability factors involved in why some of the individuals who experience trauma develop PTSD.

Since PTSD commonly occurs with other psychiatric disorders, and because of the relative frequency of traumatic events as well as the heterogeneity of presentation of PTSD, screening for traumatic events and PTSD should be standard in both psychiatric and primary care practice. In order to prevent long-term psychological effects after traumatic events, it has been recommended that disaster services should be provided for at least two years particularly to those survivors who are injured, who experience risk of death, or who witness death (Selley et al., 1997). High levels of distress during and immediately after the accident were highly associated with severe PTSD symptoms (Di Gallo et al., 1997). The individual's perception of the trauma is particularly important. The services for survivors should take these factors into account, identifying these risk groups, recognising their needs as early as possible.

Patients with severe PTSD often have problems trusting other people, including the therapist/clinician. Therefore the clinician should make special efforts to offer support and convey empathy and caring, including calling the patient between sessions. Flexibility in scheduling appointments may often be necessary.

Neuropsychological testing, particularly evaluation of memory deficits, may represent an objective assessment of patients with PTSD symptoms and should be considered as a useful approach to assist clinicians in the diagnosis and treatment of PTSD. On the other hand, it appears also that more sophisticated tests of attention and memory are required as interpretation of some study results may be constrained by potential ceiling effects of certain tests, limiting the ability to detect subtle performance alterations. These tests may also be used to predict PTSD in patients susceptible to develop the symptoms after traumatic events so that appropriate preventive treatment may be started. With these tests, screenings for PTSD can take place as early as one week (Shalev et al., 1997). It also appears that all questionnaires (e.g. Horowitz's Impact of Event Scale and Mississippi Scale for Combat-Related PTSD) are good tests, in that they are better able to predict PTSD than chance. They measure the level of psychological distress in general, rather than a particular syndrome (Shalev et al., 1997). It was also suggested that it is possible to use these questionnaires to screen for who will not go on to develop PTSD. For those who might develop it, where prediction is less certain, it may be best to use a clinician-administered instruments such as the CAPS. The inclusion of these neuropsychological evaluations may improve the prediction of PTSD and hence the effectiveness of preventive programs.

Issues relating to dissociative amnesia need clarification from more research. To demonstrate dissociative amnesia, investigators should interview and follow-up patients who experience a well-documented trauma. These patients should be free of neurological problems such as head injury or drug intoxication. The traumatic event must be too important to the individual to plausibly be lost by ordinary forgetfulness. Failure to adequately respond during the first interview may be followed by a subsequent clarification interview during which the patients should be asked whether they remember the specific event that they are known to have experienced. Such types of approaches with these criteria are required to clarify issues relating to dissociative amnesia; until then dissociative amnesia remains unproven.

With respect to pharmacological treatment, several unanswered questions remain. These include the importance of PTSD subtypes in relation to differential drug effect. A recent study emphasised the importance of screening substance abusers for PTSD because it can identify a small but substantial number of patients who might require additional treatment (Najavits et al., 1998). Guidelines for selecting the initial medication have been proposed but the optimum length of treatment as well as relapse rates over time need to be studied (The Expert Consensus Guidelines Series, 1999) (see Tab. 7.6). Whether earlier treatment intervention leads to a more favourable prognosis needs to be established. The analysis of the effects of various treatments of PTSD patients suggests that the efficacy of treatment is often limited and complete remission is rarely achieved. With respect to duration of treatment, drug effects have only been demonstrated in controlled trials of at least eight weeks' duration (Davidson et al., 1990). It is likely that pharmacotherapy should continue for several months in order to produce maximum effects. Decisions on when to discontinue treatment may be based on the degree of symptom remission, progress made in psychotherapy, stability of life situations, the extent to which the patient is coping successfully with the presence of ongoing stresses and the presence or absence of adverse effects from the drug. In pharmacotherapeutic treatment of PTSD, it may be questioned whether the drug effects in PTSD are specific to PTSD symptoms or non-specifically directed at such symptoms as depression and general tension. Several studies have noted drug effects on intrusive and avoidant symptoms of PTSD, with effects mostly occurring on the intrusive cluster (Davidson & Nemeroff, 1989). Serotonin uptake inhibitors may differ from other drugs, however, in having greater effect upon avoidant PTSD symptoms.

Pharmacological studies of PTSD have several limitations such as a limited number of controlled studies and often the results are inconsistent. Most of the information on pharmacotherapy comes from open trials and case reports. Double-blind randomised placebo-controlled studies are necessary to confirm these observations of the beneficial effects of these various psychoactive medications in PTSD. It should also be emphasised that although drug treatments may provide alleviation of intrusive recollections and arousal symptoms, drug treatment alone cannot completely alleviate the suffering in PTSD. Pharmacotherapy is primarily useful as an adjunct to the psychological treatment of PTSD. Several of these studies have been performed in male combat veterans with chronic PTSD and the length of potential remissions as well as the rate of relapse has not been assessed. It also appears that pharmacotherapy alone is rarely sufficient to cure PTSD. Given the shortcoming of unidimensional treatment approach of PTSD, it may be better to combine pharmacological and psychological treatment that may yield better positive effective long-term results.

As psychological and neurological reactions to trauma are complex and variable, effective procedures need to be developed in order to understand which individual or group of patients will develop chronic PTSD that can be persistent and difficult to treat. More research is required about who will benefit from psychological and pharmacological treatments and when the optimal time for its delivery is. Our conceptualisation of the disorder will continue to evolve both with new scientific discoveries and with changes in the professional environment within which patients suffering from PTSD are treated. Hopefully, a rational pharmacotherapy for this disorder will emerge from a better understanding of the cognitive disturbances and biological correlates of PTSD.

Table 7.6: Guideline for selecting the initial medication (The Expert Consensus Guidelines Series, 1999). SSRIs include sertraline, paroxetine, fluoxetine, fluvoxamine and citalopram

Most prominent symptom	Recommended medications	Also consider
Intrusive thoughts	SSRIs Nefazodone Venlafaxine	Tricyclic antidepressants
Flashbacks	SSRIs Nefazodone Venlafaxine	Tricyclic antidepressants
Trauma-related fears, panic and avoidance	SSRIs Nefazodone Venlafaxine	Tricyclic antidepressants Benzodiazepines (e.g., clonazepam)
General anxiety (hyperarousal, hypervigilance, startle)	SSRIs Nefazodone Venlafaxine	Tricyclic antidepressants Benzodiazepines Antiadrenergics Buspirone
Numbing/detachment from others/loss of interest	SSRI Nefazodone Venlafaxine	Tricyclic antidepressants
Dissociative symptoms		SSRIs Nefazodone Venlafaxine Tricyclic antidepressants
Sleep disturbance	Trazodone	Zolpidem Benadryl Tricyclic antidepressants Benzodiazepines
Irritability/angry outbursts	SSRI Nefazodone Venlafaxine	Mood stabilisers (e.g., divalproex) Tricyclic antidepressants Antiadrenergics
Difficulty concentrating	SSRIs Nefazodone Venlafaxine	Tricyclic antidepressants
Guilt/Shame	SSRIs Nefazodone Venlafaxine	Tricyclic antidepressants

The recent increasing use of the PET technology in the understanding of the neurological deficits in PTSD will probably help to better understand the symptoms of PTSD which may lead to the development of more precise neuropsychological tests and pharmacological treatments. Results from PET suggest that ventral anterior cingulate gyrus and right amygdala may play a role in the response of patients with PTSD to mental images of trauma-related scenes (Shin et al., 1997). Re-experiencing phenomena of PTSD, which often involve emotional visual mental imagery, may be likewise associated with increased rCBF in these regions. Given the role of Broca's area in language function, decreased rCBF in this region may be consistent with diminished linguistic processing while patients with PTSD viewed and evaluated trauma pictures. Further research is required to confirm such hypotheses.

References

American Psychiatric Committee on Nomenclature and Statistics. Diagnosis and statistical manual of mental disorders, fourth edition. Washington, DC: American Psychiatric Association, 1994

Andrade J, Kavanagh D & Baddeley A. Eye-movements and visual imagery: A working memory approach to the treatment of post-traumatic stress disorder. Br J Clin Psychol 36, 209–223, 1997

Bauer M, Priebe S, Graf KJ, Kurten I & Baumgartner A. Psychological and endocrine abnormalities in refugees from East Germany: Part II. Serum levels of cortisol, prolactin, luteinizing hormone, follicle stimulating hormone and testosterone. Psychiatry Res 51, 75–85, 1994

Beck AT, Emery G & Greenberg RL. Anxiety disorders and phobias: A cognitive perspective. New York: Basic Books, 1985

Blake DD, Weathers FW, Nagy LM et al. A clinician rating scale for assessing current and lifetime PTSD: the CAPS-1. Behav Therapist 13, 187–188, 1990

Blake DD, Weathers FW, Nagy LM, Kaloupek DG, Gusman FD, Charney DS & Keane TM. The development of a Clinician-Administered PTSD Scale. J Trauma Stress 8 (1),75–90, 1995

Blanchard EB, Buckley TC, Hickling E et al. Posttraumatic stress disorder and comorbid major depression: is the correlation an illusion? J Anxiety Disord 2, 21–37, 1998

Blanchard EB, Hickling E, Taylor A & Loos WR. Psychiatric morbidity associated with motor vehicle accident. J Nerv Ment Dis 183, 95–504, 1995

Blanchard EB, Hickling EJ, Taylor AE, Loos WR, Forneris CA & Jaccard J. Who develops PTSD from motor vehicle accidents? Behav Res Ther 34, 1–10, 1996

Blank AS. The longitudinal course of posttraumatic stress disorder. In: JRT Davidson & EB Foa (eds): Posttraumatic stress disorder: DSM-IV and beyond. Washington DC: American Psychiatric Association Press, 1993

Boudarene M & Timsit-Berthier M. Interest of events-related potentials in assessment of posttraumatic stress disorder. Annals of the New York Academy of Sciences. In: Yehuda & AC McFarlane (eds): Psychobiology of posttraumatic stress disorder. New York: The New York Academy of Sciences 821, 494–497, 1997

Bower GH. Mood and memory. Am Psychol 36, 129–148, 1981

Bremner D, Randall P, Scott TN et al. MRI-based measurements of hippocampal volume in combat-related posttraumatic stress disorder. Am J Psychiatry 152, 973–981, 1995

Bremner JD, Scott TM, Delaney RC, Southwick SM, Mason JW, Johnson DR, Innis RB, McCarthy G & Charney DS. Deficits in short-term memory in posttraumatic stress disorder. Am J Psychiatry 150 (7), 1015–1019, 1993

Bremner JD, Innis RB, Ng CK, Staib LH, Salomon RM, Bronen RA, Duncan J, Southwick SM, Krystal JH, Rich D et al. Positron emission tomography measurement of cerebral metabolic correlates of yohimbine administration in combat-related posttraumatic stress disorder. Arch Gen Psychiatry 54, 246–254, 1997

Breslau N, Schultz L & Petersen E. Sex differences in depression: a role for pre-existing anxiety. Psychiatry Res 58, 1–12, 1995

Breslau N, Kessler RC, Chilcoat HD, Schultz LR, Davis GC & Andreski P. Trauma and posttraumatic stress disorder in the Community. The 1996 Detroit Area Survey of Trauma. Arch Gen Psychiatry 55, 626–632, 1998

Breslau N, Davis GC, Andreski P, Peterson EL & Schultz LR. Sex differences in posttraumatic stress disorder. Arch Gen Psychiatry 54, 1044–1048, 1997

Breslau N, Davis GC, Andreski P, Federman B & Anthony JC. Epidemiologic findings on PTSD and comorbid disorders in the general population. In: B Dohrenwend (ed): Adversity, stress, and psychopathology. New York, NY: Oxford University Press, 319–330, 1998

Breslau N, Davis GC, Andreski P & Peterson E. Traumatic events and post traumatic stress disorder in an urban population of young adults. Arch Gen Psychiatry 48 (3), 216–222, 1991

Bryant RA, Marosszeky JE, Crooks J & Gurka JA. Posttraumatic stress disorder after severe traumatic brain injury. Am J Psychiatry 157, 629–631, 2000

Burstein A. Treatment of post-traumatic stress disorder with imipramine. Psychosomatics 25 (9), 681–687, 1984

Cahil L, Prims B, Weber M & McGaugh S. β-adrenergic activation and memory for emotional events. Nature 371, 702–704, 1994

Carroll BJ, Feinberg M, Greden JF, Tarika J, Albala AA, Haskett RF, James NM, Kronfol Z, Lohr N, Steiner M, de Vigne JP & Young E. A specific laboratory test for the diagnosis of melancholia. Arch Gen Psychiatry 38, 15–22, 1981

Carter CS, Maddock RJ & Magliozzi J. Patterns of abnormal processing of emotional information in panic disorder and major depression. Psychopathol 25, 65–70, 1992

Casella JV & Davis M. Fear enhanced acoustic startle is not attenuated by acute or chronic imipramine treatment in rats. Psychopharmacol 87, 268–282, 1985

Cassiday KL, Mc Nally RJ & Zeitlin SB. Cognitive processing of trauma cues in rape victims with post-traumatic stress disorder. Cogn Ther Res 16, 283–295, 1992

Charles G, Hansenne M, Ansseau M, Pitchot W, Machowski R, Schittecatte M & Wilmotte J. P300 in posttraumatic stress disorder. Biol Psychiatry 32, 72–74, 1995

Charney DS, Deutch AY, Krystal JH, Southwick SM & Davis M. Psychobiologic mechanisms of posttraumatic stress disorder. Arch Gen Psychiatry 50, 294–305, 1993

Charney DS, Heninger GR & Redmond DE. Yohimbine induced anxiety and increased noradrenergic function in humans: Effects of diazepam and clonidine. Life Sci 33, 19–29, 1983

Chilcoat HD & Breslau N. Posttraumatic stress disorder and drug disorders. Arch Gen Psychiatry 55, 913–917, 1998

David D, Kutcher GS & Jackson EI. Psychotic symptoms in combat-related posttraumatic stress disorder. J Clin Psychiatry 185, 434–441, 1999

Davidson JRT, Kudler HS, Smith RD, Mahorney SL, Hammett E, Saunders WB & Cavenar JO Jr. Treatment of post traumatic stress disorder with amitriptyline and placebo. Arch Gen Psychiatry 47, 259–266, 1990

Davidson JRT & Nemeroff CB. Pharmacotherapy in post traumatic stress disorder: historical and clinical considerations and future directions. Psychopharmacol Bull 25, 422–425, 1989

Davidson JRT, Roth S & Newman E. Treatment of post traumatic stress disorder with fluoxetine. J Trauma Stress 4, 419–423, 1991

Davidson JRT & Colket JT. The eight-item treatment-outcome post-traumatic stress disorder scale. A brief measure to assess treatment outcome in post-traumatic stress disorder. Int J Clin Psychopharmacol 12, 41–45, 1997

Davidson JRT, Book SW, Colket JT, Tupler LA, Roth S, David D, Hertzberg M, Mellman T, Beckham JC, Smith RD et al. Assessment of a new self-rating scale for post-traumatic stress disorder. Psychol Med 27, 153–160, 1997

Davidson JRT, Kudler HS, Saunders WB & Smith RD. Symptom and comorbidity patterns in World War II and Vietnam veterans with posttraumatic stress disorder. Compr Psychiatry 31, 162–170, 1990

Davidson JRT, Hughes D, Blazer DG & George LK. Post traumatic stress disorder in the community: an epidemiological study. Psychol Med 21 (3), 713–721, 1991

Davis LL, Nugent AL, Murray J, Kramer GL & Petty F. Nefazodone treatment for chronic posttraumatic stress disorder: An open trial. J Clin Psychopharmacol 20 (2), 159–164, 2000

Dawkins K & Furnham A. The colour naming of emotional words. Br J Psychol 80, 383–389, 1989

DeBellis MD & Putnam FW. The psychobiology of childhood maltreatment. Child Adolesc Psychiatric Clin North Am 3, 663–678, 1994

De Boer M, Op den Velde W, Falger PJR, Hovens JE, De Groen JHM & Van Duijn H. Fluvoxamine treatment for chronic PTSD: A pilot study. Psychother Psychosom 57, 158–163, 1992

De Ruiter C & Brosschot JF. The emotional Stroop interference effect in anxiety: attentional bias or cognitive avoidance? Behav Res Ther 32, 315–319, 1994

Di Gallo A, Barton J & Parry-Jones WL. Road traffic accidents: early psychological consequences in children and adolescents. Br J Psychiatry 170, 358–362, 1997

Ehlers A, Clark DM, Dunmore E, Jaycox L, Meadows E & Foa EB. Predicting response to exposure treatment in PTSD: the role of mental defeat and alienation. J Trauma Stress 11 (3), 457–471, 1998

Escobar JI, Randolph ET, Puente G, Spiwak F, Asamen JK & Hough RL. Posttraumatic stress disorder in Hispanic Vietnam veterans: clinical phenomenology and sociocultural characteristics. J Nerv Ment Dis 171, 585–596, 1983

Fairbank JA & Brown TA. Current behavioral approaches to the treatment of posttraumatic stress disorder. Behav Therapist 3, 57–64, 1987

Falcon S, Ryan C, Chamberlain K & Curtis G. Tricyclics: Possible treatment for post-traumatic stress disorder. J Clin Psychiatry 46 (9), 385–388, 1985

Falsetti SA & Resnick HS. Frequency and severity of panic attack symptoms in a treatment seeking sample of trauma victims. J Trauma Stress 10, 683–689, 1997

Famularo R, Kinscherff R & Fenton T. Propranolol treatment for childhood post traumatic stress disorder, acute type. Am J Dis Childhood 142, 1244–1247, 1988

Foa EB, Rothbaum BO & Molnar C. Cognitive-behavioral therapy of PTSD. In: MJ Friedman, DS Charney & AY Deutch (eds): Neurobiological and clinical consequences of stress: from normal adaptation to PTSD. Philadelphia: Lippincott-Raven, 483–494, 1995

Foa EB, Riggs DS & Gershuny BS. Arousal, numbing and intrusion: symptoms structure of PTSD following assault. Am J Psychiatry 152, 116–120, 1995

Foa EB & Meadows EA. Psychosocial treatments for posttraumatic stress disorder: a critical review. Annu Rev Psychol 48, 449–480, 1997

Foa EB, Steketee G & Rothbaum BO. Behavioural/cognitive conceptualisation of post-traumatic stress disorder. Behav Therapy 20, 155–176, 1989

Foy DW, Sipprelle RC, Rueger DB & Carroll EM. Etiology of posttraumatic stress disorder in Vietnam veterans: Analysis of preliminary, military, and combat exposure influences. J Consult Clin Psychol 52, 79–87, 1984

Frank JB, Giller EL, Kosten TR, Giller EL Jr & Dan E. A randomized clinical trial of phenelzine and imipramine for post traumatic stress disorder. Am J Psychiatry 145 (10), 1289–1291, 1988

Freud S. On the history of the psychoanalytic movement. Reprinted (1953–1974.) In: J Strachey (transl. and ed.): The Standard Edition of the Complete Psychological Works of Sigmund Freud, Vol. 14. London: Hogarth Press, 16, 1914

Friedman MJ & Southwick SM. Towards pharmacotherapy for PTSD. In: Neurobiological and clinical consequences of stress: from normal adaptation to PTSD. Philadelphia: Lippincott-Raven, 465–482, 1995

Friedman MJ. Toward rational pharmacotherapy for post-traumatic stress disorder. An interim report. The Am J Psychiatry 143, 3, 281–285, 1988

Friedman MJ, Charney DS & Deutch AY. Neurobiological and clinical consequences of stress: From normal adaptation to PTSD. Philadelphia: Lippincott-Raven, 1995

Gelpin E, Bonne O, Peri T et al. Treatment of recent trauma survivors with benzodiazepines: a prospective study. J Clin Psychiatry 57, 390–394, 1996

Gilbertson MW, Gurvits TV, Lasko NB & Pitman RK. Neuropsychological assessment of Vietnam combat veterans with and without PTSD. In: Yehuda & AC McFarlane (eds): Psychobiology of posttraumatic stress disorder. New York: The New York Academy of Sciences, Vol. 821, 476–479, 1997

Glod CA & Teicher MH. Relationship between early abuse, posttraumatic stress disorder, and activity levels in prepubertal children. J Am Acad Child Adolesc Psychiatry 35, 1384–1396, 1996

Glover H. Emotional numbing: a possible endorphin-mediated phenomenon associated with posttraumatic stress disorders and other allied psychopathologic states. J Traumatic Stress 5, 643–675, 1992

Glover H. A preliminary trial of nalmefene for the treatment of emotional numbing in combat veterans with post-traumatic stress disorder. Isr J Psychiatry Relat Sci 30 (4), 255–263, 1993

Goenjian AK, Pynoos RS, Steinberg AM, Narajian LM, Asarnow JR & Karayan I. Psychiatric co-morbidity in children after the 1988 earthquake in Armenia. J Am Acad Child Adolesc Psychiatry 34, 1174–1184, 1995
Goenjian AK, Yehuda R, Pynoos RS, Steinberg AM, Tashjian M, Yang RK, Najarian LM & Fairbanks LA. Basal cortisol and dexamethasone suppression of cortisol among adolescents after the 1988 earthquake in Armenia. Am J Psychiatry 153, 929–934, 1996
Green BL. Psychosocial research in traumatic stress: an update. J Trauma Stress 7, 341–362, 1994
Gross-Isseroff R, Dillon KA, Fieldust SJ et al. Autoradiographic analysis of a1-noradrenergic receptors in the human bran postmortem. Arch Gen Psychiatry 47, 1049–1053, 1990
Gurguis GNM & Uhde TW. Plasma 3-methoxy-4-hydroxyphenylethylene glycol (MHPG) and growth hormone responses to yohimbine in panic disorder patients and normal controls. Psychoneuroendocrinology 15, 217–224, 1990
Gurvits TV, Shenton ME, Hokama H, Ohta H, Lasko NB, Gilbertson MW, Orr SP, Kikinis R, Jolesz FA, McCarley RW et al. Magnetic resonance imaging study of hippocampal volume in chronic, combat-related posttraumatic stress disorder. Biol Psychiatry 40 (11), 1091–1099, 1996
Gurvits TV, Gilbertson MW, Lasko NB, Tarhan AS, Simeon D, Macklin ML, Orr SP & Pitman RK. Neurologic soft signs in chronic postraumatic stress disorder. Arch Gen Psychiatry 57, 181–186, 2000
Hales RE & Zatzick DF. What is PTSD? Am J Psychiatry 154 (2), 143–145, 1997
Hamner M, Ulmer H & Horne D. Buspirone potentiation of antidepressants in the treatment of PTSD. Depress Anxiety 5, 137–139, 1997
Harmon RJ & Riggs PD. Clonidine for posttraumatic stress disorder in preschool children. J Am Acad Child Adolesc Psychiatry 35 (9), 1247–1249, 1996
Hathaway, SR & McKinley, JC. Booklet for the Minnesota Multiphasic Personality Inventory, New York: Psychological Corporation, 1943
Heim C, Ehlert U, Rexhausen J, Hanker JP & Hellhammer DH. Psychoendocrinological observations in women with chronic pelvic pain. Annals of the New York Academy of Sciences. In: Yehuda & AC McFarlane (eds): Psychobiology of posttraumatic stress disorder. New York: The New York Academy of Sciences, Vol. 821, 456–458, 1997
Helzer JE, Robins LN & McEvoy L. Posttraumatic stress disorder in the general population: findings of the Epidemiologic Catchment Area Survey. N Engl J Med 317, 1630 – 1634, 1987
Herbert JD & Mueser KT. Eye movement desensitization: A critique of the evidence. J Behav Ther Exp Psychiatry 23, 169–174, 1992
Horowitz MJ. Stress response syndromes (2nd ed.). New York: Jason Aronson, 1986
Horowitz MJ, Wilner N & Alvarez W. Impact of Events Scale: A measure of subjective stress. Psychosom Med 41, 209–218, 1979
Horrigan JP & Barnhill LJ. The suppression of nightmares with guanfacine. J Clin Psychiatry 57 (8), (1996) 371, 1996
Jensen CF, Keller TW, Peskind ER, McFall ME, Veith RC, Martin D, Wilkinson CW & Raskind MA. Behavioral and neuroendocrine responses to sodium lactate infusion in subjects with posttraumatic stress disorder. Am J Psychiatry 154, 266–268, 1997

Jones JC & Barlow DH. The etiology of post-traumatic stress disorder. Clin Psychol Rev 10, 299–328, 1990

Kaspi SP, McNally RJ & Amir N. Cognitive processing of emotional information in posttraumatic stress disorder. Cogn Ther Res 19, 319–330, 1995

Keane TM, Fairbank JA, Caddell JM et al. Implosive (flooding) therapy reduces symptoms of PTSD in Vietnam combat veterans. Behav Ther 20, 245–260, 1989

Keane TM, Wolfe J & Taylor KI. Post-traumatic stress disorder: Evidence for diagnostic validity and methods of psychological assessment. J Clin Psychol 43, 32–43, 1987

Keane TM, Caddell JM & Taylor KL. Mississippi Scale for Combat-Related Posttraumatic Stress Disorder: Three studies in reliability and validity. J Consult Clin Psychol 56 (1), 85–90, 1988

Kessler R & McLeod J. Sex differences in vulnerability to undesirable life events. Sociol Rev (Monogr) 49, 620–631, 1984

Kessler RC, Sonnega A, Bromet E, Hughes M, Nelson CB. Posttraumatic stress disorder in the National Comorbidity Survey. Arch Gen Psychiatry 52, 1048–1060, 1995

Kilpatrick DG, Veronen LJ, Resick PA. Psychological sequelae to rape: assessment and treatment strategies. In: DM Dolays & RL Meredith (eds): Behavioral medicine: Assessment and treatment strategies. New York, NY: Plenum, 473–497, 1982

Kinzie JD. Severe post-traumatic stress syndrome among Cambodian Refugees: Symptoms, clinical course and treatment approaches. In JH Shore (ed): Disaster stress studies: New methods and findings, Washington DC: American Psychiatric Press, 123–140, 1986

Kinzie JD & Leung P. Clonidine in Cambodian patients with posttraumatic stress disorder. J Nerv Ment Dis 177 (9), 546–550, 1989

Kline NA, Dow BM, Brown SA & Matloff JL. Sertraline efficacy in depressed combat veterans with posttraumatic stress disorder. Am J Psychiatry 151, 621, 1994

Kofoed L, Friedman MJ & Peck R. Alcoholism and drug abuse in patients with PTSD. Psychiatric Quarterly 64, 151–171, 1993

Kolb LC, Burris BC & Griffiths S. Propranolol and clonidine in treatment of the chronic posttraumatic stress disorders of war. In: BA van der Kolk (ed): Post-traumatic stress disorder: psychological and biological sequelae. Washington DC: American Psychiatric Press, 97–105, 1984

Kolb LC. A neuropsychological hypothesis explaining post-traumatic stress disorder. Am J Psychiatry 144 (8), 989–995, 1987

Koren D, Arnon I & Klein E. Acute stress response and posttraumatic stress disorder in traffic accident victims: A one-year prospective, follow-up study. Am J Psychiatry 156, 367–373, 1999

Kulka RA, Schlenger JA, Fairbank JA, Hough RL, Jordan BK, Marmar CR & Weiss DS. Trauma and the Vietnam War Generation: Report of findings from the National Vietnam Veterans Readjustment Study. New York: Brunner/Mazel, 1990

LaPorta JD & Ware MR. Buspirone and the treatment of posttraumatic stress disorder. J Clin Psychopharmacol 12, 133–134, 1992

Layton BS & Wardi-Zonna K. Posttraumatic stress disorder with neurogenic amnesia for the traumatic event. Clin Neuropsychologist 9, 2–10, 1995

Lerer B et al. Cyclic AMP signal transduction in post-traumatic stress disorder. Am J Psychiatry 144, 1324–1327, 1987

Lerer B, Bleich A, Bennett ER, Ebstein RP & Balkin J. Platelet adenylate-cyclase and phospholipase C activity in posttraumatic stress disorder. Biol Psychiatry 27, 735–744, 1990

Lipper S, Davidson JRT, Grady TA, Edinger JD, Hammett EB, Mahorney SL & Cavenar JO Jr. Preliminary study of carbamazepine in post traumatic stress disorder. Psychosomatics 27, 849–854, 1986

Loughrey GC, Curran PS & Bell P. Posttraumatic stress disorder and civil violence in Northern Ireland. In: JP Wilson & B Raphael (eds): International handbook of traumatic stress syndromes. New York: Plenum, 377–383, 1993

Magdol L, Moffitt TE, Caspi A, Newman DL, Fagan J & Silva PA. Gender differences in partner violence in a birth cohort of 21-year- olds: Bridging the gap between clinical and epidemiological approaches. J Consult Clin Psychol 65 (1), 68–78, 1997

Marks I, Lovell K, Noshirvani H et al. Exposure and cognitive restructuring alone and combined in PTSD: a controlled study. Arch Gen Psychiatry 55, 317–325, 1998

Marmar CR, Weiss DS & Pynoos RB. Dynamic psychotherapy of post-traumatic stress disorder. In: MJ Friedman, DS Charney & AY Deutch (eds): Neurobiological and clinical consequences of stress: From normal adaptation to PTSD. Philadelphia: Lippincott-Raven, 495–506, 1995

McDougle C, Southwick S, St James R et al. An open trial of fluoxetine. PTSD Research Quarterly, Summer 1990, 7, 1990

McFall ME, Mackay PW & Donovan DM. Combat-related PTSD and psychosocial adjustment problems among substance-abusing veterans. J Nerv Ment Dis 179, 33–38, 1991

McFarlane AC, Weber DL & Clark CR. Abnormal stimulus processing in posttraumatic stress disorder. Biol Psychiatry 34, 311–320, 1993

McFarlane AC. The aetiology of post traumatic morbidity: predisposing, precipitating, and perpetuating factors. Br J Psychiatry 154, 221–228, 1989

McNally RJ & Shin LM. Association of intelligence with severity of posttraumatic stress disorder symptoms in Vietnam combat veterans. Am J Psychiatry 152936–938, 1995

McNally RJ, Litz BT, Prassas A, Shin LM & Weathers FW. Emotional priming of autobiographical memory in post-traumatic stress disorder. Cognition and Emotion 8, 351–367, 1994

McNally RJ, Kaspi SP, Riemann BC & Zeitlin SB. Selective processing of threat cues in posttraumatic stress disorder. J Abnorm Psychol 99, 398–402, 1990

Meichenbaum D. Cognitive behavior modification. Morristown, NJ: General Learning Press, 1974

Nagy L, Morgan III CA, Southwick SM & Charney DS. Open prospective trial of fluoxetine for posttraumatic stress disorder. J Clin Psychopharmacol 13, 107–113, 1993

Najavits LM, Gastfriend DR, Barber JP, Reif S, Muenz LR, Blaine J, Frank A, Crits-Christoph P, Thase M & Weiss RD. Cocaine dependence with and without PTSD among subjects in the National Institute on Drug Abuse Collaborative Cocaine Treatment Study. Am J Psychiatry 155 (2), 214–219, 1998

Nezu AM & Carnevale GJ. Interpersonal problem solving and coping reactions of Vietnam veterans with posttraumatic stress disorder. J Abnorm Psychol 96, 155–157, 1987

Orsillo SM, Heimberg RG, Juster HR et al. Social phobia and PTSD in Vietnam veterans. J Trauma Stress 9, 235–252, 1996

Paige SR, Reid GM & Allen MG. Psychophysiological correlates of posttraumatic stress disorder in Vietnam veterans. Biol Psychiatry 27, 419–430, 1991

Penk WE, Robinowitz R, Roberts WR, Patterson ET, Dolan MP & Atkins HG. Adjustment differences among male substance abusers varying in degree of combat experience in Vietnam. J Consult Clin Psychol 49, 426–437, 1981

Pope HG, Hudson JI, Bodkin JA & Olivia P. Questionable validity of "dissociative amnesia" in trauma victims. Br J Psychiatry 172, 210–215, 1998

Perry BD, Giller EL & Southwick SM. Altered platelet alpha2-adrenergic binding sites in posttraumatic stress disorder. Am J Psychiatry 144, 1511–1512, 1987

Peniston EG & Kulkosky PJ. Alpha-theta brainwave neuro-feedback therapy for Vietnam veterans with combat-related posttraumatic stress disorder. Med Psychother 4, 47–60, 1991

Pynoos RS, Goenjian A & Steinberg AM. A public mental health approach to the post-disaster treatment of children and adolescents. Child Adolesc Psychiatr Clin North Am 7, 195–210, 1998

Raskind MA, Dobie DJ, Kanter ED, Petrie EX, Thompson CE & Peskind ER. The α_1-adrenergic antagonist prazosin ameliorates combat trauma nightmares in veterans with posttraumatic stress disorder: A report of 4 cases. J Clin Psychiatry 61 (2), 129–133, 2000

Rauch SL, Van der Kolk BA, Fisler RE, Alpert NM, Orr SP, Savage CR, Fischman AJ, Jenike MA & Pittman RK. A symptom provocation study of posttraumatic stress disorder using positron emission tomography and script-driven imagery. Arch Gen Psychiatry 53, 380–387, 1996

Rawlins R, Williams S & Beck C. Anxiety. In: M. Chisholm (ed): Mental health psychiatric nursing. St Louis: Mosby-Year Book, 1993

Resick PA & Schnicke MK. Cognitive processing therapy for sexual assault victims. J Consult Clin Psychol 60, 748–756, 1992

Resick PA, Nisthith P & Astin M. A controlled trial comparing cognitive processing therapy and prolonged exposure: preliminary findings. Presented at the Lake George Research Conference on Posttraumatic Stress Disorder; January, Lake George, NY, 1999

Resnick H, Kimpatrick DG, Dansky B et al. Prevalence of civilian trauma and posttraumatic disorder in a representative sample of women. J Consult Clin Psychol 61, 984–991, 1993

Sapolsky RM, Krey LC & McEwen BS. Glucocorticoid-sensitive hippocampal neurons are involved in terminating the adrenocortical stress response. Proc Natl Acad Sci USA 81, 1984

Sargant WW & Slater E. The use of drugs in psychotherapy. In: WW Sargant & E Slater (eds): An introduction to physical methods of treatment in psychiatry. New York: Science House, 142–162, 1972

Salkovskis PM & Kirk J. Obsessional disorders. In: K Hawton, P Salkovskis, J Kirk et al. (eds): Cognitive behaviour therapy for psychiatric problems (eds). Oxford: Oxford Medical, 1989

Sbordone RJ. Distinguishing traumatic brain injury from posttraumatic stress disorder. The Neurolaw Letter 9, 3, 1992

Sbordone RJ & Liter JC. Mild traumatic brain injury does not produce post-traumatic stress disorder. Brain Inj 9, 405–412, 1995

Schwarzwald J, Solomon Z, Weisenberg M et al. Validation of the Impact of Event Scale for psychological sequelae of combat. J Consul Clin Psychol 55, 251–256, 1987

Selley C, King E, Peveler R, Osola K, Martin N & Thompson C. Post-traumatic stress disorder symptoms and the Clapham rail accident. Br J Psychiatry 171, 478–482, 1997

Shalev AY. Discussion: treatment of prolonged posttraumatic stress disorder: learning from experience (comment). J Trauma Stress 10, 415–423, 1997

Shalev AY, Freedman S, Peri T, Brandes D & Shar T. Predicting PTSD in trauma survivors: prospective evaluation of self-report and clinician-administered instruments. Br J Psychiatry 170, 558–564, 1997

Shalev A, Freedman S, Peri T et al. Prospective study of posttraumatic stress disorder and depression following trauma. Am J Psychiatry 155, 630–637, 1998

Shalev AY, Bonne O & Eth S. Treatment of posttraumatic stress disorder: A review. Psychosom Med 58, 165–182, 1996

Shay J. Fluoxetine reduces explosiveness and elevates mood on Vietnam combat vets with PTSD. J Traumatic Stress 5, 97–110, 1992

Shepard RH & Cooper LA. Mental images and their transformations. Cambridge, Mass.: MIT press, 1982

Shin LM, Kosslyn SM, McNally RJ, Alpert NM, Thompson WL, Rauch SL, Macklin ML & Pitman RK. Visual imagery and perception in posttraumatic stress disorder. A positron emission tomographic investigation. Arch Gen Psychiatry 54, 233–241, 1997

Shin LM, Kosslyn SM, McNally RJ, Pitman RK, Alpert NM & Rauch SL. A positron emission tomography study of combat-related post-traumatic stress disorder. Presented at the 10th Annual Meeting of the International Society for Traumatic Stress Studies; November 8, Chicago, III. Abstract, 1994

Shapiro F. Efficacy of the eye movement desensitization procedure in the treatment of traumatic memories. J Trauma Stress 2, 199–223, 1989

Solomon Z. A three year prospective study of posttraumatic stress disorder in Israeli combat veterans. J Trauma Stress 2, 59–73, 1989

Southwick SM, Yehuda R, Giller EL et al. Antidepressant treatment of PTSD: a meta-analysis. New Research Abstract 479, American Psychiatric Association, 143rd Annual Meeting, New York, NY, 1990

Southwick SM, Krystal JH, Johnson DR & Charney DS. Neurobiology of post traumatic stress disorder. In: A Tasman & MG Riba (eds): Review of psychiatry. Washington DC: American Psychiatric Press, 11, 347–370, 1992

Southwick SM, Krystal JH, Morgan AC, Johnson D, Nagy LM, Nocolaou A, Heninger G & Charney DS. Abnormal noradrenergic function in posttraumatic stress disorder. Arch Gen Psychiatry 50, 266–274, 1993

Southwick SM, Krystal JH, Bremner D, Morgan CA, Nicolaou AL, Nagy LM, Johnson DR, Heninger GR & Charney DS. Noradrenergic and serotonergic function in posttraumatic stress disorder. Arch Gen Psychiatry 54, 749–757, 1997

Spector J & Huthwaite M. Eye-movement desensitization to overcome post-traumatic stress disorder. Br J Psychiatry 163, 106–108, 1993

Spiegel DJ. Memory, trauma and psychotherapy: a cognitive science view. J Psychother Pract Res 4, 93–122, 1995

Stein MB, Yehuda R, Koverola C & Hanna C. Enhanced dexamethasone suppression of plasma cortisol in adult women traumatized by childhood sexual abuse. Biol Psychiatry 42 (8), 680–6, 1997

Stevens DR, McCarley RW & Greene RW. The mechanism of noradrenergic α_1 excitatory modulation of pontine reticular formation neurons. J Neurosci 14, 6481–6487, 1994

Stroop JR. Studies of interference in serial verbal reaction. J Exp Psychol 18, 643–662, 1935

Sutherland C, Bybee D & Sullivan C. The long-term effects of battering on women's health. Womens Health 4, 41–70, 1998

Tarrier N, Pilgrim H, Sommerfield C et al. A randomized trial of cognitive therapy and imaginal exposure in the treatment of chronic postraumatic stress disorder. J Consult Clin Psychol 67, 13–18, 1999a

Tarrier N, Sommerfeld C, Pilgrim H & Humphreys L. Cognitive therapy or imaginal exposure in the treatment of post-traumatic stress disorder. Twelve month follow-up. Br J Psychiatry 175, 571–575, 1999b

Tecce JJ & Cattanach L. Contingent negative variation (CNV). In: E Nierdermeyer & F Lopes da Silva (eds): Electroencephalography: Basic principles, clinical applications and related fields, 3rd ed. Baltimore: Williams & Wilkins, 1993

Terr LC. Childhood traumas: An outline and overview. Am J Psychiatry 148, 10–20, 1991

The Expert Consensus Guidelines Series. Treatment of posttraumatic stress disorder. 3A. Preferred psychotherapy techniques for different target symptoms. 60, Suppl 16, 1999

Thrasher SM, Dalgleish T & Yule W. Information processing in post-traumatic stress disorder. Behav Res Ther 32, 247–254, 1994

Van der Kolk BA. The drug treatment of post traumatic stress disorder. J Affect Disord 13, 203–213, 1987

Van der Kolk BA, Dreyfuss D, Michaels M, Shera D, Berkowitz R, Fisler R & Saxe G. Fluoxetine in post traumatic stress disorder. J Clin Psychiatry 55, 517–522, 1994

Van der Kolk BA. The trauma spectrum: The interaction of Biological and social events in the genesis of the trauma response. J Trauma Stress 1 (3), 273–290, 1988

Van der Kolk BA & Fisler RE. Dissociation and the fragmentary nature of traumatic memories: Overview and exploratory study. J Trauma Stress 8, 505–525, 1995

Vaughan K & Tarrier N. The use of image habituation training with post-traumatic stress disorders. Brit J Psychiatry 161, 658–664, 1992

Veronen LJ & Kilpatrick DG. Stress inoculation training for victims of rape: efficacy and differential findings. Presented at the 16th annual meeting of the Association for Advancement of Behavior Therapy, Los Angeles, Calif., 1982

Veronen LJ & Kilpatrick DG. Stress management for rape victims. In: D Meichenbaum & ME Jaremko (eds): Stress reduction and prevention. New York, NY: Plenum Press, 341–374, 1983

Vreven DL, Gudanowski DM, King LA et al. The civilian version of the Mississippi PTSD Scale: a psychometric evaluation. J Trauma Stress 8, 91–109, 1995

Weiss DS & Marmar CR. The Impact of Event Scale, Revised. In: JP Wilson & TM Keane (eds): Assessing psychological trauma and PTSD: a practitioner's handbook. New York, NY: Guildford Press, 399–411, 1997

Wells BG, Chu CC, Johnson R, Nasdahl C, Ayubi MA, Sewell E & Statham P. Buspirone in the treatment of posttraumatic stress disorder. Pharmacotherapy 11 (4), 340–343, 1991

Whalley LJ, Borthwick N, Copolov D, Dick H, Christie JE & Fink G. Glucocorticoid receptors and depression. Br Med J Clin Res Ed 292 (6524), 859–861, 1986
Williams JMG, Matthews A & MacLeod C. The emotional Stroop task and psychopathology. Psychol Bull 120, 3–24, 1996
Wolf ME, Alavi A & Mosnaim AD. Post-traumatic stress disorder in Vietnam veterans clinical and EEG findings; possible therapeutic effects of carbamazepine. Biol Psychiat 23, 642–644, 1988
Wolpe J & Abrams J. Post-traumatic stress disorder overcome by eye movement desensitization: A case report. J Behav Ther Exp Psychiatry 22, 39–43, 1991
Wonderlich SA, Brewerton TD, Jocic Z et al. Relationship of childhood sexual abuse and eating disorders. J Am Acad Child Adolesc Psychiatry 1107–1115, 1997
Woolfolk RL & Grady DA. Combat-related post-traumatic stress disorder: patterns of symptomatology in help-seeking Vietnam veterans. J Nerv Mental Dis 176, 107–111, 1988
Yehuda R, Levengood RA, Schmeidler J, Wilson S, Song Guo L & Gerber D. Increased pituitary activation following metyrapone administration in post-traumatic stress disorder. Psychoneuroendocrinology 21 (1), 1–16, 1996
Yehuda R, Boisoneau D, Lowy MT & Giller FL. Dose response changes in plasma cortisol and lymphocyte glucocorticoid receptors following dexamethasone administration in combat veterans with and without posttraumatic stress disorder. Arch Gen Psychiatry 52, 583–593, 1995
Yehuda R, Southwick SM & Giller EL. Urinary catecholamine excretion and severity of PTSD symptoms in Vietnam combat veterans. J Nerv Ment Dis, 180, 321–325, 1992
Yehuda R, Kahana B, Binder-Brynes K, Southwick S, Zemelman S, Mason M & Giller EL. Low urinary cortisol excretion in holocaust survivors with PTSD. Am J Psychiatry 152, 7–12, 1995
Yonkers KA & Ellison JM. Anxiety disorders in women and their pharmacological treatment. In: MF Jenwood, U Halbreich U & JA Hamilton (eds): Psychopharmacology and women. Washington DC: American Press, 261–285, 1996
Zeiss R & Dickman H. PTSD 40 years later: Incidence and person-situation correlates in former POWs. J Clin Psychol 45, 80–87, 1989
Zeitlin SB & McNally RJ. Implicit and explicit memory bias for threat in posttraumatic stress disorder. Behav Res Ther 29, 451–457, 1991

Chapter 8
Phobic disorders

1 Introduction

Phobias include agoraphobia, specific or simple phobia and SP (DSM-IV, 1994). Phobias are characterised by persistent and irrational fears of situations, objects, or activities that result in a compelling desire to avoid phobic stimuli. In DSM-III-R, agoraphobia came to be characterised as a secondary complication of panic and distinct from other phobias. In DSM-IV, agoraphobia, by definition, involves fear of panic attacks or limited symptom panic attacks, so the agoraphobic phenotype can no longer be separated from panic. This view is supported by a substantial body of evidence, but it remains controversial (Widiger et al., 1996). The defining feature of PD may instead be the recurrence of unexpected panic attacks and the development of anticipatory anxiety about additional attacks (Barlow et al., 1994). DSM-IV distinguishes the following subtypes of specific phobias: animal type (e.g., spiders, insects), natural environment type (e.g., storms, heights), blood-injection-injury type (e.g., seeing blood, receiving injections) and situational type (e.g., flying, enclosed spaces). The DSM-IV further notes that specific phobias frequently co-occur. In many cases, more than one subtype of specific phobia is present so that specific phobias form a heterogeneous class of anxiety disorders that frequently occur comorbidly. In a study designed to examine the structure of specific phobias, the results showed that specific phobia symptoms clustered into three factors: animal phobia, blood-injection-injury phobia and a third factor combining natural environment and situational phobias (Frederikson et al., 1996). Although the DSM-IV suggests that natural environment and situational phobias are distinct types of specific phobias, the finding that these types loaded on one factor is not surprising. We may note the strong resemblance as "fear of heights" considered as a natural environment phobia comes close to "fear of elevators" and "fear of flying" that belong to the situational phobias. Interestingly, these empirically derived types of specific phobias are largely in keeping with the typology as proposed by DSM-IV. A recent study designed to examine whether specific phobia subtypes can also be found in children confirmed that childhood-specific phobia symptoms indeed cluster into the three subtypes as described by Frederikson et al. and that these subtypes are either intercorrelated or the product of a single higher order factor (Muris et al., 1999).

The range of stimuli associated with human phobias is statistically constrained, in the sense that a disproportionate number of humans are afraid of objects such as snakes, spiders, or dogs (Marks, 1987). It appears that phobias develop more readily to some stimuli such as spiders and snakes than to other salient and dangerous objects (e.g. guns) that today account for many deaths. Whether this selectivity reflects a tendency for some phobias to be prepared *via* some evolutionary mechanism or is a consequence of other factors is still a matter of debate. A number of investigators have suggested that emotions other than fear may be implicated in the aetiology and maintenance of specific phobias (Davey, 1992; Merckelbach et al., 1993; Tolin et al., 1997). There is increasing evidence that disgust and fear underlie spider phobia. Indirect support for this position is provided by a series of studies demonstrating that common spider fear correlates with disgust sensitivity as indexed by both the Disgust Questionnaire, a questionnaire which is mainly concerned with food contamination by animal products as well as by the Disgust Scale (Davey, 1992; Haidt et al., 1994; Rozin et al., 1984). This hypothesis is further substantiated by the finding that the majority of spider phobic individuals reported that they consider their phobic stimulus (i.e. spider) as their most disgusting item (Thorpe & Salkovskis, 1998). Perhaps, spider phobia can be best be conceptualised as a fear of physical contact with a disgusting stimulus. It has been argued that certain animal fears, especially those animals considered nonpredatory (e.g., spiders, cockroaches, maggots) are mediated by a disease-avoidance process as they are perceived to be associated with dirt and disease-carrying characteristics (Rozin et al., 1993). Thus, the disease avoidance model of animal fears suggests that phobic avoidance is mediated by perceptions of contamination and disease acquisition rather than a fear of being attacked and physically harmed (Matchett & Davey, 1991). Therefore, disgust-mediated aversion in various animal phobias may be related to the prevention of disease transmission.

Although disgust may be generally involved in spider phobia, it plays a more prominent role in blood-injection-injury phobia. Clinical and experimental evidence indicates that exposure to blood-injury stimuli evokes reaction of aversions and nausea, especially among blood-injection-injury phobics who are prone to fainting (Gross & Levenson, 1993; Rachman, 1990; Kleinknecht et al., 1996). Psychophysiological data suggest that exposure to blood-injection-injury phobic stimuli often results in cardiovascular deceleration, implying activation of the parasympathetic nervous system (Thyer & Curtis, 1985; Levenson, 1992). Physiological correlates of the disgust response also reflect parasympathetic activity. The physiological mechanism of disgust contrasts with the acute sympathetic nervous system reaction (e.g., cardiovascular acceleration) associated with the fear response to phobic stimuli (Gelder & Mathews, 1968).

Specific phobias are viewed as a reaction normally generated by proximity to an avoidable major threat, or a stimulus which predicts its presence and which normally reproduces directed escape or active avoidance. The primary control centres for this are likely to lie in the medial hypothalamus and amygdala. Phobias can be transmitted by observation. For example, rhesus monkeys raised in captivity do not have fear of snakes unlike those reared in the wild. However, they rapidly acquire such a fear by watching an adult monkey behaving fearfully in the presence of a snake (Cook et al., 1985).

Agoraphobia is viewed as a reaction most frequently resulting from the conditioning of anxiety by spontaneous panic, but which may also result from excessive responsiveness to a diffuse set of poorly localizable, innate aversive spatial or social cues. The primary set of excess activity is likely to be in the septo-hippocampal system and amygdala.

2 Epidemiology

Most epidemiologic studies have found that phobias are the most common anxiety disorder in late life. Period prevalence ranges from 0% to 12% with a median rate of 3.1% (Regier et al., 1988; Lindesay et al., 1989). Agoraphobia is more common than specific phobia or SP (Manela et al., 1996; Uhlenhuth et al., 1983). In contrast with other anxiety disorders, many cases of agoraphobia in late life are new-onset cases (Lindesay, 1991). In younger individuals, agoraphobia is usually a conditioned response to panic attacks (Klein, 1980).

Simple phobia is twice as common in women as in men (Robins & Regier, 1991). Phobic objects tend to be the same for men and women (animals, heights, blood and aeroplanes), but women score somewhat higher on fear questionnaires such the Fear Survey Schedule commonly used to assess the severity of phobias (Wolpe & Lang, 1964).

3 Genetics

Some phobias in animals appear to be innate. For example, specific fears of poisonous coral snakes are found in some snake-eating birds who have never seen a snake before (Smith, 1977). Whether these reflect true phobias is perhaps questionable. A human fear of snakes in Europe constitutes a phobia but in the African or Australian culture, this fear may be realistic.

Twin studies of self-reported phobias have consistently suggested a significant role for genetic factors (Torgersen, 1979; Phillips et al., 1987; Rose & Ditto, 1983; Neale & Fulker, 1984). From these studies, the analysis of fives types of phobia (agoraphobia, SP, animal phobia, situational phobia and blood/injury phobia) showed that all phobia subtypes are moderately familial and that familial aggregation of agoraphobia, SP and animal phobia is due to genetic factors. However, for situational phobia and blood/injury phobia, the results suggest that twin resemblance might result from familial-environmental factors. A recent study designed to examine the sources of individual differences in the risks for phobias and their associated irrational fears in male twins performed personal interviews with both members of 1198 male-male twins (707 monozygotic and 491 dizygotic) (Kendler et al., 2001). The lifetime history of agoraphobia and social, animal, situational, and blood/injury phobias as well as their irrational fears was assessed. The results showed that genetic risk factors play a major role in the aetiology of phobias and their irrational fears. Family environment probably has an impact on risk for agoraphobia and SP.

Concerning the comorbidity of PD and agoraphobia, it was found that relatives of probands with agoraphobia were at an increased risk of both agoraphobia and PD, while relatives of PD probands had an increased risk of PD but not agoraphobia (Noyes et al., 1986). These findings may be interpreted as being consistent with the hypothesis that agoraphobia represents a more severe variant of PD, but subsequent studies have produced conflicting results (Mendlewicz et al., 1993; Goldstein et al., 1994).

4 Treatment

4.1 Psychological

Thus far no group investigations of phobia treatment in older samples exist. Individual case studies suggest that education, relaxation, cognitive coping strategies and imaginal and *in vivo* exposure with systematic desensitisation are generally effective in reducing anxiety and avoidance. A case study includes successful treatment of dog phobia in a 70-year-old woman using five sessions of *in vivo* exposure with dogs of increasing size (Thyer, 1981). Treatment gains were maintained at 6-month follow-up. Successful treatment of elevator phobia in four older clients using systematic desensitisation with *in vivo* exposure was described (Hussian, 1981). A case report documented successful treatment of a 68-year-old claustrophobic man using four sessions of EMDR (Lohr et al., 1996). EMDR is a form of exposure therapy in which clients re-experience and cognitively reprocess traumatic events in their imagination, while at the same time moving their eyes. For that client, subjective distress ratings decreased substantially, although heart rate did not change.

For psychological treatment of spider phobia, two methods may be considered. First, one can try to remove the intrinsically negative characteristics of spiders. Second, one can teach the phobic individuals that the chance of unwanted physical contact is in fact extremely small. The regular one-session (e.g., 2.5 h) *in vivo* exposure treatment deals with the latter dimension, as patients learn during the exposure exercises that spiders, in fact, try to avoid physical contact and are highly predictable and well controllable. A recent study designed to investigate this issue in a clinical context was performed in women with a clinically diagnosed spider phobia (de Jong et al., 2000). The first hypothesis tested was whether and to what extent a regular one-session exposure *in vivo* treatment already alters the affective valence of spiders as well as their disgusting properties. Secondly, whether the treatment of spider phobia would be more effective with respect to measures of fear, valence and disgust if a counterconditioning procedure was added was also tested. The results of this study clearly demonstrated that regular exposure treatment is already quite effective in altering the affective-evaluative component of spider phobia. Exposure with counterconditioning was not superior to the long-term treatment efficacy and was not more effective in altering the affective valence of spiders than the *in vivo* exposure treatment without counterconditioning.

4.2 Biofeedback

A study to determine whether alpha enhancement would benefit students suffering from test anxiety was performed (Garrett & Silver, 1976). Eighteen were assigned to biofeedback training and an equal number matched for level of test anxiety to an untreated control group. Half of the feedback group started with 8–13 Hz alpha-enhancement training, in which alpha in excess of 21 μV caused a feedback tone, and half started with EMG feedback. The alpha group improved alpha production from 64 to 78% of the time, and the EMG group reduced voltage from 5.84 to 3.49 μV; 83% reported being more relaxed in and out of the laboratory. Nine favoured alpha, four EMG, and five thought they were equally effective in causing relaxation. Test anxiety scores of the trained group improved (50 to 32), while those of the untrained group were essentially unchanged (48 to 47), a statistically significant difference ($p < 0.01$). This study showed that combined alpha and EMG biofeedback can reduce test anxiety.

4.3 Pharmacological

Although there has been considerable interest in phobia from a psychological perspective, there are little pharmacological data from animal studies that can be considered directly pertinent to the treatment of phobic disorders.

Clinically, BDZs alone do not appear to be beneficial in alleviating phobias other than agoraphobia. BDZs are ineffective in the treatment of specific or simple phobias (Sheehan et al., 1980). However, they can be beneficial when used in conjunction with behavioural therapies such as flooding (Marks et al., 1972; Hafner & Marks, 1976). For patients with agoraphobia, anxiolytics may increase the ease of exposure in behaviour therapy (Hafner & Marks, 1976). Clearly, more work is needed to establish whether adjunctive anxiolytics are of any use in facilitating behaviour therapy.

Recently, a study that examined the effects of long-term treatment with citalopram or clomipramine on subjective symptoms in patients with PD showed that all active treatment groups, especially the group receiving 20–30 mg per day of citalopram, effectively controlled phobic symptoms in patients with PD (Leinonen et al., 2000). Phobic symptoms were assessed using the phobia scale and the symptom checklist (SCL90) phobia-related factors (Marks & Matthews, 1979; Derogatis et al., 1973). Citalopram (20–30 mg) generally decreased phobic symptoms significantly more than placebo after month 3. Interpersonal sensitivity decreased when measured on the respective SCL-90 sub-scale. Alleviation of phobic symptoms generally continued to increase towards the end of the treatment.

5 Discussion

The subdivision of specific phobias into different subtypes seems to be relevant for clinical practice. It has been reported that each specific phobia subtype has its typical manifestation in terms of physical and cognitive symptomatology (Hugdahl & Öst, 1985; Himle et al., 1989, Antony & Barlow, 1997). For example, confrontation with the phobic stimulus elicits sympathetic activation (e.g., tachycardia) in animal phobia, but parasympathetic activation (e.g., bradycardia) in blood-injection-injury phobia. Thus, while exposure to the phobic stimulus produces heightened arousal in animal phobics, lowered arousal that may result in fainting is seen in blood-injection-injury phobias.

Given the high prevalence of phobias in older adults, the need for a reliable scale to assess specific fears is important. The Fear Survey Schedule (FSS-II) has been used to evaluate the prevalence and distribution of fears in adults age 50 and over (Liddell et al., 1991; Geer, 1965). Data suggested greater general fearfulness in women than men, and decreasing fearfulness with increasing age, additional education, and higher income. Factor analyses showed somewhat different factor structures for men and women, although factors assessing social fears, agoraphobic symptoms, animals and death and dying were identified for both genders.

It appears that diazepam enhances rather than impairs the effects of the behavioural therapies (Lister et al., 1988). This observation is of interest in view of the documented amnestic properties of the BDZs. Despite the paucity of pharmacological data, there are many behavioural studies investigating phobias in animals and in man. Such studies should soon provide a firm basis for future pharmacological research and treatment of phobias. It seems likely that the greatest contribution that can be made from animal pharmacological research may be the suggestion of treatments that benefit the patient when used in conjunction with the behaviour therapies.

References

American Psychiatric Association. Diagnostic and Statistical manual of mental disorders. 4th ed. Washington, DC: American Psychiatric Association; 1994

Antony MM, Brown TA & Barlow DH. Heterogeneity among specific phobia types in DSM-IV. Behav Res Ther 35, 1089–1100, 1997

Barlow D, Brown T & Craske M. Definitions of panic attacks and panic disorder in the DSM-IV: implications for research. J Abnorm Psychol 103, 553–564, 1994

Cook M, Mineka S, Wolkenstein B & Laitsch K. Observational conditioning of snake fear in unrelated rhesus monkeys. J Abnorm Psychol 94, 591–610, 1985

Davey GCL. Characteristics of individuals with fear of spiders. Anxiety Res 4, 299–314, 1992

De Jong PJ, Vorage I & van den Hout MA. Counterconditioning in the treatment of spider phobia: effects on disgust, fear and valence. Behav Res Ther 38, 1055–1069, 2000

Derogatis LR, Lipman RS & Covi L. SCL-90: An outpatient psychiatric rating scales – preliminary report. Psychopharmacol Bull 9, 13–28, 1973

Frederikson M, Annas P, Fisher H & Wik G. Gender and age differences in the prevalence of specific fears and phobias. Behav Res Ther 34, 33–39, 1996

Garrett BL & Silver MP. The use of EMG and alpha biofeedback to relieve test anxiety in college students. In: I Wickramasekera (ed): Biofeedback, Behavior Therapy, and Hypnosis. Chicago, IL: Nelson-Hall, 1976

Geer JH. The development of a scale to measure fear. Behav Res Ther 3, 45–53, 1965

Gelder MG & Mathews AM. Forearm blood flow and phobic anxiety. Br J Psychiatry 114, 1371–1376, 1968

Goldstein RB, Weissman MM, Adams PB, Horwath E, Lish JD, Charney D, Woods SW,

Sobin C & Wickramaratne PJ. Psychiatric disorders in relatives of probands with panic disorder and/or major depression. Arch Gen Psychiatry 51, 383–394, 1994

Gross JJ & Levenson RW. Emotional suppression: physiology, self-report and expressive behavior. J Pers Soc Psychol 64, 970 - 986, 1993

Haidt J, McCauley D & Rozin P. Individual differences in sensitivity to disgust: a scale sampling seven domains of disgust elicitors. Personality and Individual Differences 16, 701–713, 1994

Hafner J & Marks I. Exposure *in vivo* of agoraphobics: contributions of diazepam, group exposure and anxiety evocation. Psychol Med 6, 71–88, 1976

Himle JA, McPhee K, Cameron OJ & Curtis GC. Simple phobia: evidence for heterogeneity. Psychiatr Res 28, 25–30, 1989

Hugdahl K & Öst LG. Subjectively rated physiological and cognitive symptoms in six different clinical phobias. Personality and Individual Differences 6, 175–788, 1985

Hussian RA. Geriatric psychology: A behavioral perspective. New York: Van Nostrand Reinhold, 1981

Klein DF. Anxiety reconceptualized. Compr Psychiatry 21 (6), 411–427, 1980

Kendler KS, Myers J, Prescott CA & Neale MC. The genetic epidemiology of irrational fears and phobias in men. Arch Gen Psychiatry 58, 257–265, 2001

Kleinknecht RA, Thorndike RM & Walls MM. Factorial dimensions and correlates of blood, injection and related fear: cross-validation of the medical fear survey. Behav Res Ther 34, 323–331, 1996

Leinonen E, Lepola U, Koponen H, Turtonen J, Wade A & Lehto H. Citalopram controls phobic symptoms in patients with panic disorder: randomized controlled trial. J Psychiatry Neurosci 251, 24–32, 2000

Levenson RW. Autonomic nervous system differences among emotions. Psychol Sci 3, 23–27, 1992

Liddell A, Locker D & Burman D. Self-reported fears (FSS-II) of subjects aged 50 years and older. Behav Res Ther 29, 105–112, 1991

Lindesay J, Briggs K & Murphy E. The Guy's/Age Concern Survey: prevalence rates of cognitive impairment, depression and anxiety in an urban elderly community. Br J Psychiatry 155, 317–329, 1989

Lindesay J. Phobic disorders in the elderly. Br J Psychiatry 159, 531–541, 1991

Lister RG, Weingartner H, Eckardt MJ & Linnoila M. Clinical relevance of effects of benzodiazepines on learning and memory. In: I Hindmarch & H Ott (eds): Benzodiazepine receptor ligands, memory and information processing. Heidelberg: Springer, 117–127, 1988

Lohr JM, Tolin DF & Kleinknecht RA. An intensive design investigation of Eye Movement Desensitization and Reprocessing of claustrophobia. J Anxiety Disord 10, 73–88, 1996

Manela M, Katona C & Livingston G. How common are the anxiety disorders in old age? Int J Geriatr Psychiatry, 11, 65–70, 1996

Marks IM & Matthews AM. Brief standard self-rating for phobic patients. Behav Res Ther 17, 263–267, 1979

Marks IM. Fears, phobias and rituals. New York: Oxford University Press, 1987

Marks IM, Viswanathan R, Lipsedge MS & Gardner R. Enhanced relief of phobias by flooding during waning diazepam effect. Br J Psychiatry 121, 493–505, 1972

Matchett G & Davey GCL. A test of the disease-avoidance model of animal phobias. Behav Res Ther 29, 91–94, 1991

Mendlewicz J, Papdimitriou G & Wilmotte J. Family study of panic disorder: comparison with generalized anxiety disorder, major depression and normal subjects. Psychiatr Genet 3, 73–78, 1993

Merckelbach H, de Jong PJ, Arntz A & Schouten E. The role of evaluative learning and disgust sensitivity in the etiology and treatment of spider phobia. Adv Behav Res Ther 15, 243–255, 1993

Muris P, Schmidt H & Merckelbach H. The structure of specific phobia symptoms among children and adolescents. Behav Res Ther 37, 863–868, 1999

Noyes R Jr, Crowe RR, Harris EL, Hampa BJ, McChesney CM & Chaudry DR. Relationship between panic disorder and agoraphobia: a family study. Arch Gen Psychiatry 43, 227–232, 1986

Phillips K, Fulker DW & Rose RJ. Path analysis of seven fear factors in adult twin and sibling pairs and their parents. Genet Epidemiol 4, 345–355, 1987

Rachman S. Fear and courage (2nd ed.). New York, NY: W.H. Freeman and Company, 1990

Robins LN & Regier DA (eds). Psychiatric disorders in America: the epidemiologic catchment area study. New York: Free Press, 1991

Rose RJ & Ditto WB. A developmental-genetic analysis of common fears from early adolescence to early adulthood. Child Dev 54 (2), 361–368, 1983

Rose RJ, Miller JZ, Pogue-Geile MF & Cardwell GF. Twin-family studies of common fears and phobias. In: L Gedda, P Parisi & WE Nance (eds): Intelligence, personality and development. New York, NY: Alan R Liss, 169–174. Twin Research, Vol. 3, part 69B, 1981

Rozin P, Haidt J & McCauley CR. Disgust. In: M Lewis & JM Haviland. Handbook of emotions. New York, Guildford Publications, 1993

Regier DA, Boyd JH, Burke JD Jr, Rae DS, Myers JK, Kramer M et al. One-month prevalence of mental disorders in the United States: based on five epidemiologic catchment area sites. Arch Gen Psychiatry 45, 977–986, 1988

Rozin P, Fallon AE & Mandell R. Family resemblance in attitudes to food. Dev Psychol 20, 309–314, 1984

Sheehan DV, Ballenger JC & Jacobsen G. Treatment of endogenous anxiety with phobic, hysterical and hypochondriacal symptoms. Arch Gen Psychiatry 37, 51–59, 1980

Smith SM. Coral-snake recognition and stimulus generalization by naive great kiskadees (Aves: Tyrannidae). Nature 265, 535–536, 1977

Thorpe SJ & Salkovskis PM. Studies on the role of disgust in the acquisition and maintenance of specific phobias. Behav Res Ther 36, 877–893, 1998

Thyer BA & Curtis GC. On the diphasic nature of vasovagal fainting associated with blood-injury-illness phobia. J Pavlovian Biol Sci 20, 84–87, 1997

Tolin DF, Lohr JM, Sawchuk CN & Lee TC. Disgust and disgust sensitivity in blood-injection-injury and spider phobia. Behav Res Ther 35, 949–953, 1997

Torgersen S. The nature and origin of common phobic fears. Br J Psychiatry 134, 343–351, 1979

Thyer BA. Prolonged *in vivo* exposure therapy with a 70-year-old woman. J Behav Ther Exp Psychiatry 12, 69–71, 1981

Uhlenhuth EH, Balter MB, Mellinger GD, Cisin IH & Clinthorne J. Symptom checklist syndromes in the general population: correlations with psychotherapeutic drug use. Arch Gen Psychiatry 40, 1167–1173, 1983

Widiger T, Frances A, Pincus H, Ross R, First M & Davis W (eds). DSM-IV source book. Washington, DC, American Psychiatric Press, 1996

Wolpe J & Lang P. A fear survey schedule for use in behavior therapy. Behav Res Ther 2, 27–30, 1964

Chapter 9
Laboratory models of anxiety

1 Introduction

Because anxiety is a concept that describes a human subjective state, its absolute reproduction in animals is an impossible target. Since animals cannot tell us about the experience of anxiety and fear, a rich source of information that is readily obtained from humans with anxiety disorders may be missed. Therefore, it can only be modelled in animals. A model is an artificial representation of a disease or some aspects of it. Models are often evaluated on a continuum of similarity to the disease (Howard et al., 1989). In theory, the ideal model may reproduce all the features of the phenomenon under investigation and as such would be an exact reproduction rather than a model. In many instances in psychopharmacological research, a model is understood to be a screening method, validated at the standard drug correlational level. Therefore, an animal model of anxiety may be considered as an approach that registers positive for clinically proven anxiolytics and negative for drugs that are thought to be nonanxiolytic in that they usually do not relieve the symptoms of anxiety.

Animal models of anxiety are an absolute requirement for both the identification of underlying biological mechanisms and the development of novel anxiolytics. They have been used to investigate the effects of anxiolytic drugs as well as to study the neurophysiological basis of anxiety (Miczek et al., 1995). Nevertheless, until recently the main criterion for validation of an animal model of anxiety has been its sensitivity to BDZ anxiolytics. As a result, many of the existing models do not easily detect non-BDZ anxiolytics (Chopin & Briley, 1987; File, 1987; Handley & McBlane, 1993; Treit, 1991). Buspirone, an azapirone that probably exerts its clinical effects through agonist activity at the 5-HT_{1A} receptor, was developed as anxiolytic after feedback from clinical trials where it was initially tested as a potential antipsychotic. Therefore, preclinical research difficulties to develop newer animal models that must be sensitive to other classes of potential anxiolytics such as 5-HT_{1A} receptor agonists and also to the specific SSRIs which have shown some efficacy as anxiolytics in certain indications (anti-panic, anti-OCD drugs) must be recognised (Nutt & Glue, 1989). There is a clear need for new animal models that are sensitive to non-BDZ anxiolytics to address specific types of anxiety disorders, including those resistant to BDZs.

There is suggestive clinical evidence that anxiety disorders are not homogeneous in their manifestations and that different types of anxiety may prevail. The fact that anxiety, as a pathologic disease, can be subdivided into many kinds such as GAD, PD, phobias and PTSD has been further reason for studying different animal models based on the stimulus source and on the susceptibility to the effects of drugs.

State anxiety is the emotion an individual experiences when confronted with a stressful stimulus, whereas trait anxiety is an enduring feature of a subject, that is, a stable characteristic (Spielberger, 1975). Most of the animal models of anxiety use anxiogenic stimuli to provoke anxiety, such as the presentation of programmed painful stimuli (conditioned conflict tests), well-lit arenas (social interaction test, open fields, staircase), separation from the mother in infant rodents (separation vocalisations) or forced confrontation with unfamiliar environments (elevated plus-maze, holeboard, staircase, open field, light/dark choice test, etc.). Therefore, all these tests may model state anxiety.

Some evidence suggests that rodents confronted with threat stimuli such as a predator will try to avoid by "flight" or "freezing" behaviour. Animal models based on flight responses have been used to mimic the symptoms of PD. The hypothesis that in PD, panic arises when flight/fight mechanisms are aroused but no perceived route of escape is available has been used. Therefore, several models have been described which examine flight- and escape-related behaviours in rodents, and the ability of anti-panic drugs to attenuate these responses (Ashcroft et al., 1993; Griebel et al. 1996). In less threatening situations, stereotyped investigatory behaviours such as the stretched-attend posture, in which an animal moves intermittently forward with a flattened back may be observed (Blanchard et al., 1991; Grewal et al., 1997). This pattern of activity forms a cluster of information-gathering behaviours called risk assessment, which permit an anxious animal to assess and localise danger (Blanchard et al., 1990). Risk assessment may represent a conspicuous behavioural pattern seen in rodents, which can be adapted for the measurement of anxiety. Some anxiety tests that use risk assessment, such as the stretched-attend posture, as the primary dependent variable have been developed (Grewal et al., 1997; Kaesermann, 1986). A variety of other anxiety tests using Pavlovian and/or operant conditioning procedures such as the fear potentiated startle (FPS) have been used to test anxiolytic agents in rodents (Davis, 1990; Kuribara, 1994).

An ideal model would be one reproducing all features of human anxiety. It should ideally have face, construct and predictive validity (Willner, 1991). Face validity refers to the phenomenological similarity between the model and the disorder. This implies, for instance, that a model of PD produces reactions in animals that are analogous to panic attack in humans. Predictive validity refers to the sensitivity of the model to specific drug challenge. In the case of panic attacks, these models must be specifically sensitive to the effects of clinically proven, panic-modulating agents. Construct validity, which addresses the theoretical rationale of the model usually, includes etiological, neurophysiological and neuropathological aspects of the disorder. For example, a model has construct validity if the mechanism behind the pathology seems to have similar physiological substrates in the animal model and in man. In the majority of available models, the data generated are interpreted in terms of analogy rather than homology (Carey et al., 1992). In order to validate the models physiologically, changes in ACTH, corticosterone and hypothalamic noradrenaline are often measured. If the biochemical changes in pathological anxiety are the same, differing only in intensity and frequency, then these tests should normally have predictive value for the pathological state. For pharmacological validation, animal tests should be able to detect the full range of clinically accepted anxiolytic compounds as well as demonstrating opposite actions for anxiogenic drugs. Ideally they should have no false positives, nor should they be insensitive to clinically effective products.

In this chapter, the various models of anxiety currently used in preclinical research are reviewed and discussed. The validity of the various approaches in terms of their similarity to different human anxiety disorders and potentials for the discovery of new drugs in clinical treatment of anxiety are critically examined.

2 Biological animal models

Although anxiety has been an active area of research, relatively little is known about the neural substrates that regulate the aetiology of anxiety disorders. The emergence of molecular techniques that allow the alteration of genes and gene function in the intact animal is fashioning a new era in neuropsychiatric research. A transgenic mouse is often generated to study the functional consequences of gene overexpression.

2.1 GABAergic transmission and benzodiazepine receptor function

It was recently demonstrated that mice with mutation of the α1 GABA receptor subunit are insensitive to the sedative, amnesic, and anticonvulsant effects of diazepam, but remain responsive to the drug's anxiolytic effects, probably *via* action at intact α2 and α3 subunits (Rudolph et al., 1999) (see Tab. 9.1). A separate study reported that inactivating the δ subunit renders mice insensitive to the anxiolytic effects of neuroactive steroids in the elevated plus-maze (Mihalek et al., 1999). In combination with α and β subunits, the γ2 subunit is essential for the expression of the BDZ site on the $GABA_A$ receptor complex. In a recent study in which the long variant of the γ2 subunit gene was deleted, it was observed that this deletion did not alter total γ2 subunit expression but led to a compensatory increase in the short variant of the γ2 subunit (Homanics et al., 1999). However, even with this ontological compensation, γ2L subunit knockout mice exhibited heightened anxiety-like behaviour in the elevated plus-maze.

The creation of mice heterozygous for the $GABA_A$-receptor γ2 subunit has been helpful for the comprehension of the molecular basis of this disorder and is probably one of the first genetic models of an emotional disorder (Crestani et al., 1999). These mice have reduced BDZ binding, indicating a reduction in the number of γ2 subunits, and behave like patients suffering from anxiety disorders. The γ2 heterozygous mice had as much as a 35% decrease in γ2 subunits in areas such as the hippocampus, cingulate cortex and prefrontal cortex, but only about 5–15% in other areas of the brain. The hippocampus is likely to mediate the increased anxiety in the γ2 heterozygous mice. They avoid threats (unfamiliar, elevated or brightly-lit

Table 9.1: Examples of anxiety-related phenotypes in $GABA_A$ transgenic and gene knockout mice

Genetic mutation	**Anxiety-related phenotype**	**Behavioural test**	**References**
$GABA_A$ $\alpha1$ subunit mutant	No anxiety-related phenotype	Elevated plus-maze	Rudolph et al., 1999
		Light ⇔ dark exploration	
$GABA_A$ δ subunit knockout	No anxiety-related phenotype	Elevated plus-maze	Mihalek et al., 1999
$GABA_A$ $\gamma2$ subunit heterozygous knockout	Increased anxiety-like behaviour	Elevated plus-maze	Crestani et al., 1999
		Light ⇔ dark exploration	
		Free exploratory paradigm	
$GABA_A$ $\gamma2$ subunit (long-variant) knockout	Increased anxiety-like behaviour	Elevated plus-maze	Homanics et al., 1999

Table 9.2: Examples of anxiety-related phenotypes in 5-HT transgenic and gene knockout mice

Genetic mutation	**Anxiety-related phenotype**	**Behavioural test**	**References**
5-HT_{1A} receptor knockout	Increased anxiety-like behaviour	Elevated plus-maze	Ramboz et al., 1998
		Open field centre time	Heisler et al., 1998
		Elevated zero-maze	
		Novel object exploration	
5-HT_{1B} receptor knockout	Decreased anxiety-like behaviour	Elevated plus-maze	Shepherd et al., 1994
	No anxiety-related phenotype	Open field centre time	Zhuang et al., 1999
		Ultrasonic vocalisations in pups	Malleret et al., 1999
	No anxiety-related phenotype	Elevated plus-maze	Malleret et al., 1999
		Light ⇔ dark exploration	Ramboz et al., 1996
		Open field centre time	
5-HT_{2C} receptor knockout	Increased anxiety-like behaviour	Emergence test	Tecott et al., 1998
5-HT_{5A} receptor knockout	No-anxiety related phenotype	Elevated plus-maze	Grailhe et al., 1999
		Open field centre time	
		Defensive burying	7

areas), and are more likely to treat ambiguous cues as threats. Like highly anxious people, these mice are more sensitive to the anxiolytic effects of the BDZs. However, the hippocampus is implicated only in the cognitive aspects of anxiety (Davis, 1992; McNaughton, 1997). The mice may therefore model only the cognitive hippocampal aspects of anxiety disorder. The $\gamma 2$ heterozygous mice may be suitable models for anxiety, but not panic or phobia which are included in the "neurotic personality". The effects of other classes of anxiolytics such as 5-HT_{1A} agonists need also to be assessed in this model.

2.2 5-HT receptor knockouts

In view of the fact that buspirone, a partial agonist at the 5-HT_{1A} receptor, is a clinically effective anxiolytic, the anxiety-related phenotype of mice lacking the 5-HT_{1A} receptor gene has been a major discovery. A line of 5-HT_{1A} receptor knockout mice have consistently displayed heightened anxiety-like behaviour in various behavioural tests (Ramboz et al., 1998; Zhuang et al., 1999) (see Tab. 9.2). However, the recent finding that 5-HT_{1A} knockout mice are insensitive to the anxiolytic effects of diazepam also implicates changes at the level of the $GABA_A$-BDZ receptor in the anxiety-like phenotype of 5-HT_{1A} mutant mice. Reduced BDZ binding in the amygdala and cortex in 5-HT_{1A} mutant mice coupled with an insensitivity to anxiolytic doses of diazepam in the elevated plus-maze and open field test was noted (Sibille et al., 2000). It may be speculated that these changes are due to a loss of 5-HT_{1A}-mediated control over expression of $\alpha 1$ and $\alpha 2$ $GABA_A$ subunits in the amygdala in mutants. Thus, the gene knockout strategy to delete the 5-HT_{1A} receptor in the mouse adult brain could prove to be a valuable approach to study the functional roles of inter-relationship of the receptors in anxiety-related behaviour. In contrast to the confirmed anxiety-like phenotype seen in 5-HT_{1A} mutant mice, 5-HT_{1B} receptor knockout mice have displayed unaltered or decreased anxiety-like behaviour (Ramboz et al., 1996; Malleret et al., 1999).

2.3 Corticotropin-releasing hormone mutations and receptor knockouts

Dysfunction in mechanisms of the HPA axis and CRH function have been implicated in the aetiology and symptomatology of anxiety disorders. Transgenic mice overexpressing CRH exhibit heightened anxiety-like behaviour as measured by the elevated plus-maze and open field test (Stenzel-Poore et al., 1994). Recently, some studies have been performed on mutant mice lacking the CRH-R1 receptor, which has a widespread distribution in the brain (Liebsch et al., 1995, Contarino et al., 1999; Smith et al., 1998) These studies have reported dramatically reduced anxiety-like behaviour in several behavioural paradigms (see Tab. 9.3). However, studies examining the effects of CRH-R2 antisense to block receptor function in rats have not been consistent to show a significant role for the CRH-R2 receptor in anxiety-like behaviour.

Table 9.3: Examples of anxiety-related phenotypes in corticotropin-releasing hormone transgenic and gene knockout mice

Genetic mutation	Anxiety-related phenotype	Behavioural test	References
Corticotropin-releasing hormone (CRH) overexpressing transgenic	Increased anxiety-like behaviour	Elevated plus-maze	Stenzel-Poore et al., 1994
		Open field centre time	
		Light ⇔ dark exploration	Heinrichs et al., 1997
CRH knockout	No anxiety-related phenotype	Elevated plus-maze	Weninger et al., 1999
CRH R1 receptor knockout	Decreased anxiety-like behaviour	Elevated plus-maze	Smith et al., 1998
		Emergence test	
		Light ⇔ dark exploration	Contarino et al., 1999
CRH R2 receptor knockout	Increased anxiety-like behaviour	Elevated plus-maze	Bale et al., 2000
		Open field centre time	
		Emergence test	Kishimoto et al., 2000
	Decreased anxiety-like behaviour	Open field centre time	
	No anxiety-related phenotype	Light ⇔ dark exploration	Bale et al., 2000

Table 9.4: Classification of animal behavioural models currently used.

Conditioned models	Unconditioned models
Conflict procedures	Light-dark exploration
Fear-potentiated startle	Elevated plus maze
Periaqueductal gray stimulation	Defensive burying
Conditioned tasted aversion	Ultrasonic vocalisation
Conditioned place preference or aversion	Social interaction
Conditioned ultrasonic vocalisation	Defeat-induced analgesia
	Stress-induced hyperthermia

2.4 Genetically selected alcohol-preferring rats

The hypothesis that anxiety may trigger abnormal alcohol intake has been recently strengthened by the finding that genetically selected alcohol-preferring rats showed a greater innate degree of anxiety than alcohol-nonpreferring rats (Stewart et al., 1993). These results were confirmed by another study that suggests the use of Sardinian alcohol-preferring rats as a genetic model of anxiety (Colombo et al., 1995).

3 Behavioural animal models

Rats, mice and monkeys appear to be particularly suitable for behavioural anxiety tests. Animal models of anxiety can be classified into two main categories of conditioned and unconditioned models (see Tab. 9.4). Whereas conditioned models involve responses controlled by operant conditioning procedures, unconditioned models rely on natural behavioural reactions that do not require specific training. Often, unconditioned models rely on species-specific responses (e.g. social interaction, ultrasonic vocalisation) and are sometimes called "ethologically base" models. Conditioned models are often developed on the premise that aversive stimulation, either discrete or anticipated, produces a "fear"-like defensive reaction in both humans and animals. Many of the animal models of anxiety are based on the forced confrontation of rodents with unfamiliar environments, on social behaviours, or on conditioned conflict procedures (Belzung et al., 1987; Gardner, 1985; De Vry et al., 1993). These models include conflict procedures (punished lever pressing such as the Geller-Seifter conflict and Vogel drinking tests in rats) and exploratory models (elevated plus-maze test in rats and light/dark choice test in mice). Additionally, a recently developed mouse defence test battery (MDTB) was found to be useful for the screening of both anti-panic and anti-GAD drugs (Griebel et al., 1995, 1996) (see Tab. 9.5). However, as with any procedure involving behavioural suppression in control conditions, these tests are not convenient for detecting anxiogenic effects, i.e. treatments which decrease conflict responding. Although baseline conflict rates can be controlled at a high enough level to detect decreases, they usually become much more variable over time and the demonstration of anxiogenic effects a difficult issue (Hodges et al., 1987).

3.1 Anxiety

3.1.1 Elevated plus-maze

The elevated plus-maze (EPM) is one of the most widely used experimental models for the study of anxiety. It is based on the premise that environmental novelty evokes both fear and curiosity, thereby creating a typical approach-avoidance conflict (Montgomery, 1955). This model, originally developed for rats, was later adopted for use in mice (Handley & Mithani, 1984; Lister, 1987). The primary indices of anxiety are the frequency of entries and percentage of time spent by the

Table 9.5: Some animal models of anxiety disorders. Stretched attend posture (SAP).

Disorders assessed	Animal models	Description and procedure	References
Anxiety	Punished lever pressing	Animals are tested in a standard rat operant chamber fitted with a stainless steel grid floor in which electric footshocks could be delivered. Rats are trained initially to press a lever for food reward. The magnitude of footshocks is individually titrated for each rat (0.3 – 0.65 mA) to obtain stable baselines of responding. Once stable baselines are obtained, drug studies may be initiated. The drug effects are assessed on punished and unpunished response rates.	Sanger, 1995
	Punished drinking	At the beginning of the experiment, rats deprived of water before testing are placed in cages with a stainless steel grid floor. Each cage contained a drinking tube connected to an external buret. Trials start only after the animal's tongue come into contact with the drinking tube for the first time. The number of shocks was recorded automatically.	Vogel et al., 1971
	Elevated plus-maze	The maze is elevated to a height of 50 cm with two open (50 × 10 cm) and two enclosed arms (50 × 10 × 50 cm), arranged so that the arms of the same type are opposite each other, connected by an open central area (10 × 10 cm). At the beginning of the experiment, rats are placed in the centre of the maze, facing one of the enclosed arms, and observed for 4 min.	Pellow et al., 1985
	Light/dark transition	The test apparatus consists of two polyvinylchloride boxes (20 × 20 × 14 cm) covered with plexiglas. One of the boxes was darkened. A neon tube fixed on the ceiling provides the room illumination. An opaque plastic tunnel (5 × 7 × 10 cm) separates the dark box from the illuminated box. At the beginning of the experiment, a mouse was placed in the illuminated box facing the tunnel. Recording starts when the animal enters the tunnel for the first time.	Crawley, 1985 Misslin et al., 1989
	Ultrasonic distress vocalisation	In the rat, removal of the pup from its nest, mother and littemates elicits ultrasonic calling which is sensitive to treatment with anxiolytics	Winslow & Insel, 1991
	Burying behaviour	This paradigm consists of an acrylic cage with a prod emerging from one of its walls and the floor covered with bedding. Each time the animal touched the prod it received an electric shock and typically displayed the burying behaviour that consists of a rapid alternating movements of its forepaws, moving and pushing a pile of bedding over the electric prod. Two main registered parameters are the burying behaviour latency (time between the first shock and the burying behaviour display) and the cumulative burying behaviour (cumulative time the animal spends burying the prod during a 10-min test).	Pinel & Treit, 1978
	Sardinian alcohol preferring rat model.	The anxiety profile of the selectively bred alcohol-preferring sP and alcohol-nonpreferring sNP rats were assessed in an elevated plus maze. Rats were offered either water or a free choice of 10% ethanol and water for 14 consecutive days prior to the test. The results suggest a higher innate degree of anxiety in ethanol-experienced than in ethanol-naive sP rats.	Colombo et al., 1995

Table 9.5 (continued)

Disorders assessed	Animal models	Description and procedure	References
Anxiety (continued)	Canopy stretched attend posture	The SAP test apparatus comprised an elevated Perspex circular platform above which was built a canopy, dividing the platform into an inner, dimly lit covered zone, and an outer, brightly-lit exposed zone. Vehicle-treated animals exhibited a preference for exploring the covered zone and exhibited high baseline levels of SAP. Anxiolytics decreased the frequency of SAP without impairing motor activity.	Grewal et al., 1997
	Conditioned fear stress	In rodents, exposure to an environment paired with previously inescapable electric foot-shock, reliably elicits a response characterised by crouching and immobility. This termed conditioned fear stress-induced freezing behaviour and has been suggested to be used as a model of anxiety.	Fanselow & Helmstetter, 1988 Kalin et al., 1988
	Social interaction	Under bright lights or in an unfamiliar test environment, social interaction is suppressed relative to low light-familiar conditions, and this suppression is the index of anxiety.	File et al., 1984, 1985
	Hole board	The hole-board, "planche à trous" consisted of a board, 40 cm square and 1.8 cm thick, bored with 16 equally spaced holes, 3 cm in diameter. Each occurrence of a "head dip", or entry of the mouse head into the hole was measured. Number of holes explored by mice in a session is significantly increased by anxiolytics.	Boissier & Simon, 1964
Anxiety and memory	The elevated T-maze	The apparatus consisted of three arms of equal dimensions (50 × 10 cm) elevated 50 cm from the ground. One arm, enclosed by 40 cm high walls, was perpendicular to two open arms. Both inhibitory avoidance of the open arms and one-way escape from one of the open arms are measured in each animal, after drug or control injection. To assess memory, inhibitory avoidance and escape were measured again 3 days later.	Viana et al., 1994
Panic	The unstable elevated and exposed plus maze	The apparatus was a black, perspex plus-shaped maze, elevated 50 cm above the floor. All 4 arms of the maze were exposed, with only a small perspex ledge (0.5 cm high) surrounding each arm. A motor oscillated the elevated platform in the horizontal plane at a rate of 85 revs/min, with a movement amplitude of 2 cm each side of the central point. The rat was placed in the centre of the maze, the motor started after an interval of approx. 3 s, and the animal's behaviour monitored.	King, 1999
	Mouse defence test battery	The test consists of the following elements: (a). Pre-test: 3 min familiarisation period (b) Effects on flight responses: the rat avoidance test (min 4 to 6). (c) Effects on risk assessment: the chase (min 7 to 8) and the straight alley (min 9 to 11) tests. The hand-held rat is brought up to the mouse at a speed of approx. 2.0 m/s. (d) Effects on defensive threat/attack responses: the forced contact test (min 12 to 13) (e). Post-test: contextual defence. Immediately after the forced contact test, the rat is removed and the doors are opened.	Griebel et al., 1995, 1996, 1997

animal in the open arms (Rodgers & Cole, 1994). Blood corticosterone levels, which were used to assay the stress response, were significantly greater in animals confined to open arms, as were levels of defecation and freezing behaviour (Pellow et al., 1985). The reluctance of the animal to explore the open arms is probably a combination of rodent aversion for open spaces and high places (Lister, 1990). Some studies have shown that rodent aversion for open spaces is related to thigmotaxis, a natural reaction in which rats remain close to vertical surfaces (Treit et al., 1993). Despite the fact that it is one of the most commonly used animal models of anxiety, EPM may provide a wide range of contradictory results (Hogg, 1996). Some evidence for differential sensitivities between strains exist, with albino rats being more sensitive to the anxiolytic effects of 5-HT_3 receptor antagonists and 5-HT_{1A} receptor agonists than pigmented animals. Those rats that are mildly stressed by habituation to regular gentle handling have attenuated pharmacological responsiveness only, while those that have been subjected to more stressful manipulations (exposure to cat odour or surgery) have more significant changes in behaviour such as reduced open-arm exploration.

The anxiolytic effects of BDZs are attenuated in the second trial of EPM in both rats and mice. This effect is independent of the treatment on the first exposure, although it is observed only in animals that are previously habituated to regular gentle handling (File et al., 1990, 1992). The mouse EPM has been characterised extensively and appears to have reasonable predictive validity for a range of reference anxiolytic and anxiogenic drugs (Handley & McBlane, 1993; Rodgers & Cole, 1994). The inclusion of risk assessment measures in this test has been demonstrated to make it more sensitive to the effects of anxiolytic and anxiogenic drug treatment than either open arm time or percentage open arm entries (Rodgers & Cole, 1994). While locomotor activity and open arm entries tend to decrease in response to anxiogenic stimuli, an effect which can be misinterpreted as sedation, stretched-attend postures increase, thus permitting motor impairment to be dissociated from anxiogenesis (Rodgers & Cole, 1993; Shepherd et al., 1994).

An extensive series of studies examining the effects of both acute and chronic treatment with buspirone in the plus maze was conducted (Moser, 1989). An acute anxiogenic action of the drug did not disappear with 16 days of treatment. The inability of the plus-maze to detect an anxiolytic action of chronic treatment with buspirone and imipramine calls into question the general ability of the test to detect novel anxiolytics.

3.1.2 Elevated T-maze

The elevated T-Maze is derived from the EPM which has been classified as a "mixed" test of anxiety because it does not separate different types of fear (Pellow et al., 1985). This may be due to the inconsistency of the effects of 5-HT interacting drugs in the EPM (Handley et al., 1993). Therefore, the elevated T-maze was developed as an animal model of anxiety to separate, in the same rat, conditioned from unconditioned fear, which have been related to generalised anxiety and PD, respectively (Graeff et al., 1993; Viana et al., 1994). To be on an open arm seems to be an aversive experience, because rats have an innate fear of height and openness (Pellow et al., 1985; Treit et al., 1993). While inhibitory avoidance of the open arm is supposed to represent learned fear, the escape response from the open arm would represent innate fear. A recent study that investigated procedural questions raised by the use of the elevated T-maze confirms that this test generates two types of fear (Zangrossi & Graeff, 1997). It indicates that openness is the main factor motivating both inhibitory avoidance and one-way escape in this model.

The BDZ agonist diazepam and the 5-HT_{1A} ligand ipsapirone impaired inhibitory avoidance in a dose-dependent way. Therefore, inhibitory avoidance in the T-maze may be related to pathologic conditions that are responsive to 5-HT_{1A} agonists or low doses of BDZs, such as anticipatory anxiety and GAD. On the other hand, these two drugs did not affect one-way escape behaviour. These data may correlate with the ineffectiveness of these compounds in PD (Nutt, 1991). A recent study in rats confirmed that anxiolytics such as diazepam, buspirone and ipsapirone (5-HT_{1A} agonists) as well as ritanserin (5-HT_2 antagonist) selectively antagonised inhibitory avoidance while leaving one-way escape unaffected (Graeff et al., 1998). In contrast to the anxiolytic effects, the anxiogenic drugs yohimbine, trifluoromethylphenylpiperazine (TFPP) and *m*-CPP facilitated avoidance. Escape was not affected by yohimbine, but was moderately attenuated by the two 5-$HT_{2C/2B}$ agonists. The antidepressant clomipramine also had an anxiogenic-like effect on inhibitory avoidance, but did not affect escape from the open arm. It was argued that the behavioural and pharmacological results support the view that inhibitory avoidance in the elevated T-maze may be related to GAD, while one-way escape may be associated with PD.

The elevated T-maze was also suggested to serve as both a test of anxiety and memory (Viana et al., 1994). The doses of 1, 2, and 4 mg/kg diazepam and 1 and 2 mg/kg ipsapirone impaired inhibitory avoidance, an effect that may be considered as anxiolytic (Viana et al., 1994; Lucki et al., 1987; Schweitzer & Rickels, 1991). Inhibitory avoidance remained impaired 3 days later in the rats treated with 1–4 mg/kg diazepam, indicating anterograde amnesia. In rats, age appears as crucial factor as although rats at 30, 90 and 120 days of age equally learned the inhibitory avoidance, with little variation in relation to the mean number of trials required to reach criterion, the 60-day old rats exhibit a lower fear response (Sanson & Carobrez, 1999). That study highlighted the importance of controlling organismic variables such as age in order to reduce experimental variability in this model.

However, the usefulness of the T-maze in mice may not represent a good model to test new anxiolytics. A study which explored whether this test may be applied to mice as a model of anxiety showed that they do not appear to acquire inhibitory avoidance in the standard T-maze, since their latencies to leave enclosed arm did not increase along trials (Jardim et al., 1999). Mice acquire inhibitory avoidance of the open arms by decreasing and increasing time in risk assessment and freezing, respectively, along consecutive trials. They learn to avoid the open arms already at the first exposure, but this acquisition is detected through risk assessment and freezing behaviour measurement rather than latencies to leave the enclosed arm. Nevertheless, one-way escape could not be characterised. Since in the elevated T-maze important differences between mice and rats in the performance of behavioural tasks exist, species differences in the use of this test must be carefully considered. The T-maze may be applied to mice as a model of anxiety, but not as originally used for rats. The possibility to separate conditioned and unconditioned fear in this test in mice may be limited.

3.1.3 *The holeboard test*

The test assesses an animal's directed exploration (head dipping) and its locomotor activity (Boissier & Simon, 1964). A weakness of this test is that the effects of a drug on the behaviour of an animal (as in the open field test) can be critically dependent on the familiarity of the animal with the test environment (File, 1973). In mice naive to the testing apparatus, BDZs exert a biphasic effect on exploratory head dipping, low doses increasing and high doses decreasing this measure (Nolan & Parkes, 1973). If the mice have previously been familiarised with the apparatus in an undrugged state, then doses of BDZs that increase exploration in naive mice fail to modify or decrease exploratory head dipping. Despite a large number of experimental studies, it seems premature to accept the holeboard test as a valid model of anxiety. An increase in exploratory head dipping is suggested as an anxiolytic effect in animals naive to the test apparatus. However, certain drugs that appear to lack anxiolytic effects such as the BDZ-receptor antagonists flumazenil also increase directed exploration (File et al., 1982; Lister, 1988). In mice, decreases in exploration can also be noted with concomitant increases in locomotor activity following moderate doses of BDZs or ethanol (Lister, 1987). Whether this reflects a biphasic effect of anxiety on exploration needs yet to be demonstrated.

3.1.4 *Stress-induced hyperthermia*

Recently, a new animal model in mice called stress-induced hyperthermia that may reflect human anticipatory anxiety was developed (Borsini et al., 1989). This model is based on the finding that when group-housed mice are removed one by one from their home cage, the mice removed last always have a higher rectal temperature than those removed first. This mouse model with NMRI mice is reported to be very robust, reproducible and stable (Zethof et al., 1995). In this test, BDZs (diazepam, alprazolam), alcohol, and some 5-HT_{1A} receptor agonists (flesinoxan, buspirone), but not all (e.g. ipsapirone) showed anxiolytic properties. Clonidine (α_2-adrenoceptor agonist) and prazosine (α_1-adrenoceptor antagonist), at high doses only, showed some anxiolytic effects. Drugs such as antidepressants (desipramine, fluvoxamine, nomifensine, tianeptine, amitriptyline, clomipramine, imipramine), serotonergic ligands (ondansetron, ketanserin, eltoprazine) and various other classes (pentetrazol, haloperidol, apomorphine, amphetamine, dizocilpine) did not show any anxiolytic effects. However, the stress-induced hyperthermia model with mice fails to detect anxiogenic compounds (e.g. pentetrazol, *m*-CPP); this may be due to the impossibility of increasing mouse rectal temperature further than 1–1.5 °C.

Stress-induced hyperthermia appears to possess high face validity. A stress-induced temperature rise may appear as a universal phenomenon occurring in several species such as rats, rabbits and humans (Briese & Cabanac, 1991; Marazziti et al., 1992; Yokoi, 1966; Yoshiue et al., 1989). Strong indications that stress-related hyperthermia in man uses physiological and endocrinological mechanisms similar to those found in animals were suggested (Marazziti et al., 1992). CRH is involved in the regulation of a variety of responses occurring in stress and anxiety (Dunn & Berridge, 1990). However, its predictive validity is slightly weak as a potential anxiogenic effect cannot be detected. It also failed to demonstrate the anxiolytic effects of phenobarbital up to 60 mg/kg, i.p. (Zethof et al., 1995).

3.1.5 Fear potentiated startle

The FPS paradigm, in which the animal's startle response to a sudden loud tone is increased by simultaneous presentation of a brief light stimulus previously associated with shock, has been shown to be selectively sensitive to anxiolytic and anxiogenic treatment (Davis et al., 1993). Anxiolytics produce a dose-response reduction in FPS, an effect not found with, for example, antidepressants (Casella & Davis, 1985). For instance, the non-BDZ anxiolytic buspirone has an inconsistent profile on the plus-maze, but gives positive results using potentiated startle (Dunn et al., 1989; Mansbach & Geyer, 1988). This paradigm is also sensitive to putative anxiolytics such as clonidine and 5-HT_3 receptor antagonists (Davis et al., 1979; Glenn & Green, 1989).

A study which investigated the acute effects of nicotine compared to chlordiazepoxide and amphetamine in this paradigm showed that nicotine (0.1 mg/kg, s.c.) eliminated potentiation of startle in rats, an effect comparable to that of 2.5 mg/kg chlordiazepoxide (Vale & Green, 1996). On the other hand, d-amphetamine did not significantly influence potentiation of startle. It was suggested that nicotine has an anxiolytic profile in the potentiated startle paradigm that is not due to its psychostimulant properties. It was also hypothesised that the behaviour assessed in the FPS may reflect different types of anxiety and that nicotine may have specific anxiety-reducing properties, which would have implications for models of nicotine dependence and withdrawal effects.

The FPS procedure possesses face validity as humans exhibit an enhanced startle response when experiencing fears (Brown et al., 1951; Grillon et al.1993). Although this approach was initially developed using rats, it appears likely that it could be adapted as an anxiety screen in mice and human volunteers.

3.1.6 Burying behaviour test

The burying behaviour test has been previously described in detail and validated as a useful and selective model for establishing experimental anxiety (Pinel & Treit, 1978). It has been considered that burying behaviour latency inversely reflects the animals' reactivity, while the cumulative burying behaviour directly denotes the experimental anxiety levels (Pinel & Treit, 1978; Treit, 1985). The effects of anxiolytics on probe-burying can be distinguished from those of several nonanxiolytics, although the drug class-specificity of the test is sensitive to procedural variations (Treit, 1990). The suppression of burying behaviour by BDZ anxiolytics does not appear to be secondary to analgesia or to associative deficits, and can be blocked by BDZ receptor antagonists such as flumazenil (Treit, 1985, 1987; Blampied and Kirk, 1983). In addition, putative anxiogenic agents such as yohimbine have been reported to increase the duration that rats spent burying the probe (Tsuda et al., 1989).

The anxiolytic effect of buspirone (5 mg/kg), ipsapirone (5 mg/kg), indorenate (5 mg/kg) and 8-OH-DPAT (0.5 mg/kg) was established in this test (Fernandez-Guasti & Lopez Rubalcava, 1998). These results suggest that the shock probe-burying model may be a valuable method with good predictive value for the study of the anxiolytic effect of BDZ and 5-HT_{1A} agonists. However, a problem with this test is that the basic dependent variable (depth of sawdust etc. piled up) is likely to prove unsuitable for fine-grained dosage or drug comparisons.

3.1.7 Stretched attend posture test

The stretched attend posture (SAP) is a characteristic posture observed in a number of rodent species which is characterised by a forward elongation of the body exhibited when the animal is either standing still or moving slowly forward (Grant and Mackintosh, 1963). It was classified as an ambivalent element which reflects an approach-avoiding conflict and an integral component of the "risk assessment" repertoire of defensive behaviour in rodents. The novel canopy SAP test was shown to be sensitive to the effects of anxiolytics in both mice and rats and can also detect anxiogenic effects in the rat (Grewal et al., 1997). This paradigm shown to be a useful approach to study risk assessment behaviour in both rats and mice may be a sensitive rodent model of anxiety.

3.1.8 Light-dark transition test

This model initially devised for mice appears to be based on the natural tendency of rodents to avoid brightly lit areas of a compartmentalised test chamber (Crawley, 1981). This test possesses a certain degree of face validity in that light serves as anxiogenic stimulus and there is an apparent conflict between the desire to explore and the desire to avoid the brightly lit part of the apparatus. A variety of BDZ anxiolytics, including diazepam, clonazepam, flurazepam and chlordiazepoxide, produced dose-dependent increases in the number of light/dark transitions, while antidepressants (clorgyline and butriptyline) and an antipsychotic (chlorpromazine) did not increase the number of transitions (Crawley, 1985). The increase in transitions is probably not a function of generalised locomotor hyperactivity, since the same doses did not increase general locomotion in mice placed in a bare, undifferentiated cage on a locomotion meter (Crawley & Goodwin, 1980). The increased exploration was seen in either the daytime or evening phase of the circadian rhythm, in mice reused up to three times, irrespective of the number of days intervening between trials (Blumstein & Crawley, 1983). The relative potency of anxiolytics in increasing the number of mouse exploratory transitions agreed well with their relative potency in the clinical treatment of human anxiety (Crawley, 1981).

The anxiolytic effect of diazepam in this test could be counteracted by the co-administration of the BDZ receptor antagonist flumazenil, CGS 8216 and FG-7142 (Crawley et al., 1984). None of these antagonists produced effects of their own when administered in these models. These agonist-antagonist interactions suggest that the facilitation of rodent exploration in the light-dark chamber by BDZ anxiolytics is mediated by central BDZ receptor.

Low doses of buspirone produced an anxiolytic effect, increasing rodent exploration of the light chamber (Costall et al., 1989; Onaivi & Martin, 1989). The magnitude of this effect was comparable with that of diazepam. Other 5-HT_{1A} agonists such as ipsapirone (2.5–5 mg/kg) and indorenate (5–10 mg/kg) increased light-dark transitions, at doses that do not increase motor activity (Fernandez-Guasti & Lopez-Rubalcava, 1990). Furthermore, the non-specific serotonergic antagonists (e.g., pindolol, 2 mg/kg and alprenolol, 5 mg/kg) blocked the anxiolytic effect of ipsapirone and indorenate without affecting motor activity. Therefore, the light-dark exploratory test seems to be also sensitive to the anxiolytic effect of 5-HT_{1A} agonists.

Contrary to mice, rats are not useful in this model (Crawley, 1985). Their exploratory tendency appears to be considerably lower and no increases in scores on doses of diazepam from 0.05 to 2 mg/kg, with sedation at higher doses have been noted.

3.1.9 Social interaction

Several anxiolytic agents, including chlordiazepoxide, diazepam and flurazepam have been reported to antagonise the suppression of social interaction under unfamiliar, high-light conditions without producing concomitant changes in motor activity. In contrast, non-anxiolytics such as the neuroleptics (e.g., haloperidol and thioridazine) and stimulants such as amphetamine did not induce these selective effects on social interaction (File & Hyde, 1979). In a modified social interaction test version, flumazenil completely reversed the social anxiolytic effect of chlordiazepoxide while having no effect when administered on its own (Bold et al., 1985). These results indicate that the BDZ receptor complex mediates the anxiolytic and the anxiogenic effects of drugs on rodent social behaviour.

5-HT_{1A} agonists produce effects comparable with those of BDZs. Using acute administration, it was shown that buspirone (5–10 mg/kg) and gepirone (5–10 mg/kg) produced significant increases in social interaction, although buspirone also reduced motor activity (Dunn et al., 1989). Thus this test is sensitive to both BDZs and 5-HT_{1A} agonists.

However, this model raises some complex issues that need clarification. It is not known whether the drugs active in this model affect the emission or the reception of social cues, particularly as either two drugged or two non-drugged rats are always tested together. This procedure represents a serious methodological drawback. In addition, several laboratories have found it difficult to use because of the large variability of responses. It also seems that this test may not be valid for female rats, which also respond less than male rats to changes in familiarity of the test arena (Johnston and File, 1991). Nevertheless, further validation and exploration of this model may help to clarify and consolidate its status as a reliable model of anxiety.

3.1.10 Ultrasonic distress vocalisation

Rat pups separated from their mother and littermates emit high-frequency (30–50 kHz) distress calls, which in turn elicit retrieval behaviour from the mother (Noirot, 1972). An anxiolytic effect in this model is indicated by a significant decrease in high-frequency vocalisation in the absence of sedation (Engel et al., 1987). Chlordiazepoxide and diazepam inhibited ultrasonic vocalisation in rat pups at doses that did not generally disrupt behaviour, whereas muscimol, chlorpromazine, yohimbine, morphine, amphetamine, amitriptyline, haloperidol, naloxone and clonidine did not selectively suppress vocalisation (Gardner et al, 1985a, b). However, meprobamate was found to be a false negative and amitriptyline a false positive (Benton & Nastiti, 1988). Therefore, this test appears to be only partially selective and its predictive validity is rather weak.

3.1.11 A primate model

A primate model should, in principle, be more relevant clinically. Intense anxiety in patients and normal volunteers has been reported with non-convulsant doses of pentylenetetrazol (PTZ) (Rodin & Calhoun, 1970). The effects of non-convulsant doses of PTZ in rhesus monkeys living together in a social colony was also shown to produce anxiogenic effects (Palit et al., 1998). The animals exhibited hypervigilance, aggressiveness, tachypnea, piloerection and frequent change of posture and also had raised cortisol levels. These physiological and behavioural effects were antagonised by BDZs such as diazepam (1 mg/kg, i.v.) and alprazolam (0.05 mg/kg, p.o.). However, although buspirone (10 mg/kg, p.o.) blocked the behavioural effects, it did not antagonise the rise in plasma cortisol concentration. It was suggested that since PTZ induces an anxiety syndrome in the rhesus monkey which is specifically blocked by anxiolytic drugs, this model may be useful in evaluation of newer anxiolytic agents as well as in conducting studies to understand the basic mechanisms involved in the clinical manifestation of anxiety.

However a primate model of anxiety may also be problematic. It is expensive and there is no convincing evidence that monkey models are superior to rodent models in quality of data. Although the complexity of primate behaviour presents unique opportunities for modelling psychopathology, it may be disadvantageous in the practical screening of new compounds for potential psychotherapeutic action (Howard and Pollard, 1983).

3.2 Panic disorder

3.2.1 Periaqueductal gray model

In the dorsolateral periaqueductal gray (dPAG, a key area for initiating the various components of fear-induced defensive behaviour) model of panic anxiety, local stimulation is applied to the dPAG neurons. This procedure elicits intense emotional and behavioural responses reflected in animals by abrupt escape and flight reactions accompanied by characteristic anxiety autonomic changes. In particular, the local microinjection of low doses of kainic acid to excite PAG neurons elicits an alert posture (freezing and rearing), forward or backward motion, analgesia and ultrasonic vocalisations similar to those observed in rats facing an enemy. Some of these behaviours resemble, at least in part, those associated with a panic attack. They indicate that an appropriate model of PD should also consider involvement of the PAG. Indeed, direct electrical stimulation of the PAG in humans has been reported to induce very unpleasant and fearful sensations as well as physical signs of autonomic activation which are reminiscent of the symptom profile of a panic attack (Bandler, 1988). Acute systemic administration of flesinoxan enhanced the sensitivity of rats to the panic-like aversion elicited by local stimulation of the dPAG. Drugs acutely reducing (e.g. clonazepam, alprazolam) or precipitating (caffeine, yohimbine) panic attacks in patients were found to acutely and dose-dependently reduce or enhance, respectively, the aversion induced by dPAG stimulation in rats (Jenck et al., 1995). Therefore, this experimental paradigm in rats has been validated as realistically simulating several aspects of panic anxiety with objective signs of symptomatic and predictive validity using established antipanic and panicogenic drugs (Jenck et al., 1995).

This model appears to have reasonable face validity. In a remarkable analogy, the self-interruption behaviour in rats has a direct counterpart in humans since dPAG neurostimulation in man induces acute anxiety feelings such that a stimulated subject would generally not allow further stimulation and would probably interrupt if given the possibility (Nashold et al., 1969). Experimental use of clonazepam or alprazolam to alleviate discomfort in, for example, chronic pain patients stimulated in the dPAG has not been reported. However, there seems to be a good degree of pharmacological homology between the acute effects of clonazepam, alprazolam, yohimbine and caffeine in rats and their short-term effects in panic patients. However, the pharmacological specificity of this response is dependent upon the region of the dPAG stimulated, and does not always match the known pharmacotherapy of human PD (Griebel et al., 1996). Studies on the use of the dPAG stimulation model in mice appear to be lacking.

As for construct validity, previous positive conclusions on face and predictive validity suggest that dPAG neurostimulation in man and in rats as well as panic attacks in man may share in the dPAG or at other brain sites some similar brain mechanisms. PAG is a brain location involved in the response to stress and is the influence of higher centres in the limbic system including the amygdala. Emotional and vegetative symptoms of panic have been induced by stimulation of the amygdala and the hippocampal gyrus in man (Gloor et al., 1982). There are some reasons to suggest that aversive dPAG stimulation-induced aversion in animals adequately simulates at least some aspects of human PD.

3.2.2 The mouse defence test battery

Defensive behaviours constitute the reactions of animals to the host of life-threatening dangers encountered in every natural environment, i.e. predators and threatening features of the environment (Blanchard et al., 1993). Among these, flight/avoidance and defensive threat/attack responses were predominant (Griebel et al., 1995). The MDTB which permits to assess the mouse flight responses is suggested to have a face validity as a model of panic attack. This view is supported by clinical observations that PD patients often report intense desire to flee or escape from the place where the panic attack is occurring. However, the fact that the stimulus is hand held in this paradigm introduces the possibility of unconscious experimenter biases. Pharmacological assessment of the MDTB has shown that panic-modulating compounds specifically affect animals' flight responses with panicogenic treatment increasing flight and panicolytic medication challenge decreasing it (see Tab. 9.6).

Evaluation of the construct validity of the MDTB as of any other model of psychopathology is a complex issue involving the extent to which neurobehavioral defence systems are conservative and represented in much the same form across mammals. However, the MDTB appears to possess predictive and face validity. It underscores the potential usefulness of using flight responses for assessing certain aspects of anxiety, such as PD.

3.2.3 Other new behavioural models

Another new mouse model called conditioned fear stress (CFS) has also been proposed (Kamei et al., 1999). Mice exhibit a marked suppression of motility when they are replaced in the same environment in which they had previously received an electric footshock. This motor suppression may be considered as a conditioned emotional response to the environment associated with previous footshock and considered as CFS. The motor suppression in CFS is attenuated by sigma receptor agonists such as (+)-N-allylnormetazocine and dextromethorphan, whereas anxiolytics such as diazepam, chlordiazepoxide and antidepressants such as imipramine and fluoxetine are ineffective. This model may be useful for the investigation of the pathogenesis of affective disorders, particularly those considered to be treatment resistant, and for the development of novel effective pharmacological products.

The study of social emotional reactivity in the mouse was suggested as a highly relevant procedure to study the neurobiology of anxiety (Gendreau et al., 1998). In this study, it was observed that lower doses of quinpirole, a dopamine D_2-like receptor agonist, increased stationary forms of reactivity (i.e., startle, kicking, defensive posture, vocalisation) in a more pronounced manner in A/J mice reared in isolation as compared to A/J mice reared in groups. It was therefore suggested that social con-

Table 9.6: Effects of various psychoactive drugs on the flight/avoidance responses in the mouse defence test battery with their effect on panic attacks. ↑ Indicates an increase in the response; ↓ indicates a decrease in the response; (↓) indicates a decrease at motor-impairing doses only; O ineffective; BZPR: benzodiazepine receptor

Drug class	Drugs	Panic	Flight	References
BZPR full agonist	Chlordiazepoxide	(↓)	(↓)	Griebel et al., 1996
	Alprazolam (acute)	(↓)	(↓)	Griebel et al., 1996
	Alprazolam (chronic)	↓	↓	Griebel et al., 1996
BZPR antagonist	Flumazenil	↑	↑	Griebel et al., 1996
5-HT_{1A} partial agonist	Gepirone	↓/O	O	Griebel et al., 1996
Tricyclic antidepressant	Imipramine (acute)	↑	↑	
	Imipramine (chronic)	↓	↓	Griebel et al., 1996
SSRI	Fluoxetine (acute)	↑	↑	Griebel et al., 1996
	Fluoxetine (chronic)	↓	↓	Griebel et al., 1996
α_2 antagonist	Yohimbine	↑	↑	Griebel et al., 1996

texts or paradigms might be particularly useful for the investigation of drug effects on specific behavioural patterns with fear or anxiety.

3.3 Generalised anxiety disorder

Most strains of mice exhibit a preference for the novel area whereas BALB/c mice display neophobia, suggesting that this strain may be a good model for testing trait anxiety-releasing compounds (Beuzen & Belzung, 1995). Because of its chronicity, the neophobia exhibited by BALB/c mice in free exploratory paradigm may model generalised anxiety (Belzung & Berton, 1997). In a study designed to extend the testing of established and putative anxiolytics in the BALB/c mouse model, it was shown that BDZ receptor full and partial agonists, meprobamate, ethanol and NMDA antagonists are able to abolish the BALB/c neophobia (Belzung & Berton, 1997). However, drugs like BDZ receptor-selective compounds, barbiturates, 5-HT products (5-HT_{1A} agonists, 5-HT_2 and 5-HT_3 antagonists), α_2 adrenoceptor antagonists, D_2 antagonists and CCK_B antagonists are ineffective.

3.4 Obsessive-compulsive disorder

At present, there is no adequate animal model of OCD. However, a number of behavioural phenomena observed in animals might be of relevance to OCD (Insel, 1988). Some of the stereotyped behaviour exhibited by animals can give the impression that the animals are engaged in compulsive acts. Such stereotypes can be observed in nonhuman primates, particularly those that have been reared in isolation (Meyer-Holzapfel, 1968).

Recently, a novel transgenic mouse model exhibiting OCD behaviour such as biting, movement and behavioural perseverance abnormalities was created (Campbell, 1999). The abnormal behaviour expressed by these mice (D1CT mice) is caused by expression of a neuro-potentiating cholera toxin transgene in dopamine D1 receptor-expressing (D1+) neurons within the amygdalar intercalated nucleus and within cortical areas that project to orbitofrontal cortex and striatum. Therefore, based upon the parallel CNS changes in OCD and D1CT transgenic mice, and the frequent correlation of anxiety with compulsions in OCD, it has been suggested that the D1CT mice might exhibit increased basal anxiety-like behaviour associated with their OCD-like behavioural disorder.

3.5 Posttraumatic stress disorder

No animal model has yet been proposed specifically for PTSD although several lines of investigation may be of use in the search for such a model. The behavioural changes following exposure to inescapable shock have been the subject of much research and alterations in behaviour have also been found following a single exposure to a pharmacological stressor (Drugan et al., 1985). While much of this work has been discussed in terms of depression, it may have some relevance to PTSD. Therefore, there is a need to assess the effects and relevance of long-term changes produced by severe stressors in animals to PTSD and its pharmacological treatments.

3.6 Effects of antidepressants in the models

In particular clinical studies have shown that some antidepressants, either tricyclics, MAOIs or SSRIs may be more efficient than BDZs to alleviate anxiety associated with PD (Copland et al., 1992; Lydiard & Ballenger, 1987). In GAD, on chronic treatment, imipramine can be more effective than BDZs (Kahn et al., 1986). However, in animal procedures used in the study of anxiety and anxiolytics, the effects of antidepressants are not unequivocal. This is probably due to several factors, among which is the fact that these experimental approaches were developed and optimised primarily for evaluating BDZs and were further validated by their sensitivity to this class of compounds. On acute injection, antidepressants failed to induce anxiolytic effects in various procedures such as the two-compartment test, the elevated plus-maze, and the potentiated startle reflex (Cassella & Davis, 1985; Cole & Rodgers, 1995; Costall et al., 1989; File & Johnston, 1987). On chronic administration, antidepressants have been shown to exert anxiolytic-like effects in some studies. For instance, chronic treatment with antidepressants induced a release of behavioural blockade in procedures such as the conditioned suppression of drinking (Fontana et al. 1989; Fontana & Commissaris, 1988). However, negative results have been reported in the EPM (3 weeks), the fear-enhanced acoustic startle (3 weeks) and the conditioned suppression of drinking task (at least 8 weeks) (Cassella & Davis, 1985; Commissaris et al., 1990; File & Johnston, 1987). Therefore, an anxiolytic-like effect cannot be induced by all antidepressants on chronic injection, and/or not all relevant animal procedures allow the demonstration of such a property.

4 Human models

A rational way to test potential anxiolytics in humans is the use of a laboratory procedure that elicits clinically relevant anxiety symptoms in normal volunteers for the initial screening evaluation of anxiolytic drugs. The induction of higher-state anxiety levels can be elicited by laboratory procedures (e.g. simulated public speaking, real life situations like dental surgery and drug administration, for example caffeine) (Pillard & Fisher, 1978). Such approaches have some advantages as the volunteers can be easily recruited, leading to a rapid execution of the study. Other advantages include greater control and homogeneity of induced anxiety, more "pure" anxiety symptoms and a clearer profile of drug side-effects (McNair et al., 1982). Mental test procedures (e.g. Stroop colour-word test) and simulated public speaking are the most frequently experimentally-induced procedures used. In a study using situational anxiety (psychological state of patients awaiting cardiovascular examination or surgery), it was shown that drugs such as alpidem (50 and 75 mg) may induce anxiolytic effects in normal volunteers (Regnier et al., 1989).

4.1 Some models of anxiety

4.1.1 The video-recorded Stroop colour word test

A recent study which assessed the utility of the Stroop colour word test (SCVT; this test consists of submitting the volunteers to a cognitive conflicting condition in which they have to nominate the colour of a coloured word that denotes a different colour) shows that it is an effective anxiety-provoking test that can detect the effect of standard anxiolytic drugs (Stroop, 1935; Leite et al., 1999). In this study, the public simulation with a video camera was effective in raising the anxiety state of normal volunteers. This increase in anxiety was prevented by oral administration of 5 mg diazepam but not by placebo. Therefore video-SCVT may be a useful and sensible method to study potential anxiolytic drugs in normal volunteers.

4.1.2 Fear potentiated startle

Recently, a human equivalent of the "fear-potentiated startle response" paradigm has been described (Grillon et al., 1991). It has been shown that a light signal associated with the "threat" of an electric shock increases the amplitude and shortens the latency of the eye-blink response evoked by an abrupt loud white noise in human volunteers. As the effect of threat on the acoustic startle response is susceptible to both anxiogenic (e.g. yohimbine) and anxiolytic drugs (e.g. alcohol), it was proposed that the fear-potentiated acoustic startle response could be used as a laboratory model of human anxiety (Morgan et al., 1993; Grillon et al., 1994, Davis et al., 1993). A study in 12 healthy volunteers which examined whether the amplitude of the pupillary light reflex can be modified by the threat of an electric shock, using the study design of Grillon et al., showed that the anticipation of an electric shock can modify not only the startle reflex response but also the pupillary light reflex (Bitsios et al., 1996). It was argued that the inhibition of the light reflex by threat may be a suitable laboratory model of human anticipatory anxiety.

4.2 Generalised anxiety disorder

At the centre of GAD appears to be the experience of uncontrollability and distressing worry. A cognitive model of GAD has recently been advanced describing the processes involved in the development and maintenance of the psychopathology (Wells, 1995). In this model, GAD results from the usage of worrying as a coping strategy and subsequent negative evaluation of worrying. The use of worry as a strategy is supported by positive metabeliefs concerning worry, whereas the negative appraisal of worrying (worry about worry) is linked to negative metabeliefs developed out of previous experience. These beliefs centre on the themes of uncontrollability of worries and the dangerous consequences of worrying. The model presents new implications for a cognitive therapy of GAD and these are illustrated with a single case treatment study. A recent study in volunteers to test this model shows that a series of regression analyses support the hypothesis that pathological and problematic worry is directly associated with type 2 (meta-worry) rather than type 1 worry (Wells & Carter, 1999). Unfortunately, no confirmation with pharmacological intervention is described to support the model.

4.3 Panic disorder

Sodium lactate infusion is the most extensively studied laboratory method of provoking panic. Sodium lactate-induced panic has been shown to be specific to patients with a history of spontaneous panic attacks (Gorman et al., 1985; Cowley et al., 1986; Lindy et al., 1988). It provokes panic that closely resembles naturally occurring panic and may be blocked by all drugs that are known to block clinical attacks (i.e. tricyclics, MAOIs and alprazolam) (Gorman et al., 1985; Rifkin et al., 1981; Liebowitz et al., 1986).

5 Issues relevant to some non-benzodiazepine anxiolytics

5.1 5-HT receptors

The opposite and inconsistent pattern of results observed with 5-HT_{1A} receptor full agonists in different animal models or patient populations suggests that the 5-HT_{1A} receptor subtype exerts a complex control over different types of anxiety (Treit et al.,

1993). This is in accordance with the hypothesis on the complex dual action of 5-HT on the neural mechanism of anxiety where 5-HT is suggested to either facilitate or inhibit different kinds of fear *via* different receptor subtypes located in different brain regions (Deakin & Graeff, 1991). Furthermore, there is important evidence for a role of gender and pre-test stress exposure in the sensitivity of animals to 5-HT_{1A} receptor agonists (Blanchard et al., 1992; McBlane and Handley, 1994). Important species and anxiety paradigm differences, particularly for the action of 5-HT_{1A} drugs, have been addressed (Barrett et al., 1986; Broekkamp et al., 1989; Fernandez-Guasti et al., 1992). It has been shown that buspirone exhibits anxiolytic action in rats, but not in mice and hamsters (Fernandez-Guasti et al., 1992; Fernandez-Guasti & Lopez-Rubalcava, 1995). Moreover, it seems that in the anxiolytic action of these 5-HT_{1A} agonists, the noradrenergic system is involved in rats, but not in mice (Lopez-Rubalcava & Fernandez-Guasti, 1994). In relation to the differences in the anxiety paradigms, several investigators have reported anxiolysis, no effect, and even anxiogenic activity of the 5-HT_{1A} compounds, depending upon the animal model of anxiety used (Davis et al., 1988; Fernandez-Guasti & Hong, 1989; Meert & Colpaert, 1986). Thus, many variables such as route of administration, dosage, animal strain, ethnic origin, responder or non-responder, age or rating scale presumably contribute to the variability in responses to 5-HT_{1A} receptor agonists in preclinical or clinical studies.

5.2 Cholecystokinin receptors

There is now clinical evidence that systemic administration of CCK_B elicits panic-like symptoms in healthy volunteers, and potentiates the occurrence of panic attacks in PD patients (Van Megen et al., 1996). In recent years, specific and highly potent antagonists for CCK receptors have been discovered and developed (Woodruff & Hughes, 1991). However, the study of CCK receptor antagonists in animal models of anxiety suggests that classical animal models of anxiety may not be suitable for evaluation of the behavioural effects of CCK receptor antagonists, whereas tests which may model certain aspects of human panic such the MDTB appear to be more reliable tools when screening such products (Griebel et al., 1997a). In fact, in this study, whereas CCK_A (lorglumide) and CCK_B (PD 135,158 and LY 288513) antagonists were inactive in all tests, the CCK_B antagonists significantly decreased avoidance distance when the rat was first placed in the test apparatus, an effect which may be consistent with an anti-panic-like action. However, a recent placebo-controlled trial of L-365,260 (a CCK_B receptor antagonist) on naturally occurring panic attacks failed to show clinically significant differences between drug treatment and placebo (Kramer et al., 1995).

6 Discussion

Considering biological models, studies in transgenic and gene knockout mice have already produced some significant insights into the neural mechanisms underlying anxiety. Evidence that mice with either loss-of-function or gain-of-function mutations in a specific gene exhibit significant modifications in anxiety-related behaviour can have direct implications for the discovery of novel treatments for anxiety disorders. Hopefully in the next few years, this approach will be able to show its advantages in helping to bring rapidly to the market selective safe and effective anxiolytics.

Regarding currently used laboratory behavioural paradigms, no single model of animal anxiety unambiguously selects BDZs without a false positive or false negative. Nevertheless, several models such as the EPM and potentiated startle have proved highly selective for a range of compounds. They have also been shown to respond to non-BDZ anxiolytics, such as meprobamate, acting *via* the GABA-BDZ receptor. Another major issue is that research for new anxiolytics has produced a range of compounds acting on 5-HT neurotransmission, either as 5-HT_{1A} mixed agonist/antagonists, 5-HT_2 antagonists, or 5-HT_3 antagonists, whose potency in various animal models is totally absent or patchy (File, 1987). The problem becomes more serious if potent new anxiolytics are noted in the clinics but are wholly inactive in the animal screening models used. The fact that many human anxiety states and treatments are chronic, whilst the majority of studies using animal models are acute, brings another serious handicap to the validity of animal models. There are a number of unresolved conceptual issues regarding the nature of anxiety which make it difficult to develop and validate suitable animal models. Anxiety disorders are heterogeneous and many existing animal models do not clearly discriminate specific types of anxiety. The complexity of the clinical picture and lack of consensus amongst clinicians make it difficult to develop animal models for specific subtypes of anxiety disorders. Clearly, the assessment of a model is critically dependent on our knowledge of the phenomenon that is being modelled. Unfortunately, our knowledge of anxiety in humans is still rather limited. Many of the problems confronting the animal models stem from this incomplete understanding.

Animal models are often judged on their face validity, the similarity in phenomenology between the model and the human condition. In the models used, aetiology is reduced to aversive stimuli, symptoms become apparently simple behavioural responses and autonomic arousal. Although none of the currently available models exactly mimic the symptomatology of a specific anxiety disorder, these models do show a fair degree of face validity in that the aversive stimuli employed provoke fear in humans; these stimuli induce anxiety-associated behavioural and physiological modifications. Considering predictive validity, most models have been assessed on their ability to discriminate between drugs shown clinically to be anxiolytic or those that have no effect on anxiety. Nearly all these tests are sensitive to BDZ anxiolytics (see Tab. 9.7). Thus, the pharmacological approach to homology has been successful since anxiolytics such as BDZs reduce human anxiety and antagonise behavioural indices of fear in animal models. They act on a specific receptor in the brain found in humans and animals with comparable distributions. They probably represent a system whose behavioural functions must then be homologous in animals and humans (Nielsen et al., 1978). However, sensitivity of a model to BDZs does not necessarily imply that a paradigm measures anxiety. These tests may be assessing the side effects of the BDZs such as sedation and retrograde amnesia and are therefore less sensitive to changes in anxiety mediated by non-BDZ mechanisms. Conversely, a drug that has inconsistent or unreliable anxiolytic effects in humans cannot be used to validate an animal model. For example, the variation in the clinical efficacy of some 5-HT_{1A} agonists might account for some of the inconsistency of results concerning that class in some animal paradigms. Buspirone may be more effective in female than in male patients (Sheehan et al., 1988; 1990). It may not be more effective in patients with a previous history of BDZ treatment. Therefore, if anxious humans respond in a variable manner to some of the anxiolytics pertaining to this class, it is not surprising that the validation of animal models with these sort of drugs become even harder.

Tests that use exploratory drive may raise more problems in the assessment of anxiolytic effects. The difficulty of how to dissociate changes in anxiety from changes in exploratory drive is to some degree inherent in all exploration models, especially when the only parameters recorded from these tests are spontaneous locomotion behaviour. This issue becomes more crucial especially since prior test experience in these various models can alter behavioural baselines and attenuate or abolish the anxiolytic efficacy of anxiolytics (Holmes et al., 2001). However, the inclusion of risk assessment measures may increase the sensitivity of anxiety models. It also enables drug effects on anxiety to be dissociated from motor impairment. However, the methodological deficiencies inherent in principal component data analytic techniques of the risk-assessment behaviour of rodents in the anxiety tests should be carefully addressed so as to improve the model for meaningful data with an acceptable number of inclusion of indicator variables in the analysis (Wall & Messier, 2001). Ideally, anxiety should be assessed by behaviour that is performed only by anxious animals. This would normally remove ambiguity in interpretation.

Several of the behavioural tests used to detect anxiolytic activity fare quite well with regard to pharmacological validation of anxiolytic and anxiogenic drugs, but few have been able to detect an anxiolytic action of antidepressant drugs. Antidepressants are often effective in human clinical anxiety and it has been argued that anxiety and neurotic depression, while not identical, are overlapping syndromes (Gray, 1982). For example, desmethylimipramine, one of the most commonly used drugs in the treatment of depression, has been observed to decrease anxiety after chronic treatment in patients suffering from panic and generalised anxiety (Nutt & Glue, 1991; Lydiard et al., 1995). As the human clinical picture accepts overlapping syndromes and antidepressant therapy for anxiety states, animal modelling should also accept that a perfect distinction between models of anxiety and models of depression may be neither possible nor desirable. Interestingly, the anxiolytic-like effect of desmethylimipramine is observed in several animal models (e.g. ultrasonic vocalisations, exploration in the EPM and defensive burying tests) after chronic, but not acute, administration (Molewijk et al., 1996; Laino et al., 1993; Fernandez-Guasti et al., 1999). On the other hand, buspirone and the antidepressants are inactive after acute treatment in clinical studies in patients.

Whether it is possible to reproduce in animals any form of anxiety that is observed in humans is questionable. Cultural factors appear to play a role in the

Table 9.7: Comparative effects of established and putative anxiolytics in some animal models of anxiety. ++, Anxiolytic-like effect; +, anxiolytic-like effect or no effect; –, anxiogenic effect; 0, no effect; Antid. = antidepressant.

Animal model	BDZ-receptor agonist	5-HT_{1A} agonist	$5\text{-HT}_{2A/2C}$ antagonists	5-HT_3 antagonists	CCK_B antagonists	Antid.
Conflict models	++	0/+	+	0	+	0/–
Fear-potentiated	++	+		+		
dPAG	++	–		0		
Conditioned ultrasonic vocalisation	0/+	++	+	0		
Defensive burying	++	++	0	0	++	0
Ultrasonic pup vocalisation	++	++		0		
Defensive analgesia	++	++		+		
Elevated plus-maze	++	0/–	+	+/0	+	+
Social interaction	++	+/0	+	+/0		
Light-dark transition	++	+/0	+	++		–
Stress-induced hyperthermia	++	++		0		

human response to anxiety-provoking situations (Tan, 1988). In rodents, females appear less anxious than males in a number of models of anxiety whereas in humans women with anxiety disorders are encountered somewhat more frequently in the clinic than men (Showalter, 1985). All models used to date have limitations and no single paradigm adequately models all aspects of human anxiety. Therefore, a range of different approaches should be used in the assessment of potential new anxiolytics. As none of the animal models offers an absolute guarantee of the predictive value of anxiolytic in humans, there is an urgent need for new animal models for exploring chronic (trait) rather than acute (state) anxiety. The new models should, of course, be evaluated for their predictive validity in terms of sensitivity and specificity to anxiolytic and anxiogenic drugs.

Most patients requiring drug treatment for anxiety are those with a high trait anxiety due to adverse events. However, all animal tests are based on conditions that generate changes in state anxiety. Only when specific strains of rodents have been screened in animal tests of anxiety shall we know whether these strains could provide an animal analogue of differences in trait anxiety. Therefore, the genetic mouse model offers the promise of a genetic model of the anxiety-predisposed human, which may be useful in improving drug discovery. Rather than examining the effects of novel anxiolytics on normal rats, one may examine genetic models in the hope of finding new drugs selective for pathological anxiety. Transgenic mice are proving to be useful models for exploration of the pathogenesis of anxiety. The coming models adopting this technological approach may prove more fruitful in bringing novel effective anxiolytics to the clinics.

Given these various difficulties at both clinical and preclinical levels, it can be concluded that animal models of anxiety may well be able to help clarify some of these human issues. As shown by a factor analysis of animal tests of anxiety, it could also be that different tests are measuring a different state of anxiety in the rodents (File, 1987). Nevertheless, it is evident that a major criterion for judging the validity of animal models of anxiety lies in their responsiveness to chronic drug treatment known to be therapeutically effective. In addition, the utility of such models depends on their ability to predict the therapeutic activity of novel compounds undergoing development.

References

Ashcroft GW, Walker LG & Lyle A. A psychobiological model for panic: including models for the mechanisms involved in the regulation of mood and anxiety and implications for behavioural and pharmacological therapies. In: BE Leonard, J Butler, D O' Rourke & TJ Fahy (eds): Psychopharmacology of panic. Oxford: Oxford University Press, 131–143, 1993

Bale TL, Contarino A, Smith GW, Chan R, Gold LH, Sawchenko PE, Koob GF, Vale WW & Lee KF. Mice deficient for corticotropin-releasing hormone receptor-2 display anxiety-like behaviour and are hypersensitive to stress. Nat Genet 24, 410–414, 2000

Bandler R. Mechanism of aggression as reveladed by electrical and chemical stimulation. Suggestion of a central role for midbrain periaqueductal grey region. In: A Epstein & A Morrison (eds): Progress in psychobiology and physiological psychology, Academic Press, 67–154, 1988

Barrett JE, Witkin JM, Mansbach RS, Skolnick P & Weissman BA. Behavioral studies with anxiolytic drugs. III. Antipunishment action of buspirone in the pigeon do not involve benzodiazepine receptor mechanisms? J Pharmacol Exp Ther 238, 1009–1013, 1986

Belzung C & Berton F. Further pharmacological validation of the BALB/C neophobia in the free exploratory paradigm as an animal model of trait anxiety. Behav Pharmacol 8, 541–548, 1997

Belzung C, Misslin R, Vogel E, Dodd RH & Chapouthier G. Anxiogenic effects of methyl-β-carboline-3-carboxylate in a light/dark choice situation. Pharmacol Biochem Behav 28, 29–33, 1987

Benton D & Nastiti K. The influence of psychotropic drugs on the ultrasonic calling of mouse pups. Psychopharmacology 95, 99, 1988

Beuzen A & Belzung C. Link between emotional memory and anxiety states: a study by principal component analysis. Physiol Behav 58, 111–118, 1995

Bitsios P, Szabadi E & Bradshaw CM. The inhibition of the pupillary light reflex by the threat of an electric shock: a potential laboratory model of human anxiety. J Psychopharmacol 10 (4), 279–287, 1996

Blampied NM & Kirk RC. Defensive burying: Effects of diazepam and oxprenolol measured in extinction. Life Sci 33, 695, 1983
Blanchard RJ, Rodgers RJ & Weiss SM. The characterization and modeling of antipredator defensive behavior. Neurosci Biobehavior Rev 14, 463–472, 1990
Blanchard DC, Shepherd JK, Rodgers RJ & Blanchard RJ. Evidence for differential effects of 8-OH-DPAT on male and female rats in the anxiety/defense test battery. Psychopharmacology 106, 531–539, 1992
Blanchard DC, Blanchard RJ & Rodgers RJ. Risk assessment and animal models of anxiety. In: B Olivier, J Mos, JL Slangen (eds): Animal models in psychopharmacology. Basle: Birkhäuser Verlag, 117–134, 1991
Blanchard RJ, Yudko EB, Rodgers RJ & Blanchard DC. Defense system psychopharmacology: An ethological approach to the pharmacology of fear and anxiety. Behav Brain Res 58, 155–165, 1993
Blumstein LK & Crawley JN. Further characterization of a simple, automated exploratory model for the anxiolytic effects of benzodiazepines. Pharmacol Biochem Behav 18, 37–40, 1983
Boissier JR & Simon P. Dissociation de deux composantes dans le comportement d'investigation de la souris. Arch Int Pharmacodyn 147, 372–387, 1964
Bold JM, Gardner CR & Walker RJ. Central effects of nicotinamide and inosine which are not mediated through benzodiazepine receptors. Br J Pharmacol 84, 689, 1985
Borsini F, Lecci A, Volterra G & Meli A. A model to measure anticipatory anxiety in mice? Psychopharmacology 98, 207, 1989
Boissier JR & Simon P. Dissociation de deux composantes dans le comportement d'investigation de la souris. Arch Int Pharmacodyn Thér, 147, 372–387, 1964
Brambilla F, Perna G, Bussi R & Bellodi L. Dopamine function in obsessive compulsive disorder: cortisol response to acute apomorphine stimulation. Psychoneuroendocrinology 25, 301–310, 2000
Briese E & Cabanac M. Stress hyperthermia: physiological arguments that it is a fever. Physiol Behav 48, 1153, 1991
Broekkamp CLE, Berendsen HHG, Jenck F & Van Delft AML. Animal models for anxiety and response to serotonergic drugs. Psychopathology 22 (Suppl 1), 2–12, 1989
Brown JS, Kalish HI & Farber IE. Conditioned fear as revealed by magnitude of startle response to auditory stimulus. J Exp Psychol 41, 317–328, 1951
Campbell KM, de Lecea L, Severynse DM, Caron MG, McGrath MJ, Sparber SB, Sun LY & Burton FH. OCD-like behaviors caused by a neuropotentiating transgene targeted to cortical and limbic D1+ neurons. J Neurosci 19 (12), 5044–5053, 1999
Carey GJ, Costall B, Domeney AM, Jones DN & Naylor RJ. Behavioural effects of anxiogenic agents in the common marmoset. Pharmacol Biochem Behav 42, 143–153, 1992
Cassella JV & Davis M. Fear-enhanced acoustic startle is not attenuated by acute or chronic imipramine treatment in rats. Psychopharmacology 87, 278–282, 1985
Chopin P & Briley M. Animal models of anxiety: The effect of compounds that modify 5-HT neurotransmission. Trends Pharmacol Sci, 8, 383–388, 1987
Cole J & Rodgers R. Ethological comparison of the effects of diazepam and acute/chronic

imipramine on the behaviour of mice in the elevated plus-maze. Pharmacol Biochem Behav 52, 473–478, 1995
Colombo G, Agabio R, Lobina C, Reali R, Zocchi A, Fadda F & Gessa GL. Sardinian alcohol-preferring rats: A genetic animal model of anxiety. Physiol Behav. 57 (6), 1181–1185, 1995
Commissaris R, Ellis D, Hill T, Schefke D, Becker C & Fontana D. Chronic antidepressant and clonidine treatment effects on conflict behavior in the rat. Pharmacol Biochem Behav 37, 167–176, 1990
Contarino A, Dellu F, Koob GF, Smith GW, Lee KF, Vale W & Gold LH. Reduced anxiety-like and cognitive performance in mice lacking the corticotropin-releasing factor receptor 1. Brain Res 835, 1–9, 1999
Copland J, Gorman J & Klein D. Serotonin related function in panic-anxiety. A critical overview. Neuropharmacology 6: 189–200, 1992
Costall B, Jones BJ, Kelly ME, Naylor RJ & Tomkins DM. Exploration of mice in a black and white test box: Validation as a model of anxiety. Pharmacol Biochem Behav 32, 777, 1989
Cowley DS, Dager SR & Dunner DL. Lactate-induced panic in primary affective disorder. Am J Psychiatry 143, 646–648, 1986
Crawley JN, Skolnick P & Paul SM. Absence of intrinsic antagonist actions of benzodiazepine antagonists on an exploratory model of anxiety in the mouse. Neuropharmacology 23, 531, 1984
Crawley JN & Goodwin FK. Preliminary report of a simple animal behavior model for the anxiolytic effects of benzodiazepines. Pharmacol Biochem Behav 13, 167–170, 1980
Crawley JN. Exploratory behavior models of anxiety in mice. Neurosci Biobehav Rev 9 (1), 37–44, 1985
Crawley JN. Neuropharmacologic specificity of a simple animal model for the behavioral actions of benzodiazepines. Pharmacol Biochem Behav 15, 695–699, 1981
Crestani F, Loez M, Baer K, Essrich V, Benke D, Laurent JP, Belzung C, Fristchy J-M, Luscher B & Mohler H. Decreased $GABA_A$-receptor clustering results in enhanced anxiety and a bias for threat cues. Nature Neurosci 2, 833–839, 1999
Davis M, Redmond DE Jr & Baraban JM. Noradrenergic agonists and antagonists: effects on conditioned fear as measured by the potentiated startle paradigm. Psychopharmacology 65, 111–118, 1979
Davis M. The role of the amygdala in fear-potentiated startle: implications for animal models of anxiety. Trends Pharmacol Sci 13, 35–41, 1992
Davis M, Casella JV & Kehne JH. Serotonin does not mediate anxiolytic effects of buspirone in the fear-potentiated startle paradigm: Comparison with 8-OH-DPAT and ipsapirone. Psychopharmacology (Berlin) 94, 14–20, 1988
Davis M, Falls WA, Campeau S & Kim M. Fear-potentiated startle: a neural and pharmacological analysis. Behav Brain Res 58, 175–198, 1993
Deakin JWF & Graeff FG. 5HT and mechanisms of defence. J Psychopharmacol 5, 305–315, 1991
De Vry J, Benz U, Schreiber R & Traber J. Shock-induced ultrasonic vocalization in young adult rats: a model for testing putative anti-anxiety drugs. Eur J Pharmacol 249, 331–339, 1993

Drugan RC, Maier SF, Skolnick P, Paul SM & Crawley JN. An anxiogenic benzodiazepine receptor ligand induces learned helplessness. Eur J Pharmacol 113, 453–457, 1985

Dunn AJ & Berridge CW. Physiological and behavioral responses to corticotropin-releasing factor administration : is CRF a mediator of anxiety or stress responses ? Brain Res Rev 15, 71, 1990

Dunn RW, Corbett R & Fielding S. Effects of 5-HT1a receptor agonists and NMDA receptor antagonists in the social interaction test and the elevated plus-maze. Eur J Pharmacol 169, 1–10, 1989

Engel J, Hard E & Lindh AS. Effects of diazepam, ethanol and Ro- 15-1788 on ultrasonic vocalization, locomotor activity and body righting in the neonatal rat. Alcohol Alcoholism (Suppl) 1, 709, 1987

Fanselow MS & Helmstetter FJ. Conditional analgesia, defensive freezing, and benzodiazepines. Behav Neurosci 102, 233–243, 1988

Fernandez-Guasti A, Contreras CM, Martinez-Mota L, Estrada-Camarena E & Lopez-Rubalcava C. Chronic treatment with desipramine induces an estrous cycle dependent anxiolytic action in the burying behavior but not in the plus maze. Pharmacol Biochem Behav 63, 13–20, 1999

Fernandez-Guasti A, Hong E & Lopez-Rubalcava C. Species differences in the mechanism through which the serotonergic agonists indorenate and ipsapirone produce their anxiolytic action. Psychopharmacology (Berlin) 107, 61–68, 1992

Fernandez-Guasti A & Lopez-Rubalcava C. Action of ipsapirone and 8-OHDPAT on exploratory behavior in hamsters (*Mesocricetus auratus*): Effects of antagonists and p-CPA. Pharmacol Biochem Behav 50, 375–382, 1995

Fernandez-Guasti & Lopez-Rubalcava. Evidence for the involvement of the 5-HT_{1A} receptor in the anxiolytic action of indorenate and ipsapirone. Psychopharmacology 101, 354, 1990

Fernandez-Guasti A & Lopez-Rubalcava C. Modification of the anxiolytic action of 5-HT1A compounds by GABA-benzodiazapine agents in rats. Pharmacol Biochem Behav 60 (1), 27–32, 1998

Fernandez-Guasti A & Hong E. Antianxiety effect of various putative S1 receptor agonists on the conditioned defensive-burying paradigm. In: P Evans, AR Archer & T Archer (eds): Behavioral pharmacology of 5-HT. Hillsdale. NJ: Lawrence Erlbaum, 377–382, 1989

File SE. Potentiation of the effects of chlorpromazine on exploration in the rat by prior experience. Psychopharmacologia 29, 357–363, 1973

File SE, Lister RG & Nutt DJ. Intrinsic actions of benzodiazepine antagonists. Neurosci Lett 32, 165–168, 1982

File SE. The validation of animal tests of anxiety – pharmacological implications. Pol J Pharmacol Phar 36, 505, 1984

File SE. Animal models for predicting clinical efficacy of anxiolytic drugs: Social behaviour. Neuropsychology 13, 55, 1985

File SE. The search for novel anxiolytics. Trends Neurosci 10, 461–463, 1987

File S & Johnston A. Chronic treatment with imipramine does not reverse the effects of 3 anxiogenic compounds in a test of anxiety in the rat. Neuropsychobiology 17, 187–192, 1987

File SE, Andrews N, Wu PY & Zangrossi H Jr. Modification of chlordiazepoxide's behavioural and neurochemical effects by handling and plus-maze experience. Eur J Pharmacol 218, 9–14, 1992

File SE & Hyde RG. A test of anxiety that distinguishes between the actions of benzodiazepines and those of other minor tranquilisers and stimulants. Pharmacol Biochem Behav 11, 65, 1979

File SE, Mabbutt PS & Hitchcott, PK. Characterisation of the phenomenon of "one-trial tolerance" to the anxiolytic effect of chlordiazepoxide in the elevated plus-maze. Psychopharmacology (Berlin) 110, 240–244, 1993

Fontana D, Carbary T & Commissaris R. Effects of acute and chronic anti-panic drug administration on conflict behavior in the rat. Psychopharmacology (Berlin) 98, 157–162, 1989

Fontana D & Commissaris R. Effects of acute and chronic imipramine administration on conflict behavior in the rat: A potential "animal model" for the study of panic disorder? Psychopharmacology (Berlin) 95, 147–150, 1988

Gardner CR. Inhibition of ultrasonic distress vocalizations in rat pups by chlordiazepoxide and diazepam. Drug Dev Res 5, 185–193, 1985a

Gardner CR. Distress vocalization in rat pups. A simple screening method for anxiolytic drugs. J Pharmacol Methods 14, 181, 1985b

Gendreau P, Petitto JM, Gariépy J-L & Lewis MH. D_2-like dopamine receptor mediation of social-emotional reactivity in a mouse model of anxiety: Strain and experience effects. Neuropsychopharmacology 18 (3), 210–221, 1998

Glenn B & Green S. Anxiolytic profile of GR 38032F in the potentiated startle paradigm. Behav Pharmacol 1, 91–94, 1989

Gloor P, Olivier A, Quesney LF, Andermann F & Horowitz S. The role of the limbic system in experiential phenomena of temporal lobe epilepsy. Ann Neurol 12 (2), 129–144, 1982

Gorman JM, Dillon D & Fyer AJ et al. The lactate infusion model. Psychopharmacol Bull, 21, 610–614, 1985

Graeff FG, Viana MB & Tomaz C. The elevated T maze, a new experimental model of anxiety and memory: effect of diazepam. Brazilian J Med Biol Res 26 (1), 67–70, 1993

Graeff FG, Netto CF & Zangrossi H Jr. The elevated T-maze as an experimental model of anxiety. Neurosci Biobehav Rev 23 (2), 237–246, 1998

Grailhe R, Waeber C, Dulawa SC, Hornung JP, Zhuang X, Brunner D, Geyer MA & Hen R. Increased exploratory activity and altered response to LSD in mice lacking the 5-HT (5A) receptor. Neuron 22, 581–591, 1999

Grant EW & Mackintosh JH. A comparison of the social postures of some common laboratory rodents. Behaviour 21, 246–259, 1963

Grewal SS, Shepherd JK, Bill DJ, Fletcher A & Dourish CT. Behavioural and pharmacological characterisation of the canopy stretched attend posture test as a model of anxiety in mice and rats. Psychopharmacology 133, 29–38, 1997

Griebel G, Blanchard DC, Jung A & Blanchard RJ. A model of "antipredator" defense in Swiss-Webster mice: effects of benzodiazepine receptor ligands with different intrinsic activities. Behav Pharmacol 6, 732–745, 1995

Griebel G, Blanchard DC & Blanchard RJ. Predator-elicited flight responses in Swiss-Webster an experimental model of panic attacks. Prog Neuropsychopharmacol Biol Psychiatry 20, 185–205, 1996

Griebel G, Sanger DJ & Perrault G. Genetic differences in the mouse defense test battery. Aggressive Behaviour 23, 19–31, 1997

Griebel G, Perrault Gh & Sanger DJ. CCK receptor antagonists in animal models of anxiety: comparison between exploration tests, conflict procedures and a model based on defensive behaviours. Behav Pharmacol 8, 549–560, 1997a

Grillon C, Ameli R, Foot M & Davis M. Fear-potentiated startle: relationship to the level of state/trait anxiety in healthy subjects. Biol Psychiatry 33, 566–574, 1993

Grillon C, Sinha R & O'Maley SS. Effects of ethanol on the acoustic startle reflex in humans. Psychopharmacology 114, 167–171, 1994

Grillon C, Ameli R, Woods SW, Mericangas K & Davis M. Fear-potentiated startle in humans: effects of anticipatory anxiety on the acoustic blink reflex. Psychophysiology 28, 588–595, 1991

Handley SL & McBlane JW. An assessment of the elevated X-maze for studying anxiety and anxiety-modulating drugs. J Pharmacol Toxicol Meth 29, 129–138, 1993

Handley SL & Mithani S. Effects of alpha-adrenoceptor agonists and antagonists in a maze exploration model of "fear"-motivated behaviour. Naunyn-Schmiedebergs Arch Pharmacol 327, 1–5, 1984

Handley SL & McBlane JW. 5-HT drugs in animal models of anxiety. Psychopharmacology (Berlin) 112, 13–20, 1993

Heinrichs SC, Min H, Tamraz S, Carmouche M, Boehme SA & Vale WW. Anti-sexual and anxiogenic behavioural consequences of corticotropin-releasing factor overexpression are centrally mediated. Psychoneuroendocrinology 22, 215–224, 1997

Heisler LK, Chu HM, Brennan TJ, Danao JA, Bajwa P, Parsons LH & Tecott LH. Elevated anxiety and antidepressant-like responses in serotonin 5-HT1A receptor mutant mice. Proc Natl Acad Sci USA 95, 15049–15054, 1998

Hodges H, Green S & Glenn B. Evidence that the amygdala is involved in benzodiazepine and serotonergic effects on punished responding but not on discrimination. Psychopharmacology 92, 491–504, 1987

Hogg S. A review of the validity and variability of the elevated plus-maze as an animal model of anxiety. Pharmacol Biochem Behav 54 (1), 21–30, 1996

Holmes A, Iles JP, Mayell SJ & Rodgers RJ. Prior test experience compromises the anxiolytic efficacy of chlordiazepoxide in the mouse light/dark exploration test. Behav Brain Res 122, 159–167, 2001

Homanics GE, Harrison NL, Quinlan JJ, Krasowski MD, Rick CE, de Blas AL, Mehta AK, Kist F, Mihalek RM, Aul JJ & Firestone LL. Normal electrophysiological and behavioural responses to ethanol in mice lacking the long splice variant of the gamma2 subunit of the gamma-aminobutyrate type A receptor. Neuropharmacology 38, 253–265, 1999

Howard JL & Pollard GT. Are primate models of neuropsychiatric disorders useful to the pharmaceutical industry? In: KA Miczek (ed): Ethopharmacology: primate models of neuropsychiatric disorders. New York: Alan Liss, 307–312, 1983

Howard JL, Ferris RM, Cooper BR, Soroko FE, Wang CM & Pollard GT. Models of depres-

sion used in the pharmaceutical industry. In: GF Koob, C Ehlers & D Kupfers (eds): Animal models of depression. Boston: Birkhäuser, 186–202, 1989
Insel TR. Obsessive-compulsive disorder: a neuroethological perspective. Psychopharmacol Bull 24, 365–369, 1988
Jardim MC, Nogueira RL, Graeff FG & Nunes-de-Souza RL. Evaluation of the elevated T-maze as an animal model of anxiety in the mouse. Brain Res Bull 48 (4), 407–411, 1999
Johnston AL & File SE. Sex differences in animal tests of anxiety. Physiol Behav 49, 245–250, 1991
Jenck F, Moreau JL & Martin JR. Dorsal periaqueductal gray-induced aversion as a simulation of panic anxiety: elements of face and predictive validity. Psychiatry Res 57, 181–191, 1995
Kaeserman HP. Stretched attend posture, a non-social form of ambivalence, is sensitive to a conflict-reducing drug action. Psychopharmacology 89, 31–37, 1986
Kahn R, McNair D, Lipman R, Covi L, Rickels K, Downing R, Fisher S & Frankenthaler L. Imipramine and chlordiazepoxide in depressive and anxiety disorders. 2. Efficacy in anxious outpatients. Arch Gen Psychiatry 43, 79–85, 1986
Kalin NH, Sherman JE & Takahashi LK. Antagonism of endogenous CRH systems attenuates stress-induced freezing behavior in rats. Brain Res 457, 130–135, 1988
Kamei H, Noda Y & Nabeshima T. The psychological stress model using motor suppression. Folia Pharmacol Jpn (Nippon Yakurigaku Zasshi) 113, 113–120, 1999
Kishimoto T, Radulovic J, Radulovic M, Lin CR, Schrick C, Hooshmand F, Hermanson O, Rosenfeld MG & Spiess J. Deletion of crhr2 reveals an anxiolytic role for corticotropin-releasing hormone receptor-2. Nat Genet 24, 415–419, 2000
Kramer MS, Cutler NR, Ballenger JC, Patterson WM, Mendels J, Chenault A, Shrivastava R, Matzurawolfe D, Lines C & Reines S. A placebo-controlled trial of L-365,260, a CCKB antagonist, in panic disorder. Biol Psychiatry 37, 462–466, 1995
Kuribara H. Effects of SUN 8399, a potent and selective 5-HT_{1A} agonist, on conflict behavior and ambulatory activity in mice: comparison with those of buspirone, tandospirone and diazepam. Jpn J Pharmacol 64, 273–280, 1994
Leite JR, Seabra MV, Sartori VA & Andreatini R. The video-recorded Stroop color-word test as a new model of experimentally-induced anxiety. Prog Neuropsychopharmacol Biol Psychiatry 23, 809–822, 1999
Liebowitz MR, Fyer AJ, Gorman JM et al. Alprazolam in the treatment of panic disorders. J Clin Psychopharmacol 6, 13–20, 1986
Liebsch G, Landgraf R, Gerstberger R, Probst JC, Wotjak CT, Engelmann M, Holsboer F & Montkowski A. Chronic infusion of a CRH1 receptor antisense oligodeoxynucleotide into the central nucleus of the amygdala reduced anxiety-related behavior in socially defeated rats. Regul Pept 59, 229–239, 1995
Lindy DC.,Walsh BT, Gorman JM, Roose SP, Gladis M, Devlin MJ & Glassman AH. Lactate infusions in patients with bulimia. Psychiatry Res 26 (3), 287–292, 1988
Lister RG. Partial reversal of ethanol-induced reductions in exploration by two benzodiazepine antagonists (flumazenil and ZK 93426). Brain Res Bull 21, 765–770, 1988
Lister RG. The effects of ethanol on exploration in DBA/2 and C57BL/6 mice. Alcohol 4, 17–19, 1987

Lister RG. The use of a plus-maze to measure anxiety in the mouse. Psychopharmacology 92, 180–185, 1987
Lister RG. Ethologically based animal models of anxiety disorders. Pharmacol Ther 46, 321–340, 1990
Lopez-Rubalcava C & Fernandez-Gusti A. Noradrenaline-serotonin interactions in the anxiolytic effects of 5-HT_{1A} agonists. Behav Pharmacol 5, 42–51, 1994
Lydiard R & Ballenger J. Antidepressants in panic disorder and agoraphobia. J Affect Disord 13, 153–168, 1987
Lucki I, Rickels K, Gieseke MA & Geller A. Differential effects of the anxiolytic drugs, diazepam and buspirone, on memory function. Br J Pharmacol, 23, 207–211, 1987
Lydiard RB, Morton WA, Emmanuel NP, Zealberg JJ, Laraia MT, Stuart GW, O'Neil PM & Ballenger JC. Preliminary report: placebo-controlled, double-blind study of the clinical and metabolic effects of desipramine in panic disorder. Psychopharmacol Bull 29, 183–188, 1995
Mansbach RS & Geyer MA. Blockade of potentiated startle responding in rats by 5-hydroxytryptamine 1a receptor ligands. Eur J Pharmacol 156, 375–383, 1988
Marazziti DA, Di Muro A & Castrogiovanni P. Psychological stress and body temperature changes in humans. Physiol Behav 52, 393, 1992
McBlane JW & Handley SL. Effects of two stressors on behavior in the elevated X-maze: preliminary investigation of their interaction with 8-OH-DPAT. Psychopharmacology 116, 173–182, 1994
McNair DM, Frankenthaler LM, Czerlinsky T, White TW, Sasson S & Fisher S. Simulated public speaking as a model of clinical anxiety. Psychopharmacology 77, 7–10, 1982
McNaughton N. Cognitive dysfunction resulting from hippocampal hyperactivity – a possible cause of anxiety disorder? Pharmacol Biochem Behav 56, 603–611, 1997
Meyer-Holzapfel M. Abnormal behavior in zoo animals. Abnormal behavior in animal. Philadelphia: WB Saunders, 476–503, 1968
Mihalek RM, Banerjee PK, Korpi ER, Quinlan JJ, Firestone LL, Mi ZP, Lagenaur C, Tretter V, Sieghart W, Anagnostaras SG et al. Attenuated sensitivity to neuroactive steroids in gamma-aminobutyrate type A receptor delta subunit knockout mice. Proc Natl Acad Sci USA 96, 12905–12910, 1999
Molewijk HE, Hartog K, van der Poel AM, Moss J & Olivier B. Reduction of guinea pig pups isolation calls by anxiolytic and antidepressant drugs. Psychopharmacology 128, 31–38, 1996
Moser PC. An evaluation of the elevated plus maze test using the novel anxiolytic buspirone. Psychopharmacology 99, 48–53, 1989
Nielsen M, Braestrup C & Squires RF. Evidence for a late evolutionary appearance of brain-specific benzodiazepine receptors: an investigation of 18 vertebrate and 5 invertebrate species. Brain Res 141, 342–346, 1978
Noirot E. Ultrasounds and maternal behavior in small rodents. Dev Psychobiol 5, 371, 1972
Nolan NA & Parkes MW. The effects of benzodiazepines on the behavior of mice on a hole board. Psychopharmacology 29, 277–288, 1973
Meert TF & Colpaert FC. The shock probe conflict procedure: A new assay responsive to benzodiazepines, barbiturates and related compounds. Psychopharmacology (Berl) 88, 445–450, 1986

Miczek KA, Weerts EM, Vivian JA & Barros HM. Aggression, anxiety and vocalization in animals: GABAA and 5HT anxiolytics. Psychopharmacology 121, 38–56, 1995

Misslin R, Belzung C & Vogel E. Behavioural validation of a light/dark choice procedure for testing anti-anxiety agents. Behav Proc 8, 119–132, 1989

Montgomery KC. The relation between fear induced by novel stimulation and exploratory behavior. J Comp Physiol Psychology 48, 254–260, 1955

Morgan CA, Southwick SM, Grillon C, Ouellette V, Davis M, Krystal JH & Charney DS. Yohimbine potentiated acoustic startle reflex in humans. Psychopharmacology 110, 342–346, 1993

Nashold BS, Wilson WP & Slaughter DG. Sensations evoked by stimulation of the midbrain of man. J Neurosurg 30, 14–24, 1969

Nutt DJ & Glue P. Clinical pharmacology of anxiolytics and antidepressants: a psychopharmacological perspective. In: WC Bowman (ed): Psychopharmacology of anxiolytics and antidepressants. Glasgow: Pergamon, 1–15, 1991

Nutt DJ & Glue P. Clinical pharmacology of anxiolytics and antidepressants: a psychopharmacological perspective. Pharmacol Ther 44, 309, 1989

Nutt DJ. Anxiety and its therapy: Today and tomorrow. In: M Briley & SE File (eds): New concepts in anxiety. London: MacMillan Press, 1–12, 1991

Onaivi ES & Martin BR. Neuropharmacological and physiological validation of a computer-controlled two-compartment black and white box for the assessment of anxiety. Prog Neuropsychopharmacol Biochem Behav 38, 375, 1989

Palit G, Kumar R, Chowdhuryy SR, Gupta MB, Saxena RC, Srimal RC & Dhawan BN. A primate model of anxiety. Eur Neuropsychopharmacol 8, 195–201, 1998

Pellow S, Chopin P, File SE & Briley M. Validation of open:closed arm entries in an elevated plus-maze as a measure of anxiety in the rat. J Neurosci Methods 14, 149–167, 1985

Pillard RC & Fisher S. Normal humans as models for psychopharmacology therapy. In: MA Lipton, A Dimascio & KF Killam (eds): Psychopharmacology: A generation of progress. New York: Raven Press, 783–790, 1978

Pinel JPT & Treit D. Burying as a defensive response in rats. J Comp Physiol Psychol 92, 708–712, 1978

Ramboz S, Oosting R, Amara DA, Kung HF, Blier P, Mendelsohn M, Mann JJ, Brunner D & Hen R. Serotonin receptor 1A knockout: an animal model of anxiety-related disorder. Proc Natl Acad Sci USA 95, 14476–14481, 1998

Regnier F, Chastel A, L'heritier C, Magni G & Henry M. Comparaison en aveugle contre placebo de l'alpidem en dose unique (50 ou 75 mg) dans un modèle d'anxiété situationnelle. Therapie 44, 279–283, 1989

Rodgers RJ & Cole JC. The elevated plus-maze: pharmacology, methodology and ethology. In: SJ Cooper & CA Hendrick (eds): Ethology and psychopharmacology. Chichester: Wiley, 9–44, 1994

Rifkin A, Klein DF, Dillon D et al. Blockade by imipramine or desipramine of panic induced by sodium lactate. Am J Psychiatry 138, 676–677, 1981

Rodin EA & Calhoun HD. Metrazol in a "normal" volunteer population. J Nerv Ment Dis 150, 38–450, 1970

Rodgers RJ & Cole JC. Anxiety enhancement in the murine elevated plus maze by immediate prior exposure to social stressors. Physiol Behav 53, 383–388, 1993

Rodgers RJ & Cole JC. The elevated plus-maze: pharmacology, methodology and ethology. In: SJ Cooper, CA Hendrie (eds): Ethology and psychopharmacology, 6th ed. Chichester: John Wiley & Sons Ltd, 10–44, 1994

Rudolph U, Crestani F, Benke D, Brunig I, Benson JA, Fritschy JM, Martin JR, Bluethmann H & Mohler H. Benzodiazepine actions mediated by specific gamma-aminobutyric acid (A) receptor subtypes. Nature 796–800, 1999

Sanderson WC & Barlow DM. A description of patients diagnosed with DSM-III-R generalized anxiety disorder. J Nerv Ment Dis 178, 588–591, 1990

Sanger DJ. The behavioural effects of novel benzodiazepine (ω) receptor agonists and partial agonists: increases in punished responding and antagonism of the pentylenetetrazole cue. Behav Pharmacol 6, 116–126, 1995

Sanson LT & Carobrez AP. Long-lasting inhibitory avoidance acquisition in rats submitted to the elevated T-maze model of anxiety. Behavioural Brain Res 101, 59–64, 1999

Shepherd JK, Grewal SS, Fletcher A, Bill DJ & Dourish CT. Behavioural and pharmacological characterization of the elevated "zero-maze" as an animal model of anxiety. Psychopharmacology (Berl) 116, 56–64, 1994

Schweitzer E & Rickels K. Serotonergic anxiolytics: A review of their clinical efficacy. In: RJ Rodgers (ed):. 5-HT$_{1A}$ agonists, 5HT$_3$ antagonists and benzodiazepines: Their comparative behavioural pharmacology. Chichester: John Wiley & Sons Ltd, 365–376, 1991

Sheehan DV, Raj AB, Sheehan KH & Soto S. The relative efficacy of buspirone, imipramine and placebo in panic disorder: A preliminary report. Pharmacol Biochem Behav 29, 815, 1988

Sheehan DV, Raj AB, Sheehan KH & Soto S. Is buspirone effective for panic disorder? J Clin Psychopharmacol 10, 3, 1990

Showalter E. The female malady. New York: Pantheon Books, 1985

Sibille E, Pavlides C, Benke D & Toth M. Genetic inactivation of the serotonin (1A) receptor in mice results in downregulation of major GABA(A) receptor alpha subunits, reduction of GABA (A) receptor binding, and benzodiazepine-resistant anxiety. J Neurosci 20, 2758–2765, 2000

Smith GW, Aubry JM, Dellu F, Contarino A, Bilezijjian LM, Gold LH, Chen R, Marchuk Y, Hauser C, Bentley CA et al. Corticotropin releasing factor receptor 1-deficient mice display decreased anxiety, impaired stress response, and aberrant neuroendocrine development. Neuron 20, 1093–1102, 1998

Spielberger CD. The measurement of state and trait anxiety: conceptual and methodological issues. In: L Levi (ed): Emotions: their parameters and measurement. New York: Raven Press, 713–725, 1975

Stenzel-Poore MP, Heinrichs SC, Rivest S, Koob GF & Vale WW. Overproduction of corticotropin-releasing factor in transgenic mice: a genetic model of anxiogenic behavior. J Neurosci 14, 2579–2584, 1994

Stewart RB, Gatto GJ, Lumeng L, Li T-K & Murphy JM. Comparison of alcohol-preferring (P) and non-preferring (NP) rats on tests of anxiety and for the anxiolytic effects of ethanol. Alcohol 10, 1–10, 1993

Stroop JR. Interference in serial verbal reactions. J Exp Psychol 18, 643–661, 1935

Tan ES. Transcultural aspects of anxiety. In: M Roth, R Noyes & GD Burrows (eds): Handbook of anxiety. Amsterdam: Elsevier, Vol. I, 305 – 326, 1988

Tecott LH, Logue SF, Wehner JM, Kauer JA. Perturbed dentate gyrus function in serotonin 5-HT_{2C} receptor mutant mice. Proc Natl Acad Sci USA 95, 15026–15031, 1998

Treit D, Robinson A, Rotzinger S & Pesold C. Anxiolytic effects of serotonergic interventions in the shock-probe burying test and the elevated plus-maze test. Behav Brain Res 54, 23–34, 1993

Treit D. Ro-15-1788, CGS 8216, picrotoxin, and pentylenetetrazol: Do they antagonize anxiolytic drug effects through an anxiogenic action? Brain Res Bull 19, 401, 1987

Treit D. A comparison of anxiolytic and nonanxiolytic agents in the shock-probe/burying test for anxiolytics. Pharmacol Biochem Behav 36, 203, 1990

Treit D, Menard J & Royan C. Anxiogenic stimuli in the elevated plus-maze. Pharmacol Biochem Behav 44, 463–469, 1993

Treit D. Animal models for the study of anti-anxiety agents. A review. Neurosci Biobehav Rev 9, 203–222, 1985

Treit D. Anxiolytic effects of benzodiazepines and 5-HT_{1A} agonists: Animal models. In: RJ Rodgers & SJ Cooper (eds): 5-HT_{1A} agonists, 5-HT_3 antagonists and benzodiazepines: Their comparative behavioural pharmacology. Chichester: John Wiley & Sons Ltd, 107–131, 1991

Tsuda A, Ida Y, Nishimura H & Tanaka M. Anxiogenic effects of B-CCE as measured in two different conditioning paradigms. Psychobiology 17, 202, 1989

Vale AL & Green S. Effects of chlordiazepoxide, nicotine and d-amphetamine in the rat potentiated startle model of anxiety. Behav Pharmacol 7, 138–143, 1996

Van Megen HJ, Westenberg HG, Den Boer JA & Kahn RS. Cholecystokinin in anxiety. Eur Neuropsychopharmacol 6, 263–280, 1996

Viana MB, Tomaz C & Graeff FG. The elevated T-maze: A new animal model of anxiety and memory. Pharmacol Biochem Behav 49 (3), 549–554, 1994

Vogel JR, Beer B & Clody DE. A simple and reliable conflict procedure for testing anti-anxiety agents. Psychopharmacologia 21, 1–7, 1971

Wall PM & Messier C. Methodological and conceptual issues in the use of the elevated plus-maze as a psychological measurement instrument of animal anxiety-like behavior. Neurosci Behav Rev 25, 275–286, 2001

Wells A. Metacognition and worry. A cognitive model of generalized anxiety disorder. Behav Cogn Psychother 23, 301–320, 1995

Wells A & Carter K. Preliminary tests of a cognitive model of generalized anxiety disorder. Behav Res Ther 585–594, 1999

Weninger SC, Dunn AJ, Muglia LJ, Dikkes P, Miczek KA, Swiergiel AH, Berridge CW & Majzoub JA. Stress-induced behaviours require the corticotropin-releasing hormone (CRH) receptor, but not CRH. Proc Natl Acad Sci USA 96, 8283–8288, 1999

Willner P. Behavioural models in psychopharmacology. In: P Willner (ed): Behavioural models in psychopharmacology. Cambridge University Press, 1991

Winslow J & Insel TR. The infant rat separation paradigm: a novel test for novel anxiolytics. Trend Pharmacol Sci 12, 402–404, 1991

Woodruff GN & Hughes J. Cholecystokinin antagonists. Ann Rev Pharmacol Toxicol 31, 469–501, 1991

Yokoi Y. Effect of ambient temperature upon emotional hyperthermia and hypothermia in rabbits. J Appl Physiol 21, 1795, 1966

Yoshiue SH, Yoshizawa H, Ito H, Sekine M, Nakamura T, Kanamori H, Suzuki T, Yazumi J, Ogata J & Ishida M. Analysis of body temperature at different sites in patients having slight fever caused by psychogenic stress. In: P Lomax & S Schönbaum (eds): Thermoregulation: research and clinical applications. Basel: Karger, 1989

Zangrossi H & Graeff FG. Behavioral validation of the elevated T-Maze, a new animal model of anxiety. Brain Res Bull 44 (1), 1–5, 1997

Zethof TJJ, Van der Heyden JAM, Tolboom JTB & Olivier B. Stress-induced hyperthermia as a putative anxiety model. Eur J Pharmacol 294, 125–135, 1995

Chapter 10
Discussion and perspectives

Anxiety disorders tend to be chronic conditions. Women are more prone than men to essentially all anxiety disorders (Bland et al., 1988; Kessler et al., 1994; Offord et al., 1996; Robins & Regier, 1991). Epidemiological studies suggest that women have a 2-to 3-fold increase in the occurrence of PD, PTSD and GAD. Fluctuations in oestrogen and progesterone levels can substantially influence the severity and course of anxiety disorders. Future investigations that focus on gender differences may provide valuable information for effective treatment strategies for women with anxiety disorders.

Considering comorbidity and type of anxiety disorder, the epidemiological data from the ECA survey linked alcohol dependence to nearly all of the anxiety disorders except for simple phobia (Himle & Hill, 1991; Regier et al., 1990). Family studies obtained stronger effects when considering PD than when considering several anxiety disorders together (Merikangas et al., 1996; Maier et al., 1993). Similarly, the association of anxiety disorder to alcoholism relapse was more robust for PD than for several anxiety disorders considered together (Tomasson & Vaglum, 1996; LaBounty et al., 1992). Thus, while all the anxiety disorders, with the exception of simple phobia, appear to have a significant association with alcohol dependence, the strength of that association may vary between anxiety disorders. The anxiety-spectrum phenomena of shyness and behavioural inhibition in children may predict the development of alcohol problems in adolescence and young adulthood (Caspi et al., 1996; Ensminger et al., 1982). However, this effect applied only to boys.

The recognition of childhood anxiety disorders as prevalent, highly impairing conditions has been relatively recent. Obviously, childhood anxiety disorders require multiple informants and questionnaires must be interpreted in relation to the overall clinical presentation. Given the many developmental antecedents of childhood anxiety disorders, parent-blaming is unwarranted. Parents should be engaged in the treatment process.

Although differences between children and adults with OCD have been reported by several investigators, surprisingly little research has investigated differences between child- and adult-onset OCD specifically (Geller et al.,1998; Swedo et al., 1992). In fact, there is a relative paucity of research on adult-onset OCD in general, with most studies of OCD in adults including patients with both child- and adult-onset of the disorder. In contrast, much research exists on the onset of OCD in childhood or adolescence. This imbalance in the research on child- as opposed to adult-onset OCD makes it difficult to draw clear conclusions about common features that may exist between these subgroups of patients. In OCD studies in children, the use of multiple informants (e.g., parents) or other sources of data (e.g., medical records) may be helpful in obtaining accurate estimates of age on onset. Such approaches may improve our methods of clinical investigation. Furthermore, where possible, prospective studies that follow individuals soon after the onset of their obsessive-compulsive symptoms should be employed. Thus, future research should continue to examine similarities and differences between OCD subtypes to further our understanding of the nature and underlying pathology of these conditions, which may help in the management and treatment of OCD.

Both OCD and GAD are characterised by excessive and uncontrollable cognitive processes associated with negative affect. Because of these common processes, there might be considerable overlap between these two disorders. Worry, the basic characteristic of GAD and obsessions, a main feature of OCD share some similar characteristics. Both phenomena occur with greater frequency and are associated with greater perceptions of uncontrollability in clinical populations than in normal groups. Both worry and obsessions are associated with adverse mood and that some type of vulnerability factor determines why individuals develop pathological worries or obsessions and others do not. However, there is evidence that on a symptom level, GAD and OCD can in general be reliably differentiated by clinicians (Brown et al., 1993). The rate of co-occurrence of GAD and OCD seems to be rather low (Brown et al., 1993). In terms of form differences, worries typically appear in the form of thoughts whereas obsessions also consist of images and impulses. However, worry does not appear to be resisted as strongly as obsessional thinking although both phenomena are experienced as uncontrollable. The behaviour response to worry consists of avoidance and reassurance seeking and is not likely to comprise neutralisation behaviour in the form of rituals as in OCD. Of the obsessive-compulsive components, rumination was found to be most closely associated with worry (Van Rijsoort et al., 2001). However, when controlled for depressive mood, the overlap between rumination and worry dropped significantly. Therefore, worry and obsessive-compulsive symptoms are clearly different phenomena. Nevertheless, future research needs to focus on these differential characteristics in order to further define the different boundaries between OCD and GAD.

Anxiety in older adults is an understudied problem, despite evidence that anxiety symptoms and even anxiety disorders are fairly common in late life. The consequences of anxiety in late life have not been adequately researched. One follow-up study of older adults with untreated anxiety and depression suggests that anxiety in this population generally does not remit spontaneously over the course of 2–3 years (Livingston et al., 1997). Older people may not seek treatment for anxiety in particular because they may believe it is an inevitable part of the ageing process or because they may interpret somatic anxiety symptoms as manifestations of physical illness (Turnbull, 1989). One possibility to improve the body of evidence for the effectiveness of therapy with older people is for anxiety researchers to increase the upper age limits of their studies, frequently set at 60 or 65. In the treatment arena, well-controlled clinical trials addressing the utility of a range of pharmacological interventions are needed. Given the potential adverse effects of BDZs for older adults, studies evaluating the efficacy of alternative compounds such as antidepressants will be of particular value. All future pharmacological treatment trials will need to include patients with well-characterised anxiety symptoms and syndromes. Established measures of anxiety also need to be administered to document the significance and breadth of treatment effects. Potential adverse effects of these treatments as well as their interactions with other concomitant drug treatments will need to be monitored closely.

Some researchers have attempted to identify the main causes that are responsible for anxiety disorders. A few investigators have demonstrated that cigarette smoking is associated with anxiety disorders among adolescents and adults (Kanderl et al., 1997; Brook et al., 1998). Two types of hypothesis have been advanced. One hypothesis is that anxious individuals are at elevated risk for smoking initiation due to factors such as peer pressure, facilitation of social interaction and the presumed calming effects of smoking (Sonntag et al., 2000; Kassel & Shiffman, 1997). Research findings supporting this hypothesis have indicated that adolescents with symptoms of anxiety were at higher risk for smoking initiation than asymptomatic adolescents, that smoking in the presence of a distracting stimulus was associated with reduced anxiety (Sonntag et al., 2000; Kassel & Shiffman, 1997). Another hypothesis is that cigarette smoking contributes to the development of anxiety disorders due to factors including impaired respiration and the presumed anxiogenic effects of nicotine (Dilsaver, 1987; West & Hajek, 1997). In support of this hypothesis, clinical studies have indicated that cigarette smoking preceded the onset of panic attacks among patients with PD (Breslau et al., 1991; Pohl et al., 1992). A recent study designed to investigate the longitudinal association between cigarette smoking and anxiety disorders among adolescents and young adults confirmed that heavy cigarette smoking (≥20 cigarettes/day) during adolescence was associated with higher risk of agoraphobia, GAD and PD during early adulthood after controlling for age, sex, difficult childhood temperament, alcohol and drug abuse, anxiety and depressive disorders during adolescence (Johnson et al., 2000). Thus these findings suggest that cigarette smoking during adolescence may be associated with increased risk for agoraphobia, GAD and PD during early adulthood.

The efficacy of some psychological and pharmacological treatment has been shown for various anxiety disorders. It has been suggested that behavioural therapy may be considered as first-line treatment for childhood anxiety disorders. Clinical trials have shown several products to be effective pharmacological interventions in the management of anxiety disorders (see Tab. 10.1). As a general rule in the management of anxiety disorders drug therapies tend to give more rapid resolution of symptoms, while psychological approaches tend to have longer duration of effect. However, controlled clinical trials are needed to evaluate the efficacy of current pharmacological treatments, particularly the SSRIs in children and the elderly. Evidence supporting the long-term efficacy for drugs or behavioural cognitive therapy in most anxiety disorders in children, adults and elderly is lacking. This represents an important area for future research. An even more important issue that has been underemphasised but is central in evaluating the treatment response to all anxiety disorders is that not all patients, not even the majority, completely recover with either pharmacotherapy or psychotherapy. For both types of treatment, not even more than 50% could be considered fully recovered. Despite the excellent progress

Table 10.1: Medications found effective in controlled studies of treating anxiety disorders .

Disorder	**Benzodiazepine**	**SSRI**	**Azapirone**	**SNRI**	**MAOI**	**Tricyclics**
PD with or without agoraphobia	Alprazolam Clonazepam Diazepam Lorazepam	Citalopram Fluoxetine Fluvoxamine Paroxetine Sertraline	None		Brofaromine Phenelzine	Clomipramine Desipramine Imipramine
GAD	Various benzodiazepines	Paroxetine	Buspirone Ipsapirone	Venlafaxine	None	Imipramine
OCD	None	Fluoxetine Fluvoxamine Sertraline	None		None	Clomipramine
PTSD	None	Fluoxetine	None		Phenelzine	Amitriptyline Imipramine
SP	Alprazolam Clonazepam	Fluvoxamine Paroxetine Sertraline	None	Venlafaxine	Brofaromine Phenelzine Moclobemide	None

made in the last 10 years, improvements in treatments to increase cure rates are greatly needed.

Other treatment approaches such as biofeedback have often been used. EEG-biofeedback was associated with clinical improvement in GAD, phobic disorders, OCD and PTSD. A placebo effect was certainly present. Patients improved clinically when there was no change in alpha voltage compared with baseline (Rice et al., 1993; Sittenfeld et al., 1976; Mills & Solyom, 1974). However, alpha-enhancement was superior to suppression. These findings suggest that the biofeedback-induced changes in alpha and theta provided additional benefits to placebo effects. One important variable is whether the patient has high-trait or low-trait anxiety. Paradoxically, the high-trait volunteers had a better outcome. Future research in EEG-biofeedback for anxiety disorders should use multiple electrode sites, at least 5 h of training and clinical patients (rather than volunteers) with high anxiety levels.

Future perspectives

Considering a schema-based information-processing model of anxiety that involves features of automatic and strategic processing, the clinical implications of this model for the treatment of anxiety may be considered. Verbally mediated therapies for anxiety will be ineffective because the early stages of information processing are involuntary and possibly unconscious (McNally, 1995). Findings from thought suppression studies indicate that direct attempts to suppress thoughts that arise from automatic cognitive processes may be counterproductive.

Research is urgently needed to elucidate the neural substrates of anxious children's cognitive characteristics (selective attention and memory for threat, anxiety sensitivity, coping deficits) to integrate developmental and neurophysiological theories of anxiety to clarify the aetiology of specific disorders and to locate specific genes that contribute to anxiety disorders. New measures of anxiety must capture child impairment as well as anxiety symptoms and use multiple informants.

Treatment studies of anxious children and adolescents can be improved by strengthening existing clinician-rated global rating scales. The field of paediatric anxiety disorder research currently lacks a universally accepted, clinician-scored, anxiety symptom questionnaire. Even if this rating form was available, it would be most useful if it was accompanied by age-adjusted norms that could be used to set anxiety symptom thresholds for patient selection into treatment protocols. The development of such a rating scale, the availability of the norms, and the validation by an independent physiological measure would greatly improve paediatric treatment research in the area of anxiety disorders.

A clinician-scored rating scale for anxiety symptom severity is needed for monitoring changes during treatment when used in a repeated measure design. For adult treatment, HAM-A, a 14-item instrument using a 4-point Likert Scale that is treatment sensitive for adults with anxiety disorders, has been used (Hamilton, 1969, Guy, 1976).

References

Bland RC, Newman SC & Orn H. Epidemiology of psychiatric disorders in Edmonton. Acta Psychiatr Scand Suppl 338, 1–80, 1988

Breslau N, Kilbey MM & Andreski P. Nicotine dependence, major depression, and anxiety in young adults. Arch Gen Psychiatry 48, 1069–1074, 1991

Brown TA, Moras K, Zinbarg RE & Barlow DH. Diagnostic and symptom distinguishability of generalised anxiety disorder and obsessive compulsive disorder. Behav Ther 24, 227–240, 1993

Caspi A, Moffitt TE, Newman DL & Silva PA. Behavioral observations at age 3 years predict adult psychiatric disorders. Arch Gen Psychiatry 53, 1033–1039, 1996

Dilsaver SC. Nicotine and panic attacks. Arch Gen Psychiatry 56, 1141–1147, 1999

Ensminger ME, Brown CH & Kellam SG. Sex differences in antecedents of substance use among adolescents. J Social Issues 38, 25–42, 1982

Geller D, Biederman J, Jones J, Park K, Schwartz S, Shapiro S & Coffey B. Is juvenile obsessive-compulsive disorder a developmental subtype of the disorder? A review of the pediatric literature. J Am Acad Child Adolesc Psychiatry 37, 420–427, 1998

Guy W. ECDEU Assessment Manual for Psychopharmacology revised. DHEW Pub. No. (ADM) 76-338, Rockville, MD: National Institute of Mental Health, 1976

Hamilton M. Diagnosis and rating of anxiety. In: MH Lader (ed): Studies of anxiety (Br J Psychiatry Special Publication 3), 76–79, 1969

Himle JA & Hill EM. Alcohol abuse and the anxiety disorders: Evidence from the Epidemiologic Catchment Area survey. J Anxiety Disord 5 237–245, 1991

Johnson JG, Cohen P, Pine DS, Klein DF, Kasen S & Brook JS. Association between cigarette smoking and anxiety disorders during adolescence and early adulthood. JAMA 284, 2348–2351, 2000

Kassel JD & Shiffman S. Attentional mediation of cigarette smoking's effect on anxiety. Health Psychol 16, 359–368, 1997

Kessler RC, McGonagle KA, Zhao S, Nelson CB, Hughes M, Eshleman S, Wittchen H & Kendler KS. Lifetime and 12-month prevalence of DSM-III-R psychiatric disorders in the United States: results from the National Comorbidity Survey. Arch Gen Psychiatry 51, 8–19, 1994

LaBounty LP, Hatsukami D, Morgan SF & Nelson L. Relapse among alcoholics with phobic and panic symptoms. Addictive Behaviors 17, 9–15, 1992

Livingston G, Watkin V, Milne B, Manela MV & Katona C. The natural history of depression and the anxiety disorders in older people: The Islington Community study. J Affect Disord 46, 255–262, 1997

Maier W, Minges J & Lichtermann D. Alcoholism and panic disorder: Co-occurrence and co-transmission in families. Eur Arch Psychiatry Clin Neurosci 243, 205–211, 1993

McNally RJ. Automaticity and the anxiety disorders. Behav Res Ther 33, 747–754, 1995

Merikangas KA, Stevens D & Fenton B. Comorbidity of alcoholism and anxiety disorders. Alcohol Health and Research World 20, 100–105, 1996

Mills GK & Solyom L. Biofeedback of EEG alpha in the treatment of obsessive ruminations: an exploration. J Behav Ther Exp Psychiatry 5, 37–41, 1974

Offord DR, Boyle MH, Campbell D, Goering P, Lin E, Wong M & Racine Y. One-year prevalence of psychiatric disorder in Ontarions 15 to 64 years of age. Can J Psychiatry 41, 559–563, 1996

Pohl R, Yeragani VK, Balon R, Lycaki H & McBride R. Smoking in patients with panic disorder. Psychiatry Res 43, 253–262, 1992

Regier DA, Farmer ME, Rae DS, Locke BZ, Keith SJ, Judd LL & Goodwin FK. Comorbidity of mental disorders with alcohol and other drug abuse: Results from the Epidemiologic Catchment Area (ECA) Study. JAMA 264, 2511–2518, 1990

Rice KM, Blanchard EB & Purcell M. Biofeedback treatments of generalized anxiety disorder: preliminary results. Biofeedback & Self Regulation 18, 93–105, 1993

Robins LN, Regier DA (eds). Psychiatric disorders in America: The Epidemiologic Catchment Area study. New York, Free Press, 1991

Sittenfeld P, Budzynski T & Stoyva J. Differential shaping of EEG theta rhythms. Biofeedback & Self Regulation 1 (1), 31–46, 1976

Sonntag H, Wittchen HU, Hofler M, Kessler RC & Stein MB. Are social fears and DSM-IV social anxiety disorder associated with smoking and nicotine dependence in adolescents and young adults? Eur Psychiatry 15, 67–74, 2000

Swedo SE, Leonard HL & Rapoport JL. Childhood-onset obsessive compulsive disorder. Psychiatr Clin North Am 15, 767–775, 1992

Tomasson K & Vaglum P. Psychopathology and alcohol consumption among treatment-seeking alcoholics: A prospective study. Addiction 91, 1019–1030, 1996

Turnbull JM. Anxiety and physical illness in the elderly. J Clin Psychiatry 50, 40–45, 1989

Van Rijsoort S, Emmelkamp P & Vervaeke G. Assessment of worry and OCD: how are they related? Personality and Individual Differences 31, 247–258, 2001

West R, Hajek P. What happens to anxiety levels on giving up smoking? Am J Psychiatry 154, 1589–1592, 1997

Subject index

MIX
Papier aus verantwortungsvollen Quellen
Paper from responsible sources
FSC® C105338

If you have any concerns about our products,
you can contact us on
ProductSafety@springernature.com

In case Publisher is established outside the EU,
the EU authorized representative is:
Springer Nature Customer Service Center GmbH
Europaplatz 3, 69115 Heidelberg, Germany

Printed by Libri Plureos GmbH
in Hamburg, Germany